SPIRITUAL DIMENSIONS
OF NURSING PRACTICE

SPIRITUAL DIMENSIONS OF NURSING PRACTICE

REVISED EDITION

VERNA BENNER CARSON &
HAROLD G. KOENIG, editors

TEMPLETON FOUNDATION PRESS

West Conshohocken, Pennsylvania

Templeton Foundation Press
300 Conshohocken State Road, Suite 670
West Conshohocken, PA 19428
www.templetonpress.org

*Templeton Foundation Press helps intellectual leaders and others learn about science research on
aspects of realities, invisible and intangible. Spiritual realities include unlimited love, accelerat-
ing creativity, worship, and the benefits of purpose in persons and in the cosmos.*

Designed and typeset by Kachergis Book Design

LIBRARY OF CONGRESS CATALOGING-IN-PUBLICATION DATA
Spiritual dimensions of nursing practice / edited by Verna Benner Carson
and Harold G. Koenig. — Rev. ed.
    p. ; cm.
Includes bibliographical references and index.
ISBN-13: 978-1-59947-145-7 (alk. paper)
ISBN-10: 1-59947-145-0 (alk. paper)
1. Nursing—Religious aspects.   2. Nursing—Research—Moral and
ethical aspects.   I. Carson, Verna Benner.   II. Koenig, Harold George.
[DNLM: 1. Nursing Care.   2. Spirituality.   3. Nurse-Patient
Relations.   4. Religion and Medicine.
WY 87 S75951 2008]
RT85.2.C37 2008
610.73—dc22

                        2008017272

Printed in the United States of America

08   09   10   11   12   13   10   9   8   7   6   5   4   3   2   1

CONTENTS

PREFACE

There is probably nothing more certain in life than change. Change moves us along—sometimes in directions of our choosing and other times into uncharted territory. We move with trepidation as we face the unknown, and we feel excitement as we contemplate the possibilities that await us. As the initial editor of this book in 1989, change has been a constant in my own life. When the first edition was published, I was a young wife and the mother of three wonderful sons, Adam, Johnny, and Robbie. I was surrounded and supported by a large extended family who served as my constant cheering squad. I was an assistant professor of psychiatric nursing at the University of Maryland. I had not yet earned my Ph.D. In retrospect, life seemed easy.

Today many of my extended family have passed into eternity, and I still feel the loss of each one of them. However, the cheering squad is not diminished—just changed. I now have two lovely daughters-in-law and their families, three grandsons, and an ever-widening circle of friends and colleagues who provide support and encouragement. I left the University of Maryland to establish a psychiatric home care program across the country, and most recently I became the mental health director for assisted living and skilled nursing facilities with a national continuing care retirement community. I am no longer the sole editor of this book, but share this responsibility with Dr. Harold G. Koenig. Together we published two previous books and, in the process, have become dear friends.

As I reflect on the changing tapestry of my own life, I am struck by the fact that some threads are the same—maybe more brilliant in color, with greater depth and significance to me, but at their core still the same. Of course, the important thread of family and friends grows with every day—I am incredibly blessed. The thread of work is a strong and defining one. I feel called to make a difference through work—through writing, teaching, and through my interactions with others. And as the years move along, there is a heightened sense of urgency about the work: It is not mine—never has been—it belongs to God and I want to do the best job I can to please my Maker! The essential part of this work, also a thread through my life, is spirituality. Spirituality is a focus of my personal walk with the Lord, but it is also the focus of the work that I am called to do, especially in educating nurses and other health care professionals about the importance of spirituality to health care.

Spirituality defines the best in health care. Spirituality is the driving force when health professionals feel "called" to do what they do. Spirituality is the reason for inquiring about the stories of patients and families because we know that only through their stories do we capture the meaning of health and illness to those in our care. Spirituality is what motivates us to go the extra mile and keeps us going because we see that the needs are so great. Spirituality infuses the work we do with love, compassion, and a sense of gratitude for being participants in God's healing work.

Spiritual care can take many different forms; there is no one way that we touch another's spirit. This process involves recognizing and honoring the religious beliefs and practices of those in our care, but it can also be accomplished through shared laughter or tears or remembering a patient's birthday. Spiritual care can mean keeping vigil with a family as a loved one struggles to recover. It can be crying with that same family when their loved one dies. It can be supporting a chronically ill individual who is struggling to redefine his worth and personal meaning in light of the illness and its demands. It can be a gentle backrub, coupled with soothing words, that allows a worried patient to fall asleep. It can be a shared prayer or religious reading that has special meaning to the patient. Spiritual care cannot be boxed in and narrowly defined.

Spiritual care is not provided only to those who believe a certain way or who define God according to a specific doctrine. Spiritual care is for everyone. People may express their spirituality in unique ways, but everyone has a spiritual nature that can be touched through the kindness, compassion, and ministrations of another.

When the first edition of this book was published, I formulated very clear goals for the book. First, I wanted the book to address the universality of spirituality. I wanted the book to be meaningful to people who do not believe in a God, people who share my belief in Jesus Christ, and people who define their God in other ways. Second, I wanted to convey the idea that meeting spiritual needs is a form of caring and that without it nursing—indeed, all of health care—is incomplete. Third, I wanted to demystify the concept of spiritual care and spiritual needs, so health care providers could see that providing this type of care is indeed within their capabilities as well as their responsibilities. These goals are still valid as the second edition of this book is published.

Nurses are the primary focus of this book. There are opportunities to identify and meet spiritual needs in every clinical setting. Having worked in home care, I found unlimited situations where I was confronted with spiritual issues—situations that called forth my utmost sensitivity to assess, to listen, to be present, and to minister. Today when people enter the hospital it is frequently for very serious illnesses, and at such times spiritual needs move to the forefront of the thinking of many patients and families. Hospital nurses must be prepared to recognize and respond to patient concerns about dying and finding meaning amid changing life circumstances. Nurses who work in skilled nursing facilities are providing care to patients who are nearing the end of their lives and who may be cognitively impaired. It is interesting to note that one of the most effective ways to reach a patient who is seemingly lost in dementia is through prayer and the use of hymns. When all other memories seem to have vanished, these memories are retained, and when nurses are able to elicit these memories they make a profound connection with their patients. No matter what the setting, nurses have not only the opportunity, but the responsibility to recognize and respond to the spiritual in those for whom care is provided. The reward to nurses who seize these opportunities is priceless.

Although the primary focus of this book is on nurses and nursing, the applicability of the book goes beyond nursing and is quite broad. Students of nursing, medicine, and social work; physical, occupational, and speech therapists; and pastoral care professionals can all benefit from the insights within these pages. Faculty will find valuable resources that facilitate thought and discussion. However, Dr. Koenig and I also want to reach experienced health care providers who may question their ability to provide spiritual care in their daily practice. In that respect, the book has value in planning continuing education programs to help a broad range of health care providers become more knowledgeable about spiritual needs and competent in providing support and care.

The book has a number of special features that facilitate the teaching and learning process. First, the very breadth of information on the many aspects of spirituality makes it unique. Second, each chapter begins with a quote intended to stimulate reflection and to prepare the reader for the material contained within the chapter. Finally, each chapter concludes with reflective activities. These are intended to facilitate spiritual development.

In choosing contributors for this book, we did not seek people whose religious beliefs were the same as ours. In fact, the contributors represent a wide variety of religious faiths as well as professional backgrounds. In choosing contributors, we looked for those who live out the notion of touching the spirit of others in their daily lives and could present their topics with passion and conviction. We are fortunate to know such individuals and hope that you are touched by their contributions.

Verna Benner Carson

PART I

SPIRITUALITY AND THE NURSING PROFESSION

Part I introduces the reader to the concept of spirituality and its relationship to nursing. In the first chapter, spirituality is defined as a universal human dimension that expresses itself through relationships, creativity, emotions, physical modalities, religion, and worldviews. Chapter 2 reviews the findings of research related to spirituality and religion and the implications of these findings for nurses.

1

SPIRITUALITY

DEFINING THE INDEFINABLE AND REVIEWING
ITS PLACE IN NURSING

VERNA BENNER CARSON AND RUTH STOLL

> *I gave in and admitted that God was God.*
> —C. S. Lewis

In 1989, the first edition of this book was published with a focus on the importance of spirituality in nursing. At that time, because there was a paucity of research, publications, or even awareness regarding the importance of spiritual issues to health, this text was considered a seminal work. Other than texts from religious publishing houses, most health care literature had little to say about the topic of spirituality. This is not to say that there weren't doctors, nurses, social workers, and physical, occupational, and speech therapists who recognized the importance of a patient's spirituality and religious beliefs, but these practitioners may have been in the minority, and they weren't publishing their thoughts.

Today, however, the landscape is very different for all health professionals. There is a wider acceptance that health care providers, in particular nurses, need to understand the spiritual and religious beliefs, needs, and practices of patients in order to provide whole person health care. Let's take a look at a patient whose story underscores this importance.

Marcy was a married woman in her late twenties. She loved her hus-

3

band dearly and counted among her blessings a close network of family and friends. Marcy had worked as a nurse and had always felt a call to her work. Now Marcy was in almost constant pain. She was confined to her home and spent most of her day in bed as a result of serious complications of systemic lupus erythematosus. Recently, she had undergone extensive surgery but was not healing well. During a home health visit, Marcy spoke to the nurse about her up-and-down physical condition, her fears that she would not get better, her physical symptoms of unrelenting headaches and pain, and the difficulty she had dressing her large wound. Over time, Marcy shared with the nurse that, despite her loneliness and her losses, she held tight to an unshakable hope and the courage to face whatever was ahead day by day. The nurse asked Marcy how she accounted for her strength and evident courage. Without hesitation, Marcy replied, "Prayer, the Bible, my husband, and friends."

"What helps you pass the time?" asked the nurse. "What is meaningful and helps you feel worthwhile?"

Marcy confided that she had developed a new practice of "journaling." She wrote letters of encouragement to others who were homebound due to illness; she prayed with people over the telephone. Even though Marcy was confined to her home, she reached out to the broader community. This hurting patient's behavior expresses her particular spirituality. So what is spirituality?

The purpose of this chapter is to answer that question as well as to look at the relationship of spirituality to religion and worldview and how nursing approaches spirituality in clinical settings.

Spirituality Defined

Spirituality is an elusive word to define. Like the wind, we can see its effects but we can't grasp it in our hands and hold onto it. We recognize when someone is in "low" or "high" spirits, but is that spirituality? We believe that a patient's quality of life, health, and sense of wholeness are affected by spirituality, yet still we struggle to define it. Why? Most likely because spirituality represents "heart" not "head" knowledge, and "heart" knowledge is difficult to encapsulate in words.

Spirituality is described in a variety of ways: as a principle, an experience, a sense of God, the inner person. According to Mary Elizabeth O'Brien (2003, 4), "Spirituality, as a personal concept, is generally understood in terms of an individual's attitudes and belief related to transcendence (God) or to the nonmaterial forces of life and of nature." O'Brien concludes that most descriptions of spirituality include not only transcendence but also the connection of mind, body, and spirit, plus love, caring, and compassion and a relationship with the Divine (2003, 6).

Take a moment to ask yourself, "What does spirituality mean to me?" Ruth Stoll answered that question in the 1989 edition of this text. Her answer is still relevant. "It is who I am—unique, and personally connected to God. That relationship with God is expressed through my body, my thinking, my feelings, my judgments, and my creativity. My spirituality motivates me to choose meaningful relationships and pursuits. Through my spirituality I give and receive love; I respond to and appreciate God, other people, a sunset, a symphony, and spring. I am driven forward, sometimes because of pain, sometimes in spite of pain. Spirituality allows me to reflect on myself. I am a person because of my spirituality—motivated and enabled to value, to worship, and to communicate with the holy, the transcendent" (1989, 9). Dr. Stoll's definition is clearly related to a belief in God. If you find that your definition differs significantly from Dr. Stoll's, it may be because you are operating from a different worldview, a concept we will discuss later in the chapter. Dr. Stoll's definition derives from a Christian theistic worldview.

Dr. George Fitchett (2002), a chaplain and researcher, defines spirituality as having seven distinct dimensions. The first dimension is that of belief and meaning, and refers not only to the individual's beliefs, which give meaning and purpose to his life, but also to his personal story about how these beliefs are lived. The second dimension has to do with a sense of obligation to live out our professed beliefs. The third dimension deals with experiential and emotional aspects of spirituality. For instance, the experiences the individual has had in relation to the sacred, the Divine, or the demonic, and what emotional significance these experiences hold for her. The fourth dimension deals with our courage and willingness to grow spiritually, a process that entails putting aside existing beliefs and integrating new experiences. The fifth dimension relates to participation in formal and informal communities where members are able to share common beliefs, experiences, and meaning. The sixth dimension has to do with the source of authority for our beliefs. The seventh dimension focuses on where we turn for guidance when faced with painful life experiences. For instance, do we turn inward or outward to others? These seven dimensions are sometimes used to provide structure to spiritual assessments conducted by hospital chaplains (see chapter 8).

Chaplain Batchelor (2006, 8) describes spirituality as follows: "'Breath,' 'wind,' 'meaning,' 'connected'—any or all of these terms may come to mind when one tries to grasp the concept 'spirituality.'" For many, spirituality evokes reverence, peacefulness, and the very foundation for a meaningful life. It may do so either from within the framework of a particular religion or from an avowedly nonreligious perspective. For some who chafe from negative religious experiences, spirituality's distinction from organized religion is what makes spirituality attractive. For yet others, this same distinction from organized religion may invite suspicion or outright rejection of spirituality as too individualistic or New Age. Batchelor's definition covers a lot of ground and illustrates the two major ways that patients often view spirituality.

Many current definitions of spirituality tend to downplay any connections to God, but instead focus on humanistic concepts, individual feelings of well-being, and a sense of connectedness (Carson 1993, Smith and Denton 2005, Turner 1990). Plante and Sherman (2001) echo this observation in their remark that, for many, a spiritual quest for the transcendent may have nothing to do with the sacred. Increasingly, people are identifying any experience that makes them feel connected to something larger than themselves as being "spiritual." Experiences such as being captivated by a beautiful sunset, playing on a sports team, or engaging in a political campaign have not traditionally been viewed as spiritual experiences. However, ordinary activities can be imbued with spiritual meaning if these activities are linked to the Divine, "as in the case of a Jew reciting a prayer while washing her hands or a Catholic who looks upon meal preparation as a sacrament" (Emmons & Crumpler 1999, 16).

Components of Spiritual Interrelatedness

According to Shelly and Miller (2006, 96), spirituality is all about relationships—"a relationship of the whole person to a personal God and to other people (or other spirits)." The core relationship is centered on the Creator, and the significance of this relationship reverberates and shapes all other relationships. The manner in which we connect with family, friends, our communities, our workplace, and even how we relate to ourselves— all are affected by our relationship to the Divine. Art, music, crafts, cooking, woodworking, volunteer activities, and sports can all be influenced by the way a person views God's role in his life (Carson and Koenig 2004, 74; Emmons and Crumpler 1999). Even the act of finding meaning and purpose, an aspect of spirituality, is relational. When people struggle to make sense out of life and in that struggle they grapple with tough questions, such as, "Why me?" "Why now?" "What does it mean?" and "What difference do I make?" they are attempting to define the relationship of their lives to ultimate truth and reality. Nurses and other health care professionals not only witness patients and families as they grapple with these same questions; nurses grapple with the same questions thesmelves as they face the limits of their skills and abilities to make people better, to ease pain, and to create a healing environment (Carson & Koenig 2004, 74).

The integral nature of relationship to spirituality suggests both a vertical and a horizontal dimension. The vertical dimension has to do with the person's transcendent (beyond and/or outside self) relationship, the possibility of a personal relationship with a Higher Being—God—not necessarily as defined by a particular religion. The horizontal facet reflects and "fleshes out" the many ways in which a personal relationship with the Divine influences our beliefs, values, lifestyle, quality of life, and interactions with ourself, with others, and with nature. As we will see later on, a person's perception of and experience with the Transcendent will in great measure influence how that person views life and copes with crises of illness, suffering, and loss. Figure 1–1 depicts the two-dimensional nature of spirituality in a visual model.

Looking at the box, you can see that there is a continuous interrelationship between and among the inner being of the person, the person's vertical relationship with the transcendent or whatever supreme values guide

Figure 1–1   Spiritual interrelatedness, or integration, comes about through forgiveness, love, and trust, resulting in meaning and purpose and hope in life. (Redrawn by permission of Ruth I. Stoll. © Ruth I. Stoll, 1987.)

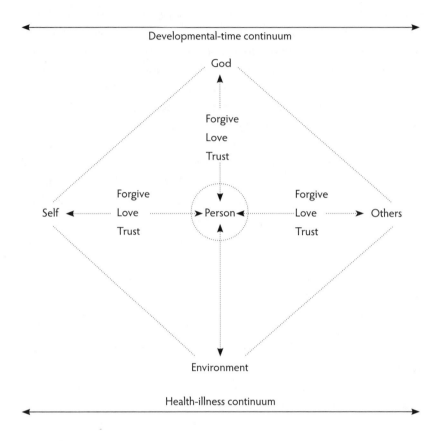

his life, and his horizontal relationships with himself, others, and the environment. These relationships are depicted by the inner dotted lines in Figure 1–1. The person's relationships are grounded in expressions of love, forgiveness, and trust, and result in meaning and purpose in life. Noted above and below the model depicting the inner person are factors that continuously influence the spiritual well-being or distress of the person (see Part IV).

Spirituality: Whole Person Perspective

A person's human spirit does not reside in a vacuum; rather, it is housed in a physical body. In other words, we are embodied spirits. The person is a whole being who is more than and different from the sum of her parts and cannot be separated into segments for diagnosis and care. The body, mind, and spirit are dynamically woven together, one part affecting and being affected by the other parts. Figure 1–2 depicts an adaptation of a model, developed by Stallwood and Stoll (1975), which serves to illustrate a person's wholeness.

The following descriptions are meant to clarify the meaning of each circle in the model and the interrelatedness of the identified parts. The outer circle represents the physical body—what is seen and experienced by others. Our bodies allow us to be in touch with the world through our senses; our abilities to touch, taste, hear, see, and smell. The second circle represents the psychosocial—the dimension that allows us to experi-

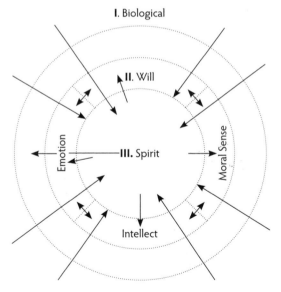

Figure 1–2 Conceptual model of the nature of humans. I. Biological: Five senses, world-conscious. II. Psychosocial: emotion, intellect, moral sense, and will. III. Spirit: God-conscious, relatedness to deity. The arrows coming from the center "Spirit" indicate the centrality of God consciousness and indicate that the spirit influences both the psychosocial and biological dimensions. The arrows coming from outside Circle I indicate that influences from the environment influence biological, psychosocial, and spirit dimensions. The double-sided arrows indicate the interactive influence among will, moral sense, intellect, and emotion. (Reprinted with permission of Macmillan Publishing Company from *Clinical Nursing*, 3rd ed., by Irene L. Beland and J. Y. Passos. Copyright © 1975 by Macmillan Publishing Company.)

ence self-consciousness and personality through our emotions, intellect, moral sense, and will. The innermost circle, the spirit, is the most difficult to comprehend because of its mystery and empirically indefinable nature. The spirit is that dimension that pervades all other dimensions of the person and allows us to be conscious of and related to God.

With all our various dimensions, we are and we function as a dynamic whole. This is depicted in the model by the broken lines and arrows. The body influences and is influenced by the psychosocial and spiritual dimensions. The psychosocial dimension expresses itself through the body, the biological dimension. The spirit expresses itself through the total being— the psychosocial and the biological dimensions.

Clinical Examples

Let's take another look at Marcy. Her example illustrates both models and explanations. Marcy's behavior demonstrates that her living spirit expresses itself through both psychosocial and biological dimensions. Marcy expresses her psychosocial dimension in tears, bodily expressions of sadness, and joy by squeezing another's hands or smiling. Marcy's will (decision maker) and power to choose are revealed in her choice of and active participation in prayer and meditation to relieve her pain and reduce her fears. Her conscience (moral sense), discernment of "shoulds" and "oughts," motivates her to maintain those practices that would encourage positive interpersonal relationships ("journaling" or letter writing and telephone calls). She reasons through her thought processes about how God was helping her, how to apply passages of scripture to her illness experience, and she shares her feelings verbally with the nurse and others. Marcy has a conscious, loving, trusting relationship with a personal God. It is the integration of the vertical relationship with her God into her being and lifestyle that gives meaning and hope to horizontal relationships with herself and with others and, in large measure, influences her outlook and her ability to cope with the tragedy of illness.

Another clinical example illustrates of a dormant spirit creatively affected by a health crisis. Sam is a sixty-year-old man with metastatic carcinoma. He has been in and out of hospitals for the past three months. At this point, he is in the hospital, lethargic but conscious. "I've had it. . . . The hardest thing is just waiting and suffering. . . . I know it sounds awful to say it, but I want to die." As the nurse explores the meaning of what it is like to die, Sam continued, "I'm really afraid to die." In answer to the nurse's question, "Is there anything I can do to help you cope with your suffering—more pain medication, a visit from the chaplain, or prayer?"Sam replied, "I'm not religious. I was brought up in a church and I went on Sundays, but I don't want to go running to God now. It's not fair of me. I've ignored God up until now. But I would appreciate the prayers—please pray for me in your own way wherever you want, but not here."

Sam's sense of isolation and fear seem to motivate him to tentatively, yet with a ray of hope, grasp onto the possibility that maybe, just possibly, there is something or someone to guide him through and bring him some relief in the last stage of life, in his experience of pain and death. This man's crisis brought awareness of a need for bonding with the Transcendent, which seemingly had not taken place yet.

A third example illustrates how the beliefs of the patient were respected in a long-term care facility. An elderly Muslim gentleman was noted to orient his wheelchair in a certain direction throughout the day. If the staff spoke to him at these times, he became visibly upset. The hospital chaplain, making rounds, discussed this situation with the nurses who identified the patient's unusual behavior. The chaplain spoke to the patient and asked him if there was a problem that the chaplain might be able to alleviate. The patient told the chaplain that throughout the day he oriented his wheelchair to the east and was engaged in praying. The chaplain explained the patient's behavior to the nursing staff, who certainly wanted to be respectful of the patient's prayer time. They reoriented his bed so it faced the east, recognizing his need to pray toward Mecca (Carson & Koenig 2004, 76).

The Universality of Spirituality and Religion

One of the major difficulties in interpreting spirituality seems to be the question of universality. Spirituality is a universal dimension within every person—religious, atheist, or humanist. However, the expression and meaning that individuals attribute to spirituality may differ significantly. Frequently, spirituality is equated with religion or even a particular doc-

Table 1–1   Comparison of Religion and Spirituality

Religion	Spirituality
Community focused	Individualistic
Observable, measurable, objective	Less visible and measurable, more subjective
Formal, orthodox, organized	Less formal, less orthodox, less systematic
Behavior-oriented, outward practices	Emotionally oriented, inward-directed
Authoritarian in terms of behaviors	Not authoritarian, little accountability
Doctrine separating good from evil	Unifying, not doctrine-oriented

Source: Adapted from H. G. Koenig et al., *Handbook of Religion and Health* (New York: Oxford University Press, 2001), 18.

trine or belief; for many, their religion provides a framework through which to express their spirituality. However, spirituality and religion are not necessarily synonymous. Spirituality is about relationships and meaning, whereas religion reflects our attempts to structure and codify spirituality. Table 1–1 offers a comparison of spirituality and religion.

Spirituality and Worldview

When the first edition of this book was published in 1989, it was safe to say that in America the predominant worldview was a Christian theistic one—not just within society as a whole but also within the health care professions. Many nurses, physicians, and other health care providers believed that the human person is created in the image of God and that the body is the "temple of the Holy Spirit" (*The Soul Bible*, 1 Corinthians 6:19). For many today, this is no longer true, so we need to examine the implications of this change.

You may be wondering what a "worldview" is. Perhaps you have never before thought in terms of a worldview. That's probably because the idea of a worldview used to be reserved for the domain of philosophers and anthropologists. But now we all need to look at this concept: The events of September 11, 2001, make this imperative. Following the terrorist attacks of 9/11, most of us pondered what could drive people to commit such horrors; what kind of religious beliefs motivate the behavior of the Islamic terrorists; or how could these terrorists justify causing the deaths of so many Americans? Many throughout the world continue to struggle with understanding the extremist beliefs that are fueling violent and dramatic events around the globe. The drive to comprehend the meaning of these events is ultimately a struggle to grasp and understand the collision of opposing worldviews.

According to James Sire (2004, 2004a), everyone has a worldview, and the better we understand our own worldview the more we grow in self-awareness, self-knowledge, and self-understanding. Sire defines a worldview as follows:

a commitment, a fundamental orientation of the heart, that can be expressed as a story or in a set of presuppositions (assumptions that may be true, partially true or entirely false) which we hold (consciously or subconsciously, consistently or inconsistently) about the basic constitution of reality, and that provides the foundation on which we live and move and have our being. (Sire 2004, 17)

Sire suggests that an understanding of our personal worldview and that of others can be achieved by answering the seven questions in Box 1–1.

So how has the worldview shifted in the United States, and how has this shift affected our understanding of spirituality? Many theorists suggest that we are living in a postmodern world that dismisses the entire concept of "ultimate truth." In fact, postmodernism fails to recognize any worldview as having any greater value or validity than another worldview, and the "truth" of a particular story is dependent not on verifiable facts but on how effective the storyteller is in convincing his listener(s). The philosophy of postmodernism dismisses the belief in the infinite value of the human being as created "a little lower than the angels . . . crowned with glory and honor" (The Soul Bible, Psalm 8:5). Today there is a greater openness to the idea of spirit with an interpretation that spirit is impersonal energy that can be manipulated. In essence, this is a belief that God or gods can be manipulated and healings produced at will. Increasingly, we hear of practitioners referring to themselves as "healers" rather than "instruments of healing," a reference that flows from the understanding that the power to heal resides in divine hands alone. This shift in belief toward spirit as

Box 1-1   Seven Basic Questions to Determine Worldview

1. What is prime reality—the really real? To this we might answer God, or the gods, or the material cosmos.

2. What is the nature of external reality, that is, the world around us? Here our answers point to whether we see the world as created or autonomous, as chaotic or orderly, as matter or spirit, or whether we emphasize our subjective, personal relationship to the world or its objectivity apart from us.

3. What is a human being? To this we might answer a highly complex machine, a sleeping god, a person made in the image of God, a "naked ape."

4. What happens to a person at death? Here we might reply personal extinction, or transformation to a higher state, or reincarnation, or departure to a shadowy existence on "the other side."

5. Why is it possible to know anything at all? This is the language of James Sire—would it be clearer to ask: How do we know anything at all? Sample answers include the idea that we are made in the image of an all-knowing God or that consciousness and rationality developed under the contingencies of survival in a long process of evolution.

6. How do we know what is right and wrong? Again, perhaps we are made in the image of a God whose character is good; or right and wrong are determined by human choice alone or what feels good; or the notions simply developed under an impetus toward cultural or physical survival.

7. What is the meaning of human history? To this we might answer, to realize the purposes of God or the gods, to make a paradise on earth, to prepare a people for a life in community with a loving and holy God, and so forth.

Used with permission: J. W. Sire, *The Universe Next Door* (Downers Grove, Ill.: InterVarsity Press, 2004), 20–21.

impersonal energy has led to practices that involve channeling or manip-
ulating spirits, as well as the use of therapeutic touch that seeks to alter
the body chi (life energy in Chinese medicine), shamanistic practices, and
those of magic and the occult. These practices can take place even within
traditional Christianity.

How do individuals reconcile the inconsistencies between more traditional religious beliefs and pagan practices? In a postmodern world, there
is no need to reconcile these inconsistencies. The spiritual world today is
like a huge smorgasbord that allows those interested to take a bit of this
and a bit of that, no matter whether the various aspects are philosophically
compatible. With this approach, one might profess a belief in reincarnation that is totally incompatible with other religious beliefs that the individual holds just as strongly. In Christianity, as in Islam, time is linear. A
person gets one chance in this life to "do it right." That person may find
herself making the same mistake over and over again, and asking, "Will I
ever learn?" And, although she may repeat the same mistake, the circumstances are different. Christians believe that Jesus came once, was crucified
once, rose from the dead once, and ascended into heaven once. There is no
need for Jesus to repeat these events. Contrast this view of time and history with the perspective held in the Eastern philosophies, in which time
is viewed as circular and death does not lead to heaven or hell but rather
to reincarnation as either a lower life form or a more advanced human
being, depending on the quality of the person's prior life. While reincarnation may be viewed by some as incompatible with Christianity, Judaism,
and Islam, there are those who profess a belief in these faith traditions who
find the belief in reincarnation appealing. An individual's worldview need
not be internally consistent.

This shift in worldview is particularly apparent in nursing—more so
than in the other health care professions. Shelly and Miller (2006) point
to a movement in current nursing theories that encourages spirituality but
not spirituality connected to a personal God. The nursing interventions
that grow out of these theories embrace energy therapies. Prayer is frequently viewed as "merely good intentions on the part of the nurse healer
toward the ill person" (Shelly & Miller 2006, 50). Furthermore, Shelly and
Miller (2006) posit that this move in nursing is linked to a pervasive sense
of powerlessness. For nurses who believe in God, there is power in know-

ing that in their role as health care providers, their knowledge, compassion, and very presence speak of God's infinite knowledge, compassion, and presence to the ill person. However, once a nurse moves away from a grounding in a Christian or Jewish theistic worldview, the sense of being an instrument of God's power also wanes and the nurse feels helpless to alleviate pain and suffering. The energy therapies offer personal power in place of God's power.

Physicians rarely feel powerless; they have an arsenal of procedures and medications to draw upon. As a group, they are not as vulnerable to the appeal of the energy therapies, although they may feel pressured to recommend, or at least not criticize, nontraditional therapies sought by their patients.

What are the different worldviews? Sire (2004) identifies eight, including postmodernism (previously discussed), theism (Christian, Jewish, and Muslim), deism, naturalism, nihilism, existentialism (atheistic and theistic), Eastern pantheistic monism, and New Age. The following discussion provides an overview of theism, Eastern pantheistic monism, and New Age as the most relevant worldviews for the purpose of this text.

Theism

A belief in a personal God and ruler of the world that dominated thought in the Western world through the end of the seventeenth century. Christianity had so permeated the ideas and discourse that even if individuals did not believe in Christ or behaved as Christians should, they lived in a world where Christian ideas of God, the individual's relationship to God, sin, justice, heaven, and hell filtered through all thought.

CHRISTIAN THEISM

A belief in a personal (triune Father, Son, and Holy Spirit) God who is infinite, transcendent (or beyond us); God is all knowing; God is sovereign over the entire universe; God is good and from God's goodness we have an absolute standard of righteousness; God created an orderly and open universe from nothing; God spoke it into existence. We are created in God's image, which means we have personality, intelligence, morality, creativity, self-transcendence, and sociability. We are able to know the world around us and Godself because God created us with the ability to do so and the Divine takes an active role in communicating with us. Human beings were created good but through the sin of Adam and Eve the image of God within was damaged. That image is capable of being restored through the work of Christ, through whom God redeemed the human race and began the work of restoring people to goodness. Because God gives us free will, we may reject the Divine's redemptive actions. Death is either a gateway to heaven with God or a gateway to eternal separation from God; and last, ethics is transcendent and based on God's character, which is good and loving (Sire 2004, 6–41). Marcy's story represents the Christian theistic worldview.

JEWISH THEISM

Very similar to Christian theism—G-d is personal but not triune; G-d is the G-d of the universe, creator and all-powerful. Jewish theism does not believe that Jesus is the Son of God, the Messiah. Jews still await the coming of the Messiah. Jews believe that human beings are created to be responsible for their actions and as such they have free will—freedom to be obedient or disobedient to the universal law established by G-d as reflected in the Torah or "the law"—what Christians call the first five books of the Old Testament. Throughout the history of the Jewish people there have been times when the Israelites obeyed G-d's commandments and were faithful to G-d; at other times they failed to be faithful to this ideal and were disobedient. Jews believe that they have a unique relationship with G-d and that this relationship is expressed in a corporate life that encompasses every aspect of life, both public and private (Monk et al. 2003).

ISLAMIC THEISM

Known as one of the three great Abrahamic faiths. Like Judaism and Christianity, Islam was founded by a descendant of Abraham. Adherents to Islam believe in "Allah," the Arabic name for God. Allah is the source of all creation, personal, transcendent, and immanent. They hold to a strict monotheistic view of Allah in contrast to the triune nature of God held by Christians. They believe that Muhammad the prophet was a messenger of Allah who received revelations over a period of twenty-three years from the Angel Gabriel. The Qur'an ("The Reading" in Arabic) is the holy book that includes the messages brought to Muhammad; these messages were written down by others throughout the twenty-three years of revelation and compiled into the Qur'an after Muhammad's death. Islam holds that Muhammad completed a long succession of prophets, including Abraham, Moses, and Jesus, each of whom refined and restated the message of God. Followers of Islam (meaning submission to God, peace, safety, purity) are called Muslims. Muslims believe in a heaven and hell, a Day of Judgment, the return of Jesus (however not as the Son of God), predestination, and free will.

Eastern Pantheistic Monism

This foundational worldview undergirds Hinduism, Buddhism, and Taoism. We will look at Hinduism as the exemplar of Eastern pantheistic monism and offer descriptions of Buddhism and Taoism in chapter 4.

HINDUISM

Underlying belief is that only one impersonal element makes up reality. In this worldview the soul of each and every human being is called the Atman and the Atman is the same as Brahman, which is the Soul of the whole cosmos. In other words, each person is God. However, God is defined differently in pantheistic terms; God is infinite and impersonal, the ultimate reality. God is the cosmos. Getting to oneness with Brahman can be achieved through multiple paths; the focus of the journey is not on ideas or developing a relationship with the One, but on techniques such as chanting, meditation, or repetition of prayers or acts of genuflection. All these techniques lead the individual to connect to Brahman, the One. History is cyclical. Issues of morality are dealt with in the notion of karma that posits that our current fate and life's circumstances are the result of past actions; it is inextricably tied to reincarnation, which holds that no soul ever passes out of existence and it may take many years for a soul to find its way back to the One. The reason for doing good is to help our soul and to eliminate or minimize the suffering of our soul at a later time. The motivation for good deeds is to attain unity with the One. Death ends the existence of an individual so that, even though the Atman (individual soul) survives, there is no personal and individual immortality (Sire 2004, 141–61).

New Age

Begun in the 1970s, New Age beliefs are now integrated within many other belief systems. The human being is the prime reality, but the nature of the self is not always agreed upon—the self could be an idea, or a spirit, or a psychomagnetic field—but whatever it is, the self is at the center. Everything external to the self exists for the self. The self represents the cosmos and it is manifested in the dimension of the visible universe that can be accessed through ordinary consciousness and the invisible universe that can be accessed through altered states of consciousness; that is, through meditation, trance, ritualized dance, and the like (Sire 2004, 184). The invisible universe is referred to in a variety of ways: Mind at Large, expanded consciousness, alternative consciousness, Universal Mind, and so on. Within this invisible universe, the laws of the visible universe are suspended: Time and space are elastic, individuals experience power surges that can be transmitted to others, physical healings are said to occur, and distinctive personal beings exist. These beings are identified by many names, including demons, spirits, angels, guides, helpers, or guardians. Physical death is not the end of the self but signals the transition to another state. Ethics is not emphasized within New Age thinking because decisions of right and wrong reside within the self (Sire 2004, 162–210).

Pluralism

As the preceding discussion of worldviews makes absolutely clear, we live in a pluralistic world. Our views (whatever they may be) are not universally held by others and, indeed, may be vehemently opposed. Your notion of spirituality and religiousness may derive from a theistic (or nontheistic) worldview, and you may be confronted with patients and families who represent a range of worldviews. How do you communicate with those whose worldviews are not only different from your own but in direct opposition to yours? Certainly, this is a challenging task. It begins with the acknowledgment that it is never our job as nurses and other health care professionals to change the beliefs of the patients and families for whom we provide care. Our job is to help them meet their spiritual needs (as they perceive them), and that requires us to ask the right questions; to listen respectfully to the answers; to locate and provide spiritual/religious resources; to refer patients to professional chaplains, when indicated; to modify the environment, as needed; to be still in the face of questions; to be willing to share our own spiritual journey if that is appropriate; and even to pray, especially if the patient requests it. The "how to" for assessing and intervening to meet spiritual needs is discussed in chapter 6, "Spirituality: Identifying and Meeting Spiritual Needs."

Clinical Approaches to Spirituality

The bulk of the writing regarding the importance of spirituality comes from hospital chaplains, medicine, and nursing, with increasing awareness of this in the literature of social work as well as in physical, occupational, and speech therapies.

Professional Chaplains

Professional chaplains, when available, are the experts in dealing with spiritual and religious concerns in the hospital. They straddle two worlds—the world of hospital care and the world of religion. This places them in a unique position of being able to communicate with health care providers and to give direction to these providers as they grapple with spiritual and religious concerns that arise out of interactions with patients and families. Chaplains also support these same health care providers who struggle with their own spiritual and religious concerns. On the website for the Association of Professional Chaplains, www.professionalchaplains.org, there is a white paper titled "Professional Chaplaincy: Its Role and Importance in Healthcare," which readers are encouraged to consult. This reference identifies five reasons that the role of the hospital chaplain is essential in meeting spiritual needs, not only of patients and families but also of staff and the organization as a whole:

1. Patients and families want this care and have a right to such services.
2. Illnesses frequently produce fear and loneliness that lead to spiritual crises requiring spiritual interventions.

3. When a cure is not possible, spiritual care plays an important role in helping patients and families find meaning in their circumstances.

4. Spiritual care is vital to organizations because it helps address the spiritual needs of employees.

5. Spiritual care is important in health care organizations when staff and families are confronted with ethical issues.

Professional chaplains have extensive training in providing spiritual care to hospitalized patients, families, and staff. Certified chaplains complete four years of college, three years of divinity school (master's of divinity), one or two years of clinical pastoral education, pass a written examination, pass an oral examination, and must be recommended by their denomination. Community clergy typically do not have this kind of training, and are not able to address the special spiritual needs that arise when patients are hospitalized with disabling and often life-threatening illnesses— at least not the way chaplains are. The Association of Professional Chaplains has a strategic plan, a code of ethics, and a best practices focus that all members of this organization must adhere to (Association of Professional Chaplains 2007). Professional chaplains are required to obtain continuing education units (CEUs) each year in order to stay updated on the latest research, patient education, and clinical practices. When anything but the simplest of spiritual concerns arise, the chaplain needs to be involved. Increasingly, professional chaplains are being included as part of the multidisciplinary health care team, together with doctors and nurses.

Medicine

Physicians, too, need to be aware of and concerned about patients' spiritual needs. There are at least five reasons why (Koenig 2007):

1. Many patients are religious, and religious beliefs help them to cope.

2. Religious beliefs influence medical decisions, especially when patients are seriously ill, and in some instances may conflict with medical treatments.

3. Religious beliefs and activities are related to better health and quality of life.

4. Many patients would like physicians to address their spiritual needs.

5. Calling on physicians to address spiritual needs is not new; it is rooted in the long historical relationship between religion, medicine, and health care (Koenig 2002, 5).

These reasons do not necessarily compel physicians to address spiritual and religious concerns. In fact, whether or not this is an appropriate area for physicians to explore is passionately debated. The groundwork for this debate was laid in 1999 when psychologist Richard Sloan of Columbia University wrote a paper that was published in *The Lancet*. He followed with another paper that appeared in the *New England Journal of Medicine*. In both of these papers Sloan criticized research studies on religion and health for weak methodology. Furthermore, he stated that religion and medicine don't mix and that encouraging patients toward spiritual practices may actually be harmful. Although encouraging patients to become more religious or prescribing religion to nonreligious patients is not what we recommend, being aware of each patient's beliefs, and supporting those beliefs, is very much a part of holistic medical practice.

Even when physicians believe that spirituality and religion are appropriate areas for inquiry with patients, this does not guarantee that they actually engage in this discussion with their patients. In a 2006 cross-sectional study published in *Medical Care*, 1,144 physicians out of 2,000 potential respondents completed a survey that examined this very issue. Ninety-one percent of the physicians said that it is appropriate to discuss religious /spiritual issues if the patient initiates the discussion; 73 percent said that, when patients initiate a discussion of religious/spiritual issues, they encourage the patient's own religious/spiritual beliefs and practices. However, there was less agreement about when physicians should inquire about religious/spiritual issues, with only 55 percent saying that it is usually or always appropriate. Forty-three percent said it is appropriate to share their own religious beliefs or experiences if the patient asks; 14 percent said it is never appropriate to share personal religious beliefs. Fifty-three percent said that praying with patients is appropriate only if the patient asks, while 17 percent said that praying with patients is never appropriate. The study also found that physicians, especially Protestant physicians, who identified themselves as more religious or spiritual, were more likely to initiate a discussion about religious and spiritual issues, to share their own religious and spiritual beliefs and practices, and to pray with patients (Curlin et al. 2006).

One reason physicians give for not addressing the spiritual component is a basic lack of know-how in this area. Over the last fifteen years, this lack of know-how has begun to be addressed in medical education. Today over 100 of the 141 U.S. and Canadian medical schools offer some type of course on spirituality and health. Some of these courses are electives and reach only a small number of medical students, but, according to Puchalski (2006), increasingly these courses are required (70 percent).

Nursing

Nursing approaches spirituality differently from medicine and has developed three diverse but interrelated approaches: spiritual distress, spiritual needs, and spiritual well-being. Each approach has its strengths. Each sheds light on a different facet of spirituality, but none provides a total picture. Because of the complexity and multidimensionality of spirituality, it is uniquely experienced and interpreted by each person. Only a person himself is able to provide another with unique perceptions of his own spirituality. Nurses and others depend on a patient's self-report and validation of observed behaviors to understand his sense of spirituality.

SPIRITUAL DISTRESS

Spiritual distress is a nursing diagnosis approved by the North American Nursing Diagnosis Association (NANDA). Spiritual distress is defined as follows: "Impaired ability to experience and integrate meaning and purpose in life through a person's connectedness with self, others, art, music, literature, nature or a power greater than oneself" (NANDA International 2005, 186). Defining characteristics of spiritual distress are shown in Box 1–2. The risk factors for spiritual distress are shown in Box 1–3.

SPIRITUAL NEEDS

A second nursing approach to spirituality in patients is that of spiritual needs. This approach is derived from a Christian theistic worldview. Stallwood and Stoll (1975) defined spiritual needs as "any factors necessary to establish and/or maintain a person's dynamic personal relationship with God (as defined by that individual) and out of that relationship to experience forgiveness, love, hope, trust and meaning and purpose in life" (1088).

Box 1–2   Defining Characteristics of Spiritual Distress

Connections to Self

Expresses lack of:
Hope
Meaning and purpose in life
Peace/serenity
Acceptance
Love
Forgiveness of self
Courage

Anger

Guilt

Poor Coping

Connections with Others

Refuses interactions with spiritual leaders
Refuses interactions with friends, family
Verbalizes being separated from their support system
Expresses alienation

Connections with Art, Music, Literature, Nature

Inability to express previous state of creativity (singing/listening
    to music/writing)
No interest in nature
No interest in reading spiritual literature

Connections with Power Greater than Self

Inability to pray
Inability to participate in religious activities
Expresses being abandoned by or having anger toward God
Inability to experience the transcendent
Requests to see a religious leader
Sudden changes in spiritual practices
Inability to be introspective/inward turning
Expresses being without hope, suffering

Used with permission: NANDA International, *Nursing Diagnoses: Definitions & Classification 2005–2006* (Philadelphia: NANDA International, 2005), 186.

> **Box 1–3   Risk Factors for Spiritual Distress**
>
> **Physical**
>   Physical illness
>   Substance abuse/excessive drinking
>   Chronic illness
>
> **Psychosocial**
>   Low self-esteem
>   Depression
>   Anxiety
>   Stress
>   Poor relationships
>   Separate from support systems
>   Blocks to experiencing love
>   Inability to forgive
>   Loss
>   Racial/cultural conflict
>   Change in religious rituals
>   Change in spiritual practices
>
> **Developmental**
>   Life change
>   Developmental life changes
>
> **Environmental**
>   Environmental changes
>   Natural disasters
>
> Used with permission: NANDA International, *Nursing Diagnoses: Definitions & Classification 2005–2006* (Philadelphia: NANDA International, 2005), 188.

Stallwood and Stoll (1975) used a two-dimensional approach to spiritual needs, although clearly based on a relationship with God (as defined by that person). Shelly (2000) mirrors the Stallwood and Stoll definition, but clarifies that understandings of spiritual needs may differ widely, with some defining spiritual needs as involving the arts and creativity and others viewing spiritual needs from a psychosocial perspective and focusing on social systems and mental health (Shelly 2000, 29).

The nurse is seen as the "instrument" to encourage the patient to experience God's meeting of these spiritual needs. Lack of opportunity to carry out her usual religious practices while ill or hospitalized may cause the patient to experience spiritual needs (Shelly 2000).

SPIRITUAL WELL-BEING

The National Interfaith Coalition on Aging (NICA) developed an initial definition of spiritual well-being: the "affirmation of life in a relationship with God, self, community and environment that nurtures and celebrates wholeness" (Cook 1980, xiii). The NICA stated that spiritual well-being indicates wholeness and "expresses dependence on the source of life, God the creator." To have spiritual well-being is "to say yes to life in spite of negative circumstances . . . occurring within the context of one's relationship with God, self, community and environment. God is seen as Supreme Being, creator of life, the source and power that wills well-being. All people are called upon to respond to God in love and obedience. Realizing we are God's children, we grow toward wholeness as individuals and we are led to affirm our kinship with others in the community of faith and the entire human family . . . yes to life is the acknowledgment of the destiny of life" (Cook 1980, xiii–xiv).

Subsequently, Ellison (1983) sought to delineate further the components of spiritual well-being. He believed that the NICA's definition comprised both a vertical religious dimension, referring to a person's sense of well-being in relation to God, and a horizontal existential dimension, referring to his sense of meaning, purpose, and satisfaction with life. Spiritual well-being is not a state but, rather, is indicative of the presence of spiritual health in the person. Therefore, spiritual well-being is identified as behavioral expressions of spiritual health. Some statements that a person might report as an indicator of spiritual well-being are as follows:

Religious component (God)	I believe that God loves me and cares for me.
	I have a personally meaningful relationship with God.
	My relationship with God helps me not to feel lonely.

Meaning in life and satisfaction	I feel that life is a positive experience.
(Sociopsychological)	I feel very fulfilled and satisfied with life.
	I believe there is some real purpose for my life. (Paloutzian and Ellison 1982, 232)

Ellison and Paloutzian (1983) developed the twenty-item Spiritual Well-Being (SWB) scale containing two subscales: Religious Well-Being and Existential Well-Being. This scale has been used by many nurse researchers to examine the relationship between SWB and a variety of constructs, such as hope, hardiness, pain management, chronic illness, cancer, the needs of the geriatric patient, and the like (Carson & Green 1992; Carson, Soeken, & Grimm 1988; Chow 2005; Fehring, Miller, & Shaw 1997; Hendricks-Ferguson 2006; Landis 1996; Mickley & Soeken 1993; Mickley, Soeken, & Belcher 1992; Soeken & Carson 1987).

Each of these nursing approaches to understanding a person's spirituality suggests behaviors indicative of health or illness. These behaviors occur within the person's inner being and yet are all relational in nature—with God (or a Higher Being), oneself, others, and the environment. These behavioral characteristics are a sampling of the person's spirituality and should not be construed as comprehensive and definitive. Yet they do indicate a sense of spiritual well-being or distress. A person's inner state of being and relationships will influence and perhaps significantly govern the quality and fulfillment of her needs, goals, and aspirations in life. Our spirituality obviously fluctuates because of alterations—positive and negative—in feelings, thoughts, physical health, and situations. It is therefore important for nurses to be cognizant of a spiritual wellness–illness continuum of behaviors.

We must also recognize that people express their unique spirituality in diverse ways. In addition, the meanings these behavioral characteristics have to the person and how they impact on each one's day-to-day functioning give further evidence of spiritual health or distress.

Social Work

Increasingly there is interest among social workers in the importance of spirituality to the issues that they address with individuals, families, and communities. Issues such as substance abuse, family abuse and violence, poverty, and social justice all are identified as having spiritual and religious components that need to be addressed in order to help the client. This trend is seen not just in the United States with organizations such as the National Association of Christian Social Workers (www.nacsw.org), the Center for Spirituality and Integral Social Work at the Catholic University of America (http://csisw.cua.edu), and the Society for Spirituality and Social Work at Arizona State University (http://ssw.asu.edu/spirituality/sssw), but also in Canada in the Canadian Society for Spirituality and Social Work (http://people.stu.ca/~jcoates/cnssw/). Research conducted in the United States as well as the UK demonstrates that there is little to no course content in most social work curricula to teach social work students how to assess or intervene to meet spiritual need (Furman, Benson, Grimwood, & Canda 2004; Gilligan 2003; Gilligan & Furness 2005). In these same studies, a significant percentage of the respondents said they believe that including religion and spirituality in direct practice is compatible with social work's mission.

Therapies

Physical and occupational therapists are beginning to look at the importance of spirituality as part of their practices as well. There is an organization called Christian Physical Therapists International (http://www.cpti.org/). This is a relatively new focus for physical therapists. In a 2004 study conducted with physical therapists, 245 questionnaires were sent out, with 136 questionnaires returned. Ninety-six percent of the respondents agreed or strongly agreed that spirituality is an important component of health care. However, over 50 percent never discussed spiritual issues with patients, and 42 percent believed that the discussion of spiritual needs is inappropriate for the physical therapist (Oakley, Katz, Sauer, & Dent 2004). Although many of the programs that prepare physical therapists to become doctors of physical therapy are currently including content on spirituality, spirituality is not part of the standard curriculum to become a physical therapist.

Judging by the number of journal articles dealing with the role of the occupational therapist (OT) in meeting spiritual needs, this is an area of interest to occupational therapists both in the United States and Canada. However, a finding replicated in several studies is that the majority of occupational therapists report that their academic training did not prepare them to address the spiritual needs of patients (Collins, Paul, & West-Frasier 2001; Engquist, Short-DeGraff, Gliner, & Oltjenbruns 1997; Taylor, Mitchel, Kenan, & Tacker 2000; Zorzes 2004). Notwithstanding the lack of preparation, OTs report using spiritual interventions. Collins, Paul, & West-Frasier (2001) sent 396 questionnaires to OTs randomly selected from the American Occupational Therapy Association (AOTA) database, and 206 (52 percent) usable questionnaires were returned. The most frequently reported interventions were praying for a patient (74 percent), using spiritual language or concepts (57 percent), and discussing with patients ways that the therapist's own religious beliefs are helpful (53 percent). Taylor, Mitchel, Kenan, & Tacker (2000) also used a survey design, sending out questionnaires to 250 randomly selected members of the AOTA; 112 completed surveys were returned. The therapists were presented with eight topics and asked how often they address these topics with patients. The results were as follows: 63.4 percent of respondents occasionally or very frequently discuss the meaning or purpose of illness, belief and faith, religious values, and fears of death or dying; 61.6 percent discuss the following topics at least occasionally: attitudes about giving and receiving love, and meditation or quiet reflection; 51.8 percent discuss prayer at least occasionally; 48.2 percent discuss attitudes about forgiveness at least occasionally; and 41 percent discuss the role of God in illness at least occasionally. Also interesting to note, there is an association of Christian OTs called the International Occupational Therapists for Christ, Inc. (http://www .otforchrist.org).

Summary

This chapter has offered an overview of spirituality and laid the foundation for an understanding and appreciation of the significance of spirituality to health and wholeness. Spirituality is an abstract, multifaceted concept, comprising numerous components interacting at many levels of awareness. Spirituality is affected by personal experience, religion, culture, and worldview. The connections that link our internal spirit and its outward expressions are many (see Boxes 1–1 and 1–2). Our spirituality ebbs and flows—sometimes in an even flow, sometimes in trickles, and infrequently in tumultuous "peak experiences." Our experience of the Divine, however perceived, and of the ultimate values that govern and shape our lives is not static. Each person longs to experience the integrity of a life lived in a rich, woven tapestry. As health care providers—chaplains, physicians, nurses, social workers, and therapists—we are challenged to honor the integrity of the lives of our patients and their families and to respond to the spiritual needs that contribute to the weaving of their personal tapestries. Furthermore, we need to acknowledge our own personal spiritual journeys, and not confuse them with our patients' journeys, for it is in the continuous recognition of and meeting our own spiritual needs that we will be able to assist patients in maximizing their own spiritual well-being as they perceive it. In addition to the respectful and competent meeting of health care needs, one of the greatest gifts that any of us can offer patients is a rich, living spiritual connection, if the patient desires. This gift of one's true self given in care to the patient experiencing a health crisis will inevitably help to support the patient's spiritual well-being.

In the next chapter you will read about the contributions made by research to our understanding of spirituality/religion and health.

Reflective Activities

1. Consider how you might describe your own spirituality. Try to write a description or share it with a trusted friend.
2. Identify how you express your spirituality in behavioral terms and which of those behaviors indicate expressions of spiritual well-being or spiritual distress.
3. Have you observed how a patient's illness or other health care crises affect his spirituality? If so, reflect on those observations and how the patient might have been helped by your intervention.
4. What difference does spirituality make in your lifestyle? In your relationships? In your role as a health care provider?
5. How can you nurture your own spiritual well-being?

REFERENCES

Association of Professional Chaplains. (2007). See *About APC* at website http://www.professionalchaplains.org/. Accessed February 2, 2007.

Batchelor, G. (2006). Professional chaplains and spirituality. *Atlanta Hospital News* 1(7): 8.

Carson, V. B. (1993). Spirituality: Generic or Christian. *Journal of Christian Nursing* 10(1): 24–27.

Carson, V. B., & Green, H. (1992). Spiritual well-being: A predictor of hardiness in the AIDS patient. *Journal of Professional Nursing* 8(4): 209–20.

Carson, V. B., & Koenig, H. G. (2004). *Spiritual Caregiving: Healthcare as a Ministry.* Philadelphia: Templeton Foundation Press.

Carson, V. B., Soeken, K. L., & Grimm, P. M. (1988). Hope and its relationship to spiritual well-being. *Journal of Psychology and Theology* 16: 159–67.

Chow, R. K. (2005). Life's quest for spiritual well-being. *Geriatric Nursing* (September/October): 80–83.

Clinton, T. (editor). (2001). *The Soul Care Bible.* Nashville: Thomas Nelson Publishers.

Collins, J. S., Paul, S., & West-Frasier, J. (2001). The utilization of spirituality in occupational therapy: Beliefs, practices, and perceived barriers. *Occupational Therapy in Health Care* 14: 73–92.

Cook, T. C. (1980). Preface. In Thorson, J. A., & Cook, T. C. (eds.), *Spiritual Well-Being of the Elderly.* Springfield, Ill.: Charles C. Thomas.

Curlin, F. A., Chin, M. H., Sellergren, S. A., Roach, C. J., and Lantos, J. D. (2006). The association of physicians' religious characteristics with their attitudes and self-reported behaviors regarding religion and spirituality in the clinical encounter. *Medical Care* 44(5): 446–52.

Ellison, C. W. (1983). Spiritual well-being: Conceptualization and measurement. *Journal of Psychological Theology* 11: 330–40.

Emmons, R. A., & Crumpler, C.A. (1999). Religion and spirituality: The roles of sanctification and the concept of God. *International Journal for the Psychology of Religion* 9(1): 17–24.

Engquist, D. E., Short-DeGraff, M., Gliner, J., & Oltjenbruns, K. (1997). Occupational therapist's beliefs and practices with regard to spirituality and therapy. *American Journal of Occupational Therapy* 51(3): 173–80.

Fehring, R. H., Miller, J. F., & Shaw, C. (1997). Spiritual well-being, religiosity, hope, depression, and other mood states. *Oncology Nursing Forum* 24(4): 663–71.

Fitchett, G. (2002). Assessing spiritual needs: a guide for caregivers. Lima, Ohio: Academic Renewal Press.

Furman, L. D., Benson, P. W., Grimwood, C., & Canda, E. (2004). Religion and spirituality in social work education and direct practice at the millenium: A survey of UK social workers. *British Journal of Social Work* 34(6): 767–92.

Gilligan, P. A. (2003). It isn't discussed. Religion, belief and practice teaching: Missing components of cultural competence in social work education. *Journal of Practice Teaching in Health and Social Work* 5(1): 75–95.

Gilligan, P. A., & Furness, S. (2005). The role of religion and spirituality in social work practice: Views and experiences of social work students. *British Journal of Social Work* (October 3). http:/bjsw.oxfordjournals.org/cgi/content/short/bch252v1. Accessed September 2, 2006.

Hendricks-Ferguson, V. (2006). Relationships of age and gender to hope and spiritual well-being among adolescents with cancer. *Journal of Pediatric Oncology Nursing* 23(4): 189–99.

Koenig, H. G. (2002/2007). *Spirituality in Patient Care: Why, How, When, and What*. Philadelphia: Templeton Foundation Press.

Landis, B. J. (1996). Uncertainty, spiritual well-being and psychosocial adjustment to chronic illness. *Issues in Mental Health Nursing* 17(3): 217–23.

Mickley, J. R., & Soeken, K. (1993). Religiousness and hope in Hispanic and Anglo-American women with breast cancer. *Oncology Nursing Forum* 20: 1171–76.

Mickley, J. R., Soeken, K., & Belcher, A. (1992). Spiritual well-being, religiousness and hope among women with breast cancer. *Image: Journal of Nursing Scholarship* 24(4) (Winter): 267–72.

Miller, J. F (1985). Assessment of loneliness and spiritual well-being in chronically ill and healthy adults. *Journal of Professional Nursing* 3: 79–85.

Monk, R. C., Hofheinz, W. D., Lawrence, K. T., Stamey, J. D., Alfeck, B., & Yamamori, T. (2003). *Exploring Religious Meaning*, 6th ed. Upper Saddle River, N.J.: Prentice Hall.

NANDA International (2005). *NANDA Nursing Diagnoses: Definitions & Classification 2005–2006*. Philadelphia: NANDA International.

Oakley, E., Katz, G., Sauer, K., & Dent, B. (2004). Physical therapists' perception on spirituality and patient care: Beliefs, practices and perceived barriers. *Journal of the American Physical Therapy Association* (June 30–July 3). www.apta.org/am/abstracts/pt2004/abstractspt2004.cfm?pubNo=PO-RR-113-TH. Accessed September 2, 2006.

O'Brien, M. E. (2003). *Spirituality in Nursing: Standing on Holy Ground*, 2nd ed. Boston: Jones and Bartlett Publishers.

Paloutzian, R. F., & Ellison, C. W. (1982). Loneliness, spiritual well-being, and the quality of life. In L. A. Peplau and D. Perlman (eds.), *Loneliness: A Sourcebook of Current Theory, Research and Therapy*. New York: John Wiley & Sons.

Plante, T. G., & Sherman, A. C. (2001). *Faith and Health: Psychological Perspectives*. New York: Guilford Press.

Puchalski, C. (2006). Spirituality and medicine: Curricula in medical education. *Journal of Cancer Education* 21(1): 14–18.

Shelly, J. A. (2000). *Spiritual Care: A Guide for Caregivers*. Downers Grove, Ill.: InterVarsity Press.

Shelly, J. A., & Miller, A. B. (2006). *Called to Care: A Christian Worldview of Nursing*, 2nd ed. Downers Grove, Ill.: InterVarsity Press.

Sire, J. W. (2004). *The Universe Next Door*, 4th ed. Downers Grove, Ill.: InterVarsity Press.

———. (2004a). *Naming the Elephant: Worldview as a Concept*. Downers Grove, Ill.: InterVarsity Press.

Smith, C., & Denton, M. L. (2005). *Soul Searching: The Religious and Spiritual Lives of American Teenagers*. New York: Oxford University Press.

Soeken, K. L., & Carson, V. B. (1987). Responding to the spiritual needs of the chronically ill. *Nursing Clinics of North America* 22: 603–11.

Stallwood, J., & Stoll, R. (1975). Spiritual dimensions of nursing practice. In I. L. Beland & J. Y. Passos (eds.), *Clinical Nursing*, 3rd ed. New York: Macmillan.

Stoll, R. I. (1989). The essence of spirituality. In Verna Benner Carson (ed.), *Spiritual Dimensions of Nursing Practice*. Philadelphia: W. B. Saunders Company.

Taylor, E., Mitchel, J. E., Kenan, S., & Tacker, R. (2000). Attitudes of occupational therapists toward spirituality in practice. *American Journal of Occupational Therapy* 54: 421–26.

Turner, S. (1990). Lean, green, and meaningless. *Christianity Today* (September 24): 26–27.

Zorzes, J. (2004). How Are Occupational Therapists Addressing Spirituality in Their Practice? http://www.rehab.queensu.ca/cats/PDFs%5C21.pdf. Accessed February 25.

2

RELIGION, SPIRITUALITY, AND HEALTH

UNDERSTANDING THE MECHANISMS

HAROLD G. KOENIG

Restore me to health and make me live!
—Isaiah 38:16

Introduction

Growing attention has been paid to the possible health benefits of religion over the past two decades. In this chapter I will give an overview of research linking religion and health, and explore mechanisms by which religion may influence physical health outcomes, information that should be helpful to nurses. Before proceeding, however, it is important to define the terms *religion*, *spirituality*, and *humanism* as I will be using them. Investigators often use these terms to describe the same thing, and yet it is important to keep the meaning of these words distinct.[1] *Religion* involves public and private practices and rituals, beliefs, and a creed with dos and don'ts. It is community-oriented and responsibility-oriented. Nevertheless, it can also be divisive, since different religions teach different things that may conflict with one another (as seen in the last chapter). Because these teachings are held so deeply and passionately, conflict may spark the persecution—or harming—of people of one religion by those of another. Because of this potential for divisiveness, *religion*, or religiosity, is an unpopular term. However, it is relatively easy to define, measure, and quantify.

Spirituality, on the other hand, involves a quest for the sacred. In this author's opinion, in order to be called spiritual, it must have a relationship to the Transcendent. The Transcendent may be God, Allah, Jesus, a Higher Power, Brahman, Krishna, or Ultimate Reality. Spirituality is more personal and individual-focused than religion. It is inclusive and less divisive, and, consequently, is more popular than religion. However, because spirituality is so individualistic, it is difficult to define and measure for research purposes, except for simple self-ratings (for example, on a scale of 1 to 5, how spiritual are you?).

Humanism is a third term that needs to be defined and distinguished from religion and spirituality. There are forms of Christian humanism and secular humanism. Secular humanism involves human experiences that lack a connection to the Transcendent, to a Higher Power, or to Ultimate Truth, where the focus is on the human self as the ultimate source of power and meaning. This, in my opinion, should not be called spirituality, although opinions vary in this regard. Most authorities, but not all, agree that religion is a component of spirituality, and a person can be spiritual but not religious; others argue that spirituality is a subset of deeply religious people. Because it is easier to measure, religion has been the focus of most research.

Religion and Neurosis

The neurotic aspects of religion (called a "universal obsessional neurosis" by Freud) are often emphasized,[2] and there is little doubt that religion has been associated with neurotic tendencies. Religion may be used to justify hatred, aggression, and prejudice against people who are different. It may be used to gain power and control over others, most prominently illustrated in religious cults. Religion can foster rigid thinking by emphasizing the rules rather than the spirit of its doctrine. It can reward individuals for obsessive practices, such as repetitive prayer or other repetitive rituals.

Religion may foster anxiety, fear, or excessive guilt over real or imagined sins in the sensitive individual who is prone to such emotions. Religion may be used in a magical or unrealistic manner to deny the facts of a situation, encouraging people to pray for miraculous healing rather than seeking medical attention, thereby delaying diagnosis and/or effective treatment. From a psychological standpoint, religion may be used defensively to avoid addressing issues or avoid making important changes in behavior that is necessary for mental health and well-being. Bizarre religious beliefs are common in the thoughts of psychotic persons, and 25 percent to 40 percent of patients with schizophrenia experience religious delusions.[3] Religion may also interfere with mental health care; religious communities may encourage members to stop taking their medications, discourage them from seeking needed psychotherapy, and foster negative attitudes toward mental health professionals. Some religious teachings may not be healthy for certain individuals who are psychologically fragile and may misinterpret those teachings.

Religion and Coping with Illness

While in some instances religion can be used in a neurotic way, or may exacerbate guilt or anxiety in vulnerable patients, it does not usually do so. Religious beliefs are often used to cope with or make sense of stressful experiences or life changes. This is especially true for medical or psychiatric patients. When sickness strikes and threatens to affect a person's life, that person may pray or read religious scriptures for hope and consolation, or the religious community may mobilize support around that person.

Numerous studies document a high prevalence of religious activity as a coping behavior by patients undergoing serious medical problems. These studies have been done in patients with arthritis,[4] heart or pulmonary disease,[5] chronic pain,[6] end-stage kidney disease,[7] cancer,[8] sickle-cell disease,[9] and AIDS/HIV,[10] and with severely ill children or adolescents.[11] Among hospitalized patients, one study reported that nearly 90 percent scored themselves 5 or higher on a visual analog scale indicating how much they depended on religion to cope.[12] A score of 0 on this scale indicated "not at all," 2 or 3 meant "a little bit," 5 indicated "a moderate extent," 7–8 indicated "a large extent," and 10 signified "the most important factor that kept the person going" (over 40 percent of 337 patients specified 10). In fact, prayer is among the most common alternative medicine modalities that people engage in when self-treating their medical problems (25–35 percent of Americans).[13] Stress, in general, tends to precipitate coping strategies involving religion. In a random sample of the U.S. population after 9/11, no fewer than 9 out of 10 Americans turned to religion to cope.[14]

How Religion Influences Coping

How might religious beliefs and practices enable a person under stress to cope better? First, religion provides a positive worldview. In the Christian tradition, for example, God is seen as all-powerful, everywhere present, loving, caring, and responsive to individual needs. There is the belief in an afterlife both for the individual and for departed loved ones that makes death seem less threatening, and separation seem less permanent. Furthermore, there are religious rituals and traditions that bring comfort to the bereaved person or the family of the deceased person. The scientific, secular worldview sees the world and humans in it as having evolved by accident, and death being the final end of the deceased person and eternal separation from him.

Second, the religious worldview sees the lives of each human as having unique meaning and purpose. Humans were created by God with a purpose in mind, and can relate to and work with God in achieving God's purpose. Regardless of what situation a person finds herself in, God can use that person and her situation so that some good might result. As the scripture says, "And we know that all things work together for good to them that love God, to them who are the called according to his purpose."[15] The secular, scientific worldview sees each human's life as the result of mere chance, without any ultimate purpose or meaning. These differences regarding purpose and meaning become particularly important for the disabled, sick, or suffering person. Religion helps to interpret such suffering in meaningful ways, whereas the secular worldview sees no purpose or meaning in suffering.

Third, religion facilitates psychological integration of difficult life experiences or traumas. For example, a person has a stroke that prevents him from working and makes him dependent on others for his most basic needs. In order to integrate this dramatic life change and move on with life, he must make sense of what has happened in a way that is consistent with his understanding of himself and the world. Religion helps people to do that by providing explanations and reasons that give meaning to the event and helps to maintain a cohesive worldview. This helps the person to psychologically integrate the event and move on with life, as opposed to being stuck in a traumatized, psychologically unintegrated state from which he cannot escape.

Fourth, religion gives people hope that motivates them to keep trying, and helps them to see a way out of seemingly impossible situations that would otherwise imprison and paralyze them. Having hope gives people the energy to press on and not give up. It is an antidote to depression.

Fifth, religion empowers the patient. Religious beliefs and practices give patients something they can do (either cognitively or behaviorally) to cope with their illness. As noted above, activities such as praying to God provide the patient with an indirect form of control over her illness, thereby giving her something to do that she believes will influence the outcome. If a patient believes that God is the creator and all-powerful, cares about her, and listens to personal prayer, then praying to God for relief or healing constitutes a powerful activity that represents a kind of self-care. Rather than helplessly depending on her doctor's attention, prescriptions, and goodwill, the praying patient takes things into her own hands. This gives her a sense of control over her situation, albeit a form of indirect control through her ability to influence God.

Sixth, religion provides role models for suffering. For example, the Judeo-Christian scriptures provide many stories of people who were depressed, sick, or going through some other kind of tragedy or loss. Job, David, Elijah, Jeremiah, or even Jesus dying on the cross ("My God, my God, why hast thou forsaken me?"[16]) illustrates this point. The book of Job demonstrates best how the Bible provides role models for coping. The first verse says that, "There was a man in the land of Uz, whose name was Job; and that man was perfect and upright, and one that feared God, and eschewed evil."[17] Even though Job was "perfect and upright," many tragedies befell him. He lost his job and possessions, he lost all his children, he lost his health (he was covered with boils), and he lost his mental health (he became quite depressed). His response was like that of many patients who have had one negative life experience after another, whose prayers seemingly go unanswered: He got angry at God, and accused God of punishing him unjustly. Patients ask "Why me?" and wonder what they have done to deserve this. Like Job, often they have done nothing wrong, but in the overall scheme of things (which is understood completely by God alone), these experiences are a necessary part of life. The book of Job sends the message that it is OK to be angry at God, but just remember that God knows more than you do about the past, present, and eternal future.

Seventh, religion provides social constraints and guidance for decision making that ultimately reduces stress. When patients experience the stress of illness and change, they may treat the psychological pain with alcohol, prescription drugs (sedatives or anti-anxiety drugs), or analgesics (pain killers), resulting in a substance abuse problem on top of the other problems they were having. Nearly one hundred scientific studies have now documented an inverse correlation between religious involvement and use of drugs or alcohol.[18] Likewise, patients may be tempted to give up, become overly busy to avoid the issues, withdraw socially from others, or become involved in risky sexual practices as a way to relieve their stress. These kinds of responses ultimately increase stress or worsen medical and mental health problems. Religious beliefs discourage such responses to stress and encourage activities such as prayer, altruism, reading of the scriptures, or seeking support from the religious community. These responses are much healthier than the other ones. Thus, religion helps patients make better decisions, which contribute to health rather than detract from it.

Eighth, religion provides answers to the big questions in life that are outside the realm of medicine and science: Where did I come from? Why am I here? Where am I going? Throughout human history, religions around the world have provided answers to such questions that usually encourage healthy, prosocial kinds of behaviors—doing good for others, treating others right, forgiving others for hurts inflicted, and respecting our own body.

Finally, religion provides social support, both human and divine. The largest source of support for older adults outside of their immediate family is members of their religious organizations.[19] One study of older medical patients found that over half indicated that 80 to 100 percent of their five closest friends came from their churches, mosques, or synagogues.[20] Numerous studies report that people who are more religiously involved perceive their social support to be greater (nineteen of twenty studies cited in the Handbook of Religion and Health).[21] Besides human support, the religious person also experiences divine support and guidance through a relationship with God, and this is particularly important when human support is lacking or not readily available. Patients report that by praying to God they feel less lonely and more cared for. [22]

Religion is an especially helpful coping behavior among patients with medical illness because, unlike most other coping resources, it is not lost with physical illness or disability. As long as the person is conscious and can mobilize religious beliefs, religious coping is possible. Even when she is unconscious, members of her faith community may pray for her and otherwise rally around her and her family, enabling everyone to cope better with the situation.

Research on Religion and Mental Health

Despite a potential to exacerbate mental illness and neurosis, religious involvement has been found in a number of studies to be linked with better mental health—greater well-being,[23] less depression,[24] faster recovery from depression,[25] less anxiety,[26] and better outcomes in schizophrenia.[27] Religious involvement has been shown to be particularly important for mental health among people who are stressed in some way over their circumstances.

A number of studies of medical inpatients have shown a lower prevalence of depression among those who were more religiously involved[28] and a faster speed of remission from depression.[29] For example, a study of 850 older men found that religious coping during hospitalization was related to fewer depressive symptoms and, significantly, predicted fewer depressive symptoms after an average two- to three-month follow-up.[30] Another prospective study of 87 depressed older medical inpatients found that those with higher intrinsic religiosity scores recovered significantly faster than those with lower scores, even after controlling for other predictors of recovery.[31] A more recent study of 865 depressed medical inpatients found that those who were the most religious (14 percent of the sample who attended religious services weekly, prayed daily, read the Bible several times per week, and scored high on intrinsic religiosity) went into remission from their depression over 50 percent faster than other patients.[32]

Religious beliefs and practices may be particularly important for people undergoing the most severe of stressors, for example, those with posttraumatic stress disorder (PTSD). One study involved 1,385 veterans who had experienced active combat in Vietnam, Korea, or World War II, and who were being treated in outpatient or inpatient PTSD programs.[33] This study was conducted by the VA's National Center for PTSD and Yale University School of Medicine. Investigators discovered that those who had experienced a loss of religious faith as a result of their traumatic experiences needed much more intensive VA mental health services. A weakened religious faith predicted greater use of VA mental health services even after severity of PTSD symptoms and level of social functioning were controlled for. Investigators concluded that the use of mental health services was driven more by a weakened religious faith than by clinical symptoms or social factors, and that pastoral care resources are needed in clinics that serve veterans with PTSD.

A number of randomized controlled trials (RCTs) have examined the effects of religious psychotherapy for anxiety or depressive disorder in religious patients. For example, mindfulness meditation (Buddhist practice) has been used effectively to treat generalized anxiety disorder (GAD) and panic disorder.[34] Likewise, supplementing traditional treatments with religious practices or religious cognitive therapy (in the Muslim and Tao religious traditions) has been shown to speed the remission of anxiety disorder among believers,[35] but not among nonreligious patients.[36] One of the best clinical trials was done for depressive disorder in Christian patients. In that study, Propst and colleagues randomly assigned religious patients to secular cognitive-behavior therapy (CBT), religious cognitive therapy, pastoral counseling, or no treatment.[37] Patients receiving the religious CBT recovered the fastest from depression.

Prior to the year 2000, there had been nearly 480 quantitative studies (out of a total of 724 published studies) that found religious persons had greater well-being, hope, and optimism; more purpose and meaning in life; less depression and faster recovery from depression; lower rates of suicide; less anxiety and fear; greater marital satisfaction and stability; less substance abuse; and, among youth, less delinquency.[38]

Since 2000, there has been a surge in research and articles discussing the research in mental health journals. A search of *religion and spirituality*, using the online database PsycInfo (which contains over a million articles dating back to the early 1800s) found that during the five-year period between 1971 and 1975 only 776 articles studied or discussed religion and mental health (only 9 of which addressed spirituality). In a recent five-year period (2001 to 2005), over 5,000 articles appeared, 2,757 involving spirituality and 3,170 involving religion. The proportion of studies examining religion or spirituality compared to those examining psychotherapy during the 1971–1975 period was only 24 percent, compared to 46 percent in the 2001–2005 period. Thus, religion/spirituality and mental health is receiving increasing attention in the scientific literature.

If religious or spiritual beliefs and practices have a positive impact on mental health, help people to cope better with stress, and serve to reduce negative emotions, then this may help explain how religious involvement influences physical health via mind-body mechanisms.

Mind-Body Relationship

The fight-flight response helps to explain the physiological changes that occur in the body when an individual experiences stress (whether physical, psychological, or social stress).[39] Psychological stress activates areas of the brain (the hypothalamus and the locus coeruleus), which in turn influence hormone levels in the body (cortisol, epinephrine, norepinephrine) and autonomic nervous system functions. These changes alter immune and cardiovascular activities, which may increase the risk of contracting disease or adversely affecting disease outcomes.[40]

A number of studies have demonstrated the negative effects of psychological stress on the body. For example, Rosenkranz and colleagues conducted laboratory experiments in which they induced negative moods in their subjects and measured immune responses, finding that negative emotions were associated with a reduced immune response.[41] Examining the effects of caregiver stress on interleukin-6 levels (an indicator of immune function), Kiecolt-Glaser and colleagues found that immune functioning in caregivers remained impaired for as long as two to three years after the death of the patient.[42] Given the role that immune functioning plays in the prevention and containment of cancer, it is not surprising that Brown and colleagues found that depression was associated with a shorter survival rate during a ten-year follow-up.[43]

Cardiovascular function has also been adversely affected by negative emotions as demonstrated by a twelve-year follow-up of 817 patients undergoing coronary artery bypass graft (CABG) surgery. Blumenthal and colleagues found that patients who were depressed at the time of their CABG surgery had double the mortality of nondepressed patients after controlling for number of grafts, diabetes, smoking, left ventricular ejection fraction, and previous myocardial infarction.[44]

Finally, psychological stress also appears to affect the aging process. Epel and colleagues showed that women undergoing high stress experienced a more rapid shortening of the telomeres inside their cells.[45] The telomere, the end part of the DNA molecule, facilitates DNA replication when the cell divides. With each division, the telomere shortens. When the telomere has been used up, the DNA can no longer replicate and the cell dies. Investigators found that the telomere shortening in stressed women was equivalent to their cells aging ten years faster than less stressed women.

Religion's Effects on Physical Health

One mechanism by which religious involvement may influence physical health is through the psychoneuroimmunological processes described above. If religious involvement helps people to cope better with stress, reduces anxiety, and prevents or speeds remission from depression, then it may help to neutralize the effects that these and other negative emotions have on physical health. A number of studies suggest that this is indeed the case, and have found correlations between religious involvement and immune or endocrine function,[46] mortality from cancer,[47] blood pressure,[48] heart disease,[49] stroke,[50] mortality in general,[51] and mortality after surgery.[52]

Recent studies continue to show this association between religious activity and health outcomes, shedding light on psychosocial, behavioral, and physiological pathways. For example, Lutgendorf and colleagues at the University of Iowa examined the effects of attendance at religious services on interleukin-6 (IL-6) levels in 556 older adults.[53] They showed that frequent church attenders had IL-6 levels that were 66 percent lower than those for nonattenders; this also translated into a 68 percent reduction in mortality over twelve years of follow-up. This study replicated a 1997 study at Duke University that also found lower IL-6 levels in older adults who attended religious services more often.[54]

With regard to cardiovascular pathways, King and colleagues conducted a cross-sectional survey of a nationally representative sample of 556 people with diabetes.[55] The primary outcome measure was the presence of elevated C-reactive protein (CRP), which is a strong predictor of coronary artery disease. Religious service nonattenders were over twice as likely as attenders to have elevated CRP. After adjusting for demographic variables, health status, smoking, social support, mobility, and body mass index, the association between religious attendance and CRP remained significant, providing evidence for another biological mechanism by which the effects of religion may be conveyed.

Similarly, Masters and colleagues reported that cardiovascular reactivity (a predictor of greater cardiovascular morbidity) was the same among more intrinsically religious older adults as it was for younger adults in general, suggesting that devout religious commitment may help to slow the decline in cardiovascular function that occurs with increasing age.[56] Likewise, surgical complications appear to be less common among more religious older adults having heart surgery, as reported by Contrada and colleagues from Rutgers University.[57] These investigators studied religious involvement and other psychosocial factors in 142 patients about a week prior to surgery. Those with stronger religious beliefs had fewer complications and shorter hospital stays, the former effect mediating the latter.

Research also suggests that religious involvement may delay or slow the progression of memory impairment with cognitive disorders in later life. Kaufman and Freedman, from Baycrest Centre for Geriatric Care in Toronto, reported at the 2005 American Academic of Neurology meeting in Miami that religious behavior was associated with slower progression of cognitive impairment in Alzheimer's disease.[58] Controlling for baseline cognitive function, age, gender, and education, patients scoring higher on self-rated spirituality ($p=0.01$) and private religious practices ($p=0.003$) had a significantly slower rate of cognitive decline. This study replicated an earlier study, conducted at Yale University, that examined cognitive functioning among 2,812 older men and women from New Haven, Connecticut. Religious attendance in 1982 predicted significantly less cognitive impairment in 1985 (36 percent less), although the effect weakened by the 1988 follow-up.[59]

Health behaviors and religious involvement may be additive in their effects on cancer mortality. Enstrom followed 2,290 white participants in the Alameda County (California) study between 1974 and 1987.[60] He found that weekly religious attendance and nonsmoking status predicted a 37 percent reduction in the standard mortality ratio (SMR) from cancer. When he examined frequent attenders who also exercised regularly and slept seven to eight hours at night, this reduced the SMR an additional 39 percent. Thus, the risk of dying from cancer during the follow-up period was 76 percent lower for those who attended religious services frequently and lived a healthy lifestyle.

Activity levels may also be higher among more religiously involved older persons because of religion's influence on fear related to falling. Fear of falling is strongly related to reduced activity levels and increased risk of hip and other fractures. Reyes-Ortiz and colleagues found in a sample of 1,341 older Mexican Americans that were followed over the course of three years that fear of falling was significantly lower (27 percent) among frequent church attenders, and this effect was independent of gender, poorer objective lower body performance, history of falls, arthritis, hypertension, and urinary incontinence.[61]

A number of recent studies also suggest that religious involvement is related to greater longevity. Hill and colleagues used data from the Hispanic Established Populations for Epidemiological Studies in the Elderly (EPESE) to predict the risk of all-cause mortality during an eight-year follow-up, finding that weekly church attenders had a 32 percent reduction in the risk of mortality as compared to nonattenders, even after controlling for multiple physical and psychosocial predictors of mortality.[62] Using the data on 14,456 participants involved in five other sites where the EPESE study was conducted, Bagiella and colleagues (including Richard Sloan) found that after controlling for a range of other mortality predictors, weekly religious attendance was associated with a 22 percent reduction in mortality during the follow-up period.[63] The importance of this study is that these well-known critics of the relationship between religion and health were trying to disprove the relationship between religious involvement and longevity, and ended up confirming what others had found.

Effects of religion on physical health are not limited to studies of Christian populations or to the United States. A fascinating study from Israel found that simply living in a more religious community influences the longevity of all participants. Jaffe and colleagues examined data from the Israel Longitudinal Mortality Study that involved 141,683 people over age forty-five from 882 different areas of the country.[64] After controlling for demographic and socioeconomic characteristics, both men and women living in religiously affiliated neighborhoods had lower mortality rates than others (25 percent lower for men; 14 percent lower for women). For men, the effect on mortality of living in a religious neighborhood behaved in a dose-response manner (i.e., as percentage of affiliated persons increased, mortality decreased in a linear fashion). Another study from this area of the world examined the relationship between religiosity and blood pressure among Kuwaiti Muslims. Controlling for body mass index, socioeconomic status, smoking, gender, and age, the investigator found that both systolic and diastolic blood pressures were inversely associated with religious commitment and religious activities.[65]

Finally, la Cour and colleagues from Denmark reported the first European study to look at the effects of religiousness on mortality.[66] They followed 734 elderly Danish people for twenty years. Frequent church attenders were 27 percent less likely to die during follow-up. After controlling for gender, education, medical and mental health, social relations, help given and received, and health behaviors, the association weakened but remained statistically significant (18 percent reduction in mortality). Effects were stronger in women than in men, as several other studies have found.

Possible Mechanisms

There are at least five mechanisms by which religious involvement could influence physical health and medical outcomes: (1) psychological-social influences, (2) behavioral and lifestyle factors, (3) genetic and inherited influences, (4) central nervous system factors, and (5) supernatural or superempirical effects. I will now discuss each of these.

Psychosocial Factors

The possible influence of religion on physical health through psychological and social factors has already been discussed above. There is ample evidence that religious involvement could influence immune, endocrine, and cardiovascular functioning by reducing psychological stress, enhancing positive emotions (optimism, hope, joy), preventing psychiatric disorders (or speeding their resolution), enhancing social support, and reinforcing "other"-directed attitudes and activities (forgiveness, altruism, giving support to others). Religious doctrines emphasize these experiences and behaviors; subjects report that religion helps them to cope; and studies show that religious people cope better, have more positive emotions, and fewer psychiatric disorders, and are more involved in prosocial activities. These, in turn, have been associated with better immune, endocrine, and cardiovascular functioning, which are directly linked with positive health outcomes.

I would like to further elaborate on possible mechanisms of religion's effects on health through cardiovascular pathways. Not only may religious involvement reduce blood pressure or prevent its rise, it may also affect vascular compliance, degree of plaque buildup in coronary/carotid arteries, degree of heart rate variability, and cardiovascular reactivity tied to sympathetic and parasympathetic nervous system activity. There are studies that suggest connections between religious activity and blood pressure, coronary artery disease mortality, and cardiovascular reactivity. However, no studies have yet examined relationships between traditional religious activities and vascular compliance (flexibility of blood vessel walls), heart rate variability, or plaque buildup in coronary or carotid arteries. If religious activity reduces stress level, enhances immune function (and susceptibility to viral infections that may be responsible for plaque formation), and influences inflammatory markers (such as C-reactive protein), then vascular compliance and artery plaque levels could be likewise affected. These are areas of high priority for future research.

Behavior and Lifestyle

A second reason why religious people may be healthier is that they live healthier lifestyles. There are dozens of studies that show that religious involvement is associated with less cigarette smoking.[67] If this were the only effect that religion had, then religious people would have lower levels of chronic lung disease and lung cancer, lower blood pressure, fewer strokes, less coronary artery disease, and fewer myocardial infarctions. However, not only do religious people smoke less, but when they are young they are also less likely to abuse alcohol and use other drugs, such as marijuana and cocaine. In addition to this, religious young adults eat a better diet, exercise more, and sleep more than less religious youth, as well as involve themselves in fewer high-risk behaviors (i.e., are more likely to wear seat belts, refrain from premarital sexual activity, etc.).[68] A recent systematic review of forty-six studies of adolescents (ages ten to twenty) between 1998 and 2003 found that in 84 percent of studies religious or spiritual involvement was related to significantly better health attitudes and behaviors.[69] Given the importance of adolescent attitudes toward health and health behaviors in establishing lifelong patterns of healthy living, it is significant that seven of eight recent studies found positive effects for religion/spirituality.

Genetic-Inherited Predispositions

Recent research suggests that general "tendencies toward spiritual experience" might have a genetic basis. Dean Hamer, chief of gene structure at the National Cancer Institute, is the author of *The God Gene*, in which he notes that certain genes, such as the dopamine D-sub-4 receptor gene (DRD4), may transmit such tendencies.[70] Likewise, Comings and colleagues studied 81 college students and 119 patients from an addiction treatment unit who were given temperament and character scales and provided blood samples for genetic analysis.[71] Results suggested that the DRD4 gene (with high concentrations in the frontal cortex) may play a role in "spiritual acceptance."

A number of studies of identical twins and fraternal twins, raised either together or apart, provide further evidence that there may be at least a partial genetic basis (0–44 percent) for religious or spiritual involvement. For example, Abrahamson and colleagues found that there was no genetic transmission (0 percent) of religiousness/spirituality and that it was entirely based on environmental (i.e., learning) or miscellaneous other factors.[72] In contrast, L. B. Koenig and colleagues found that the transmission of religiousness from one generation to another was determined in part by genetic factors (up to 44 percent), and the rest was determined by environmental or other factors; her sample was primarily middle-aged white males (the least religious group in the population).[73] Kendler and colleagues found in a study of female twins in Virginia that genetic transmission of religiousness varied from 0 percent to 29 percent, depending on the particular type of religious involvement assessed.[74] Thus, twin studies provide inconsistent evidence that religious involvement may be genetic in origin.

Why might tendencies toward spiritual experience, spiritual acceptance, or religiousness be encoded in our genes? Why is anything encoded in our genes? Because it has survival value. If religion/spirituality helps people to cope with stress, and if stress impairs physiological functioning and leads to greater mortality, then people who have genetically linked traits toward greater religiousness/spirituality would be more likely to survive and pass those genes onto their children, leading to the greater survival of those genes in the population. Therefore, by natural selection, people with genes favoring the trait of greater religiousness/spirituality would increase in number and those genes would ultimately become part of the human genome. This is consistent with what studies are showing concerning the relationship between religion and health. Although science is unable to prove this, is it possible that God purposely created humans with a need for spiritual experience encoded within their genes? Or did this simply evolve?

Central Nervous System Phenomena (Neuroscience)

The field of neuroscience seeks to identify neurological bases for psychological and social phenomena, including religious or spiritual experiences. For years it has been known that mystical-type experiences are more common among people with temporal lobe epilepsy (TLE).[75] Although some researchers have challenged this notion because their research finds no connection between religious involvement and TLE,[76] the earlier findings support the argument that the temporal lobes of the brain may be the organs responsible for spiritual experiences. Could the temporal lobes serve as "receivers," capturing spiritual information from transcendent sources, or has such a part of the brain simply evolved because being spiritual/religious provides an advantage that has enabled humans to survive and outcompete other species? The answer to these questions in the end may be a matter of faith, rather than fact.

In 1997, V. S. Ramachandran and colleagues presented "supporting" experimental evidence at a national meeting of neurologists (published as an abstract) that the temporal lobes are responsible for religious experience.[77] This was a very small study, and yet because of the popular interest in the subject, it received international media attention. They compared skin conduction responses (SCRs) in three groups of people: three people with TLE, ten normal highly religious people, and eight normal people not screened for religiosity. The three patients with TLE were selected for participation based on their responses to Bear-Fedio Personal Inventory and Personal Behavior Surveys designed to diagnose the interictal (between seizure) behavior syndrome in TLE patients. These measures, however, are themselves biased toward selecting TLE patients with religious/spiritual tendencies because some questions on these scales ask about religiousness and mystical states.

The experimental design of this study involved subjects reading four categories of words (neutral, religious, sexual, violent), while their skin conduction responses were measured. The results indicated that normal people were highly responsive to sexual words, but minimally responsive to violent or religious words. Two of three TLE patients were highly responsive to religious words (almost exactly the same as highly religious normal subjects were, but minimally responsive to violent or sexual words; the third person showed minimal response to sexual words, moderate response to religious words), and the greatest response to violent words.

Based on these findings, the researchers concluded, "These results clearly demonstrate that in TLE patients there can be selective enhancement and reduction of SCRs to very specific categories of stimuli; our patients exhibited large responses to words pertaining to religion and God with an actual decrement in responsivity to other categories that would ordinarily be evocative to normal people, such as to sexually loaded words." These results hardly "clearly" demonstrate anything, especially since temporal lobe injury (usually the cause of TLE) is typically associated with decreased libido and loss of sexual interest, helping to explain the blunted response to sexually loaded words in TLE patients in this study. They concluded that a "God module" exists in the temporal lobes and may have evolved to "encourage tribe loyalty and conformist behavior." This conclusion is an extraordinary extension of the findings, which are marginal and nowhere even close to statistically significant. This explains why the findings were not published in a peer-reviewed neurology journal and appeared only in abstract form at the above neuroscience meeting.

Even if the temporal lobes are the centers for mystical-type religious or spiritual experiences, this does not necessarily mean that they represent the part of the brain responsible for religious involvement and behavior, which are much more complex and are likely to be accounted for by multiple areas of the brain working together. Remember that LSD and other hallucinogens also elicit mystical-type spiritual experiences, and likely do so by affecting the limbic system in the brain (which the temporal lobes are part of). Thus, much further work is needed before sufficient scientific evidence will be available to designate any particular part of the brain as the "God module."

With the advent of neuroimaging techniques such as SPECT scans, PET scans, MRI scans, and most recently, functional MRI (fMRI) scans, some researchers have taken pictures of the brain of people who are meditating or praying in order to identify the parts of the brain that are most active during religious/spiritual practices or experiences. Best-known for this work is Andrew Newberg at the University of Pennsylvania. His book, *Why God Won't Go Away: Brain Science and the Biology of Belief*, summarizes his findings using these imaging techniques and his interpretation of what these findings mean. As other researchers above, he argues that certain parts of the brain consistently "light up" on the brain scans of Buddhist monks when meditating and Catholic sisters when praying.

While this is fascinating research, these scans (especially the SPECT and PET images) do not provide the kind of resolution needed to definitively say that any particular part of the brain is responsible for spiritual/

religious phenomena. Nevertheless, it is likely that future research may be able to answer this question. Certainly for humans to experience any-thing—anything at all—such experiences, including spiritual experiences, must be perceived or produced in some part of the brain. People who are in a coma do not have any kind of religious or spiritual experiences, or at least cannot report such experiences.

To what extent the neuroscience of spiritual or religious experience adds anything to our knowledge about the relationship between religion and health, or the mechanism of this relationship, is not clear. However, it is likely that future research will continue to try to locate what part of the brain is responsible for such experiences. Remember, however, that reli-gious or spiritual experience is very different from having faith, developing a personal connection with God, and living out a godly and faithful life-style, which may in the end be the real keys to understanding the relation-ship between religion and health.

Supernatural-Superempirical

This mechanism seeks to explain the relationship between religion and health in terms of supernatural phenomena. The argument is that religious people are healthier because God (or some other force outside of the cur-rently understood natural universe) supernaturally and unexplainably heals them of their diseases and maintains their health. This explanation does not depend on the laws of science, but in fact breaks them. People with dis-eases that would ordinarily lead to death (such as cancer) are healed sud-denly in ways that are unexplainable in terms of medicine or biology.

All the research demonstrating a relationship between religion and health that has been discussed above depends on known, natural process-es—psychological, social, physiological, or behavioral mechanisms—that science can study. These are no doubt very complex phenomena, but not so complex that scientific research cannot study them, just as research has been conducted to study other psychological and social phenomena and their health consequences.

The study of supernatural or superempirical processes, however, falls into a completely different area of research that is more closely associated with parapsychology than it is with historically based religion or spirituality. Such scientific studies have as their aim establishing "proof" of the existence of supernatural forces and effects. These include studies of intercessory prayer, healing at a distance by "healers," distant effects of human intentionality, extrasensory perception (ESP), or psychokinesis (ability to move options at a distance by thoughts only). The studies in this category have no scientific basis or known scientific mechanism (psychological, social, or behavioral) that could explain the findings. If they did end up providing proof of such phenomena, then much of what we know about the physical universe would have to change—a huge leap not based on any previous understanding of physics, mathematics, or biology, and one that would have no precedent in modern times. Hundreds of years of research of such phenomena (particularly ESP or psychokinesis) have yet to produce anything that science has accepted as credible or useful.

The type of research that has received the most attention in the media of late are studies of intercessory prayer (IP), directed at increasing the rate of healing or reducing complications following surgery. These are double-blind, randomized, controlled studies of subjects receiving intercessory prayer without knowing that they are receiving it, by people praying who are located at a distance who don't know the subjects in the study. So neither the people praying nor the prayed-for subjects know who is being prayed for.

A study by cardiologist Randolph Byrd in the late 1980s was most influential in bringing attention to this subject. There had been numerous IP studies prior to Byrd's study, but his study appeared in the *Southern Medical Journal* and received worldwide media coverage.[78] Byrd reported that patients in the group that was prayed for experienced significantly fewer complications in the coronary care unit (CCU) than patients who were not prayed for.

Many studies have attempted to replicate this finding. However, the two most recent and best-designed studies at Duke and Harvard were not successful in doing so. Mitchell Krucoff, a cardiologist at Duke, designed an IP study involving nearly 750 patients undergoing coronary artery bypass surgery, half randomized to IP from a variety of different religious groups (Christian and non-Christian) and half randomized to the control group that was not to receive prayer. The results, appearing in *The Lancet* in 2005, showed no difference between groups.[79] In the second study led by investigators at Harvard, IP had no effect on complications after CABG, although those who were told that they were being prayed for had slightly more complications.[80] This was a multicenter, double-blind, randomized control trial with 1,205 patients randomly assigned to Christian groups praying for them (601 being told that they would receive IP) and 597 assigned to a control group that was not prayed for. There was no difference in complication rate (primary endpoint) between those prayed for (52 percent) and those not prayed for (51 percent), although there was a trend for those prayed for to have more major events (secondary endpoint) (18 percent vs. 13 percent). Those who were told they were being prayed for had slightly but significantly more complications (59 percent vs. 52 percent).

In general, these kinds of studies are fraught with scientific and theological problems. If a research study is incapable of studying a phenomenon, that study cannot determine whether it is effective or not. A scientific experiment, such as those performed in these studies, cannot determine whether prayer is effective or not—particularly if there are good reasons to suspect that it is not capable of accurately measuring and statistically controlling for confounding variables. And there are many confounding variables in such studies. Did they measure "God's will" for individuals in the study (or did God simply suspend Divine will for these patients' lives so that they could participate in the study)? Is God's first priority to keep humans physically healthy (and therefore only responds to prayer by healing physically)? Did investigators measure the sincerity of prayers said by the patient, their loved ones, the hospital staff, and the intercessors, or whether patients in the control group were also prayed for by these individuals? Did they measure complications or outcomes after thirty days (God may have decided to heal people after the thirtieth day)? The answers are no, no, and no. Without measuring such powerful confounding variables, what can one expect to find? Nothing, absolutely nothing, and that is what these studies found.

In the Harvard study, it is not at all unexpected that the patients who knew that they were being prayed for did worse. The increased complication rate was due almost entirely to atrial fibrillation, a cardiac arrhythmia that can be brought on by adrenaline. When told by researchers/health professionals that, "Oh, by the way, you are one of the people that will be getting the prayer," how might such patients respond? They probably pan-icked or became more anxious, thinking, "Wow, my condition must be pretty bad if I'm the one who's getting and needs the prayer!" No surprise that these patients did worse. It is unlikely this would have occurred if family members or friends had told patients that they were praying for them. That would likely have provided comfort and hope. However, when health professionals/researchers tell patients that they are in need of prayer, that's a different matter. Health professionals must explain why they are bringing up matters related to spirituality and make sure the patient understands that this area is not being addressed because the patient is so severely ill that she is nearing the end.

In summary, IP studies such as those described above have no scientific grounds on which to explain an effect, and also have little or no theological grounds. It tells us nothing about the relationship between religion and health, or about the efficacy of IP in terms of prayer to a Christian, Jewish, or Muslim God. It does suggest, however, that positive human intentions have no effect at a distance. Another reasonable conclusion might be that the highly constrained and reductionistic scientific method is simply the wrong tool for studying supernatural phenomena.

Future Directions

The most fruitful area of future research will likely focus on understand-ing the psychosocial, behavioral, and physiological (immune, endocrine, cardiovascular) mechanisms by which religious belief, practice, and com-mitment influence physical health and medical outcomes. There is much that we do not know about these mechanisms, and because they are scien-tifically grounded, this is an area for scientific study—as with any psycho-logical or social phenomena. There are rational grounds for such effects, based on what we know about the impact that psychological, social, and behavioral factors have on health, and much more data are needed on how religious factors affect biological functioning and disease course. Once a biological mechanism has been firmly established, then both scientists and health professionals will be better able to accept this research field as one worthy of study and clinically relevant. Research that focuses on clinical applications will also be a high priority. What impact does taking a spiritual history or praying with a patient have on the clinician-patient relationship and on medical outcomes? What impact does spirituality have on the health professional's well-being, satisfaction with work, relationship with patients, and effectiveness of treatments? Almost no research has been done on such subjects.

Trying to understand the role that genetics plays in transmitting religious or spiritual tendencies, and delineating the parts of the brain that are involved in religious experience, are less important to focus on, given our limited funding resources and the lack of clinical application that such research is likely to have. This does not mean that such areas of research should not be pursued for their own value in furthering our biological understanding of such phenomena. However, again, with limited research dollars, learning how religion/spirituality impacts health and how religious or spiritual interventions affect medical outcomes and the clinician-patient relationship simply take precedence.

Studies designed to document supernatural or superempirical spiritual phenomena are a waste of time and valuable research dollars. Sufficient research has now been done to demonstrate that such matters are far too complex for reductionistic scientific research designs. Such studies only serve to worsen the reputation of more credible research on religion and health that is based on solid scientific and theological principles. Funding agencies (particularly those without religion and health researchers available to review the proposals) often become confused between these two types of research, and may reject more credible proposals because of the misconception that all such studies are trying to prove the supernatural. Thus, studies of the supernatural are actually impeding the field of religion and health research, and are therefore dead-ends in terms of future research.

Summary

Although for a long time health professionals have considered religion to be unrelated to health, or even associated with neurosis or mental illness, recent research suggests that this is not usually true. In fact, the majority of studies suggest the opposite. Religion helps people to cope with illness through a number of plausible psychological and social mechanisms, and is related to less depression, less anxiety, and fewer emotional problems, and is associated with more positive emotions, such as hope, optimism, and well-being. Because of its relationship with mental health, greater social support, and healthier lifestyle, religion is expected to be related to better health overall and faster recovery from illness. Religious people experience fewer heart attacks, are more likely to recover from open heart surgery, experience less disability and slower cognitive decline as they grow older, and generally live longer (especially if they're involved in religious community activities). These effects may be mediated by immune, endocrine, and cardiovascular effects, genetic factors, central nervous system influences, or supernatural mechanisms. All but supernatural mechanisms are likely subjects of scientific study, and such research promises to ultimately identify the pathways by which religion influences health. Given the prevalence of religious activities in the United States and around the world, and the importance that religion has for many people, this research has enormous public health and clinical significance.

Reflective Activities

1. Are you a religious person, a spiritual person, both, or neither? If spiritual, what does this mean for you?
2. Who are the most deeply religious or spiritual people that you know? How satisfied are they with their lives?
3. When you are in deep, serious prayer, notice what happens to your pulse and rate of breathing.
4. When you are worshiping and singing during religious services, how do you feel emotionally? What about physically?
5. Why might there be a "God gene" (i.e., an inherited predisposition toward religious or spiritual experience)?
6. Think of ten things that might influence how God responds to your prayer for the physical health of another person.

Acknowledgments

Support for the writing of this chapter provided by the Center for Spirituality, Theology and Health, Duke University Medical Center, Durham, North Carolina.

NOTES

1. Moreira-Almeida, A., & Koenig, H. G. (2006). Commentary: Retaining the meaning of the words religiousness and spirituality. *Social Sciences and Medicine* 63 (4): 843–45; in particular, see Koenig, H. G. (2008). Concerns about measuring spirituality in research. *Journal of Nervous and Mental Disease* 196 (5): 349–55.

2. Freud, S. (1927). Future of an Illusion. In J. Strachey (ed. and trans.), *Standard Edition of the Complete Psychological Works of Sigmund Freud*. London: Hogarth Press, 1962.

3. Koenig, H. G. (2006). Schizophrenia and psychotic disorders. In F. Lu & J. Peteet (eds.), *Religion and Psychiatric Disorders in DSM-V*. Washington, DC: American Psychiatric Publishing, Inc.

4. Cronan, T. A., Kaplan, R. M., Posner, L., Lumberg, E., & Kozin, F. (1989). Prevalence of the use of unconventional remedies for arthritis in a metropolitan community. *Arthritis & Rheumatism* 32: 1604–7.

5. Ai, A. L., Dunkle, R. E., Peterson, C., & Bolling, S. F. (1998). The role of private prayer in psychological recovery among midlife and aged patients following cardiac surgery (CABG). *Gerontologist* 38: 591–601; Matthees, B. J., Anantachoti, P., Kreitzer, M. J., Savik, K., Hertz, M. I., & Gross, C. R. (2001). Use of complementary therapies, adherence, and quality of life in lung transplant recipients. *Heart & Lung* 30: 258–68.

6. Keefe, F. J., et al. (2001). Giving with rheumatoid arthritis: The role of daily spirituality and daily religious and spiritual coping. *Journal of Pain* 2: 101–10.

7. Tix, A. P., & Frazier, P. A. (1997). The use of religious coping during stressful life events. *Journal of Consulting and Clinical Psychology* 66: 411–22.

8. Schnoll, R. A., Harlow, L. L., & Brower, L. (2000). Spirituality, demographic and disease factors, and adjustment to cancer. *Cancer Practice* 8: 298–304.

9. Cooper-Effa, M., Blount, W., Kaslow, N., Rothenberg, R., & Eckman, J. (2001). Role of spirituality in patients with sickle cell disease. *Journal of the American Board Family Practitioners* 14: 116–22; Harrison, M. O., Edwards, C. L., Koenig, H. G., & Bosworth, H. B. (2005). Religiosity/spirituality and pain in patients with sickle cell disease. *Journal of Nervous and Mental Disease* 93(4): 250–57.

10. Avants, S. K., Warburton, L. A., & Margolin, A. (2001). Spiritual and religious support in recovery from addiction among HIV-positive injection drug users. *Journal of Psychoactive Drugs* 33: 39–45.

11. Stern, R. C., Canda, E. R., & Doershuk, C. F. (1992). Use of non-medical treatment by cystic fibrosis patients. *Journal of Adolescent Health* 13: 612–15; Silber, T. J., & Reilly, M. (1985). Spiritual and religious concerns of the hospitalized adolescent. *Adolescence* 20: 217–24.

12. Koenig, H. G. (1998). Religious beliefs and practices of hospitalized medically ill older adults. *International Journal of Geriatric Psychiatry* 13: 213–24.

13. Eisenberg, D. M., Davis, R. B., Ettner, S. L., Appel, S., Wilkey, S., Van Rompay, M. & Kessler, R. C. (1998). Trends in alternative medicine use in the United States,

1990–1997: Results of a follow-up national survey. *Journal of the American Medical Association* 280(18): 1569–75.

14. Schuster, M. A., et al. (2001). A national survey of stress reactions after the September 11, 2001, terrorist attacks. *New England Journal of Medicine* 345: 1507–12.

15. Romans 8:28, KJV.

16. Matthew 27:46, KJV.

17. Job 1:1, KJV.

18. Koenig, H. G., McCullough, M. E., & Larson D. B. (2001). *Handbook of Religion and Health*. New York: Oxford University Press.

19. Cutler, S. J. (1976). Membership in different types of voluntary associations and psychological well-being. *The Gerontologist* 16: 335–39.

20. Koenig, H. G., Moberg, D. O., & Kvale, J. N. (1988): Religious activities and attitudes of older adults in a geriatric assessment clinic. *Journal of the American Geriatrics Society* 36: 362–74.

21. Koenig, McCullough, & Larson. (2001).

22. Koenig, H. G. (2002). An 83-year-old woman with chronic illness and strong religious beliefs. *Journal of the American Medical Association* 288(4): 487–93.

23. Koenig, H. G., Kvale, J. N., & Ferrel, C. (1988). Religion and well-being in later life. *The Gerontologist* 28: 18–28.

24. Koenig, H. G., Cohen, H. J., Blazer, D. G., Pieper, C., Meador, K. G., Shelp, F., Goli, V., & DiPasquale, R. (1992). Religious coping and depression in elderly hospitalized medically ill men. *American Journal of Psychiatry* 149: 1693–1700.

25. Koenig, H. G., George, L. K., & Peterson, B. L. (1998). Religiosity and remission from depression in medically ill older patients. *American Journal of Psychiatry* 155: 536–42.

26. Koenig, H. G., Ford, S., George, L. K., Blazer, D. G., & Meador, K. G. (1993). Religion and anxiety disorder: An examination and comparison of associations in young, middle-aged, and elderly adults. *Journal of Anxiety Disorders* 7: 321–42.

27. Verghese, A., John, J. K., Rajkumar, S., Richard, J., Sethi, B. B., & Trivedi, J. K. (1989). Factors associated with the course and outcome of schizophrenia in India: Results of a two-year multicentre follow-up study. *British Journal of Psychiatry* 154: 499–503; Chu, C. C., & Klein, H. E. (1985). Psychosocial and environmental variables in outcome of black schizophrenics. *Journal of the National Medical Association* 77: 793–96.

28. Koenig, H. G., Hays, J. C., George, L. K., & Blazer, D. G. (1997). Modeling the cross-sectional relationships between religion, physical health, social support, and depressive symptoms. *American Journal of Geriatric Psychiatry* 5: 131–43.

29. Braam, A. W., Beekman, A. T. F., Deeg, D. J. H., Smith, J. H., & van Tilburg, W. (1997). Religiosity as a protective or prognostic factor of depression in later life: Results from the community survey in the Netherlands. *Acta Psychiatrica Scandinavia* 96: 199–205.

30. Koenig, Cohen, Blazer, Pieper, Meador, Shelp, Goli, & DiPasquale. (1992).

31. Koenig, George, & Peterson. (1998).

32. Koenig, H. G. (2007). Religion and remission of depression in medical inpatients with heart failure/pulmonary disease. *Journal of Nervous and Mental Disease* 195: 389–95.

33. Fontana, A., & Rosenheck, R. (2004). Trauma, change in strength of religious faith, & mental health service use among veterans treated for PTSD. *Journal of Nervous & Mental Disease* 192: 579–84.

34. Kabat-Zinn, J., Lipworth, L., & Burney, R. (1985). The clinical use of mindfulness meditation for the self-regulation of chronic pain. *Journal of Behavioral Medicine* 8: 163–90; Kabat-Zinn, J., Massion, A. O., Kristeller, J., Peterson, L. G., Fletcher, K. E., Pbert, L., Lenderking, W. R., & Santorelli, S. F. (1992). Effectiveness of a meditation-

based stress reduction program in the treatment of anxiety disorders. *American Journal of Psychiatry* 149: 936–43.

35. Azhar, M. Z., Varma, S. L., & Dharap, A. S. (1994). Religious psychotherapy in anxiety disorder patients. *Acta Psychiatrica Scandinavica* 90: 1–3; Zhang, Y., et al. (2002). Chinese Taoist cognitive psychotherapy in the treatment of generalized anxiety disorder in contemporary China. *Transcultural Psychiatry* 39(1): 115–29; Azhar, M. Z., & Varma, S. L. (1995a). Religious psychotherapy in depressive patients. *Psychotherapy & Psychosomatics* 63: 165–73; Xiao, S., Young, D., & Zhang, H. (1998). Taoistic cognitive psychotherapy for neurotic patients: A preliminary clinical trial. *Psychiatry & Clinical Neurosciences* 52 (supplement): S238–41.

36. Razali, S. M., Hasanah, C. I., Aminah, K., & Subramaniam, M. (1998). Religious-sociocultural psychotherapy in patients with anxiety and depression. *Australian & New Zealand Journal of Psychiatry* 32: 867–72.

37. Propst, L. R., Ostrom, R., Watkins, P., Dean, T., & Mashburn, D. (1992). Comparative efficacy of religious and nonreligious cognitive-behavior therapy for the treatment of clinical depression in religious individuals. *Journal of Consulting and Clinical Psychology* 60: 94–103.

38. Koenig, McCullough, & Larson. (2001).

39. Cannon, W. B. (1941). The emergency function of the adrenal medulla in pain and the major emotions. *American Journal of Physiology* 33: 356.

40. Rabin, B. S. (1999). *Stress, Immune Function, and Health: The Connection.* New York: Wiley-Liss & Sons.

41. Rosenkranz, M. A., Jackson, D. C., Dalton, K. M., Dolski, I., Ryff, C. D., Singer, B. H., Muller, D., Kalin, N. H., & Davidson, R. J. (2003). Affective style and in vivo immune response: neurobehavioral mechanisms. *Proceedings of the National Academy of Sciences of the United States of America* 100(19): 11148–52.

42. Kiecolt-Glaser, J. K., Preacher, K. J., MacCallum, R. C., Atkinson, C., Malarkey, W. B., & Glaser, R. (2003). Chronic stress and age-related increases in the proinflammatory cytokine IL-6. *Proceedings of the National Academy of Sciences of the United States of America* 100(15): 9090–95.

43. Brown, K. W., Levy, A. R., Rosberger, Z., & Edgar, L. (2003). Psychological distress and cancer survival: A follow-up 10 years after diagnosis. *Psychosomatic Medicine* 65: 636–43.

44. Blumenthal, J. A., et al. (2003). Depression as a risk factor for mortality after coronary artery bypass surgery. *Lancet* 362: 604–9.

45. Epel, E. S., et al. (2004). Accelerated telomere shortening in response to life stress. *Proceedings of the National Academy of Sciences of the United States of America* 101(49): 17312–15.

46. Koenig, H. G., Cohen, H. J., George, L. K., Hays, J. C., Larson, D. B., & Blazer, D. G. (1997). Attendance at religious services, interleukin-6, and other biological indicators of immune function in older adults. *International Journal of Psychiatry in Medicine* 27: 233–50; Lutgendorf, S. K., Russell, D., Ullrich, P., Harris, T. B., & Wallace, R. (2004). Religious participation, interleukin-6, and mortality in older adults. *Health Psychology* 23(5): 465–75; Sephton, S. E., Koopman, C., Schaal, M., Thoreson, C., & Spiegel, D. (2001). Spiritual expression and immune status in women with metastatic breast cancer: An exploratory study. *Breast Journal* 7: 345–53; Dedert, E. A., Studts, J. L., Weissbecker, I., Salmon, P. G., Banis, P. L., & Sephton, S. E. (2004). Private religious practice: Protection of cortisol rhythms among women with fibromyalgia. *International Journal of Psychiatry in Medicine* 34: 61–77; 50. Woods, T. E., Antoni, M. H., Ironson, G. H., & Kling, D. W. (1999). Religiosity is associated with affective and immune status in

symptomatic HIV-infected gay men. *Journal of Psychosomatic Research* 46: 165–76; McClelland, D. C. (1988). The effect of motivational arousal through films on salivary immunoglobulin A. *Psychology and Health* 2: 31–52; Lutgendorf, S. (1997). IL-6 level, stress, and spiritual support in older adults. Psychology Department, University of Iowa and Iowa City. Personal communcation, May 1997.

47. Enstrom, J. E. (1989). Health practices and cancer mortality among active California Mormons. *Journal of the National Cancer Institute* 31: 1807–14.

48. Koenig, H. G., George, L. K., Cohen, H. J., Hays, J. C., Blazer, D. G., & Larson, D. B. (1998f). The relationship between religious activities and blood pressure in older adults. *International Journal of Psychiatry in Medicine* 28: 189–13.

49. Goldbourt, U., Yaari, S., & Medalie, J. H. (1993). Factors predictive of long-term coronary heart disease mortality among 10,059 male Israeli civil servants and municipal employees. *Cardiology* 82: 100–21.

50. Colantonio, A., Kasl, S. V., & Ostfeld, A. M. (1992). Depressive symptoms and other psychosocial factors as predictors of stroke in elderly. *American Journal of Epidemiology* 136: 884–94.

51. McCullough, M. E., Hoyt, W. T., Larson, D. B., Koenig, H. G., & Thoresen, C. (2000). Religious involvement and mortality: A meta-analytic review. *Health Psychology* 19: 211–22; Powell, L. H., Shahabi, L., & Thoresen, C. E. (2003). Religion and spirituality: Linkages to physical health. *American Psychologist* 58(1): 36–52.

52. Oxman, T. E., Freeman, D. H., & Manheimer, E. D. (1995). Lack of social participation or religious strength and comfort as risk factors for death after cardiac surgery in the elderly. *Psychosomatic Medicine* 57: 5–15; Contrada, R. J., et al. (2004). Psychosocial factors in outcomes of heart surgery: The impact of religious involvement and depressive symptoms. *Health Psychology* 23: 227–38.

53. Lutgendorf, S. K., Russell, D., Ullrich, P., Harris, T. B., & Wallace, R. Religious participation, interleukin-6, and mortality in older adults. *Health Psychology* 23(5): 465–75.

54. Koenig, H. G., Cohen, H. J., George, L. K., Hays, J. C., Larson, D. B., Blazer, D. G. (1997). Attendance at religious services, interleukin-6, and other biological indicators of immune function in older adults. *International Journal of Psychiatry in Medicine* 27: 233–50.

55. King, D. E., Mainous, A. G., 3rd, & Pearson, W. S. (2002). C-reactive protein, diabetes, and attendance at religious services. *Diabetes Care* 25(7): 1172–76.

56. Masters, K. S., Hill, R. D., Kircher, J. C., Benson, T. L., & Fallon, J. A. (2004). Religious orientation, aging, and blood pressure reactivity to interpersonal and cognitive stressors. *Annals of Behavioral Medicine* 28(3): 171–78.

57. Contrada, R. J., Goyal, T. M., Cather, C., Rafalson, L., Idler, E. L., & Krause, T. J. (2004). Psychosocial factors in outcomes of heart surgery: The impact of religious involvement and depressive symptoms. *Health Psychology* 23: 227–38.

58. Kaufman, Y., Anaki, D., Binns, M., Freedman, M. (2007). Cognitive decline in Alzheimer's disease: Impact of spirituality, religiosity, and QOL. *Neurology* 68: 1509–14.

59. Van Ness, P. H., & Kasl, S. V. (2003). Religion and cognitive dysfunction in an elderly cohort. *Journal of Gerontology* (Social Sciences) 58B(1): S21–29.

60. Enstrom. (1989).

61. Reyes-Ortiz, C. A., et al. (2006). Higher church attendance predicts lower fear of falling in older Mexican-Americans. *Aging and Mental Health* 10(1): 13–18.

62. Hill, T. D., Angel, J. L., Ellison, C. G., & Angel, R. J. (2005). Religious attendance and mortality: An 8-year follow-up of older Mexican Americans. *Journal of Gerontology B: Psychological Sciences and Social Sciences* 60(2) (March): S102–9.

63. Bagiella, E., Hong, V., & Sloan, R. P. (2005). Religious attendance as a predictor

of survival in the EPESE cohorts. *International Journal of Epidemiology* 34: 443–51.

64. Jaffe, D. H., Eisenbach, Z., Neumark, Y. D., & Manor, O. (2005). Does living in a religiously affiliated neighborhood lower mortality? *Annals of Epidemiology* 15(10): 804–10.

65. Al-Kandari, Y. Y. (2003). Religiosity and its relation to blood pressure among selected Kuwaitis. *Journal of Biosocial Science* 35: 463–72.

66. la Cour, P., Avlund, K., & Schultz-Larsen, K. (2006). A twenty-year follow-up of 734 Danish adults born in 1914. *Social Science and Medicine* 62(1): 157–64.

67. Koenig, McCullough, & Larson. (2001).

68. Wallace, J. M., & Forman, T. A. (1998). Religion's role in promoting health and reducing the risk among American youth. *Health Education and Behavior* 25: 721–41.

69. Rew, L., & Wong, Y. J. (2006). A systematic review of associations among religiosity/spirituality and adolescent health attitudes and behaviors. *Journal of Adolescent Health* 38: 433–42.

70. Hamer, D. *The God Gene: How Faith Is Hardwired into Our Genes.* (2004). New York: Doubleday.

71. Comings, D. E., Gonzales, N., Saucier, G., Johnson, J. P., & MacMurray, J. P. (2000). The DRD4 gene and the spiritual transcendence scale of the character temperament index. *Psychiatric Genetics* 10(4): 185–89.

72. Abramson, A. C., Baker, L. A., & Caspi, A. (2002). Rebellious teens? Genetic and environmental influences on the social attitudes of adolescents. *Journal of Personality & Social Psychology* 83: 1392–1408.

73. Koenig, L. B., McGue, M., Krueger, R. F., & Bouchard, T. J. (2005). Genetic and environmental influences on religiousness: Findings for retrospective and current religiousness ratings. *Journal of Personality* 73: 471–88.

74. Kendler, K. S., Gardner, C. O., & Prescott, C. A. (1997). Religion, psychopathology, and substance use and abuse: A multimeasure, genetic-epidemiologic study. *American Journal of Psychiatry* 154: 322–29.

75. Dewhurst, K., & Beard, A. W. (1970). Sudden religious conversions in temporal lobe epilepsy. *British Journal of Psychiatry* 117: 497–507; Bear, D. M., & Fedio, P. (1977). Quantitative analysis of interictal behavior in temporal lobe epilepsy. *Archives of Neurology* 34: 454–67; Bear, D., Levin, K., Blumer, D., Chetham, D., & Ryder, J. (1982). Interictal behavior in hospitalized temporal lobe epileptics: Relationship to idiopathic psychiatric syndromes. *Journal of Neurology, Neurosurgery, and Psychiatry* 45: 481–88; Fedio, P. (1986). Behavioral characteristics of patients with temporal lobe epilepsy. *Psychiatric Clinics of North America* 9: 267–81.

76. Tucker, D. M., Novelly, R. A., & Walker, P. J. (1987). Hyperreligiosity in temporal lobe epilepsy: Redefining the relationship. *Journal of Nervous and Mental Disease* 175: 181–84.

77. Ramachandran, V. S., Hirstein, W. S., Armel, K. C., Tecoma, F., & Iragui, V. (1997). The neural basis of religious experience. Poster presented at the Annual Meeting of the Society of Neurosciences, New Orleans, October 27 (Abstract #519.1, Volume 23).

78. Byrd, R. C. (1988). Positive therapeutic effects of intercessory prayer in a coronary care unit population. *Southern Medical Journal* 81(7): 826–29.

79. Krucoff, M. W, et al. (2005). Music, imagery, touch, and prayer as adjuncts to interventional cardiac care: The Monitoring and Actualisation of Noetic Trainings (MANTRA) II randomised study. *Lancet* 366(9481) (July 16–22): 211–17.

80. Benson, H., et al. (2006). Study of the therapeutic effects of intercessory prayer (STEP) in cardiac bypass patients: A multicenter randomized trial of uncertainty and certainty of receiving intercessory prayer. *American Heart Journal* 151: 934–42.

PART II

SPIRITUALITY, RELIGION, AND HEALTH CARE

EXAMINING THE RELATIONSHIPS

No book dealing with spirituality and health would be complete without a discussion of religion and its impact on health care. Although organized religion is not the sole expression of spirituality, for many people it remains an important one. Nurses as well as other health care providers need to be aware of the importance that religious beliefs play in the lives of many patients and families and also how those beliefs may affect health care. Religious beliefs frequently impact directly on such areas as diet, hygiene, and the rituals that surround birth and death.

Chapters 3 and 4 examine a sampling of religions that reflect both a theistic and a pantheistic worldview. Chapter 5 presents situations where an individual's religious beliefs and medical treatment are in conflict. In such situations, where spiritual distress is experienced by the patient, by the family, and by the nurse or other members of the health care team, it is essential for nurses and other health care providers to recognize and implement appropriate interventions.

3

THEISM AND HEALTH CARE

VERNA BENNER CARSON

> [S]pirituality is not a religion. Spirituality has to do with experience;
> religion has to do with the conceptualization of that experience. Spirituality
> focuses on what happens in the heart; religion tries to codify and capture
> that experience in a system.
>
> —Thomas Legere

The three major religions with a theistic worldview—Judaism, Christianity, and Islam—all began in the Mediterranean region. These religions are all monotheistic in belief, and the sacred scriptures of these groups focus on the importance of one God who personally created the world and who reveals himself through events in human history (Monk et al. 2003). Important to these theistic religions are their moral codes, which reject stealing, lying, slander, covetousness, and adultery, and stress honoring one's parents, honesty, kindness, and generosity as important social concerns.

Despite the similarities among Judaism, Christianity, and Islam, each religion has its own style, its own inner dynamics, its own special meanings, and its own unique approach to spiritual life. In essence, even though each represents a theistic worldview, each also interprets theism in a unique manner, thus creating variants on a theistic worldview. Therefore, each religious group must be seen from the perspective of a person within that faith in order to fully grasp the meaning of life for that individual (Josephson & Peteet 2004). Furthermore, the adherents of a particular

65

faith do not necessarily all believe the same thing. An individual's belief system may derive from a number of sources, including folk religion, family beliefs, and conclusions drawn from personal experience.

Even in today's humanistically oriented society, religion is important to many Americans. In a 2006 Gallup poll (Gallup 2007), 73 percent of Americans espoused a belief in God; 84 percent stated that religion is fairly to very important to them; 63 percent are members of a house of worship; and 40 percent claim to have attended a religious service in the past seven days. The religious belief in a higher power offers a source of strength to people to help them deal with life's important events—birth, illness, suffering, and death. A health crisis may strengthen, shatter, or awaken an individual's need to develop or change beliefs and faith.

Nurses are in a unique position to deal with people of various religious backgrounds. When illness challenges patients' beliefs, nurses can step in to support patients' beliefs and values and, with the professional chaplain's help, guide patients to identify and use religious and spiritual resources. It is not necessary for the nurse to hold similar religious beliefs as the patient or to agree with the beliefs of the patient in order to meet the patient's spiritual needs with acceptance and understanding.

In writing this chapter, I contacted many clergy. Each of them stressed that in today's complex society, it cannot be assumed that they and their congregations always know whenever one of their parishioners is ill or hospitalized. Since all religious groups desire to minister to their members in times of illness and hospitalization, responsibility for notification of the clergy should be a responsibility shared by the patient, family, and friends, as well as nurses and other health care professionals who have the patient's permission to do so.

This chapter offers a framework of knowledge for nurses and other health care providers so that the spiritual needs of patients can be met with greater sensitivity and understanding. The major religious groups with a theistic worldview are presented with a brief look at the beliefs and practices that have an impact on health care. This chapter is not intended to provide an exhaustive review of theistic religions, but rather to offer a broad sweep. Readers interested in greater depth are encouraged to seek out literature specific to a particular religion and particular religious practices. For instance, the website of the Professional Chaplains Association (http://www.professionalchaplains.org) contains an excellent learning module on cultural and spiritual sensitivity. The reader is reminded that within a specific faith tradition, not every person holds the same beliefs or even recognizes the common practices of that faith. There is no substitute for asking the patient and family what it is that they believe and practice.

Judaism

IMPACT OF BELIEFS AND PRACTICES ON HEALTH CARE

Nurses need to be familiar with the beliefs and practices of the Orthodox Jew as well as Conservative, Reform, and Reconstructionist Jews, especially in the areas of diet, birth rituals, male and female contact, and death. Jews believe in one G-d who created the universe and all that is in it. Jews believe in the importance of honoring commitments, fulfilling obligations, and carrying out duties. The sanctity of life takes precedence over all religious obligations (Wintz & Cooper 2003). See Table 3–1 for specific information.

Table 3–1   Jewish Beliefs and Practices Affecting Health Care

Religious Group	Beliefs and Practices
Observant Jews (Orthodox Judaism, and some Conservative and Reconstructionist groups)	**Birth:** For observant Jews, babies are named by the father. Male children are named eight days after birth, when ritual circumcision is done. A mohel (a person specially trained in performing religious circumcision) performs the circumcision. Circumcision may be postponed if the infant is in poor health. Female babies are usually named during the reading of the Holy Torah in synagogue. Nurses need to be sensitive to the wishes of the parents when caring for babies who have not yet been named.
	Care of women: A woman is considered to be in a ritual state of impurity whenever blood is coming from her uterus, such as during menstrual periods and after the birth of a child. During this time, her husband will not have physical contact with her. When this time is over, she will immerse herself in a pool of living waters (a lake, a river, an ocean, or a special facility in which these living waters are placed called a mikvah). Health care providers need to be aware of this practice and be sensitive to the husband and wife because the husband will not touch his wife before she immerses in the mikvah. He cannot assist her in moving in the bed, so the health care provider will have to do this. An Orthodox Jewish man will not touch any women other than his wife, daughters, and mother.

(table continues)

(Table 3–1 continued)

Religious Group	Beliefs and Practices

(Observant Jews, continued)

Dietary rules: (1) Kosher dietary laws include the following: No mixing of milk and meat at a meal; no consumption of food or any derivative thereof from animals not slaughtered in accordance with Jewish law; no consumption of pork products or shellfish; use of separate cooking utensils for meat and milk products; if a patient requires milk and meat products for a meal, the dairy foods should be served first, followed later by the meat. (2) During Yom Kippur (the Day of Atonement), a twenty-four-hour fast is required, but exceptions are made for those who cannot fast for medical reasons. (3) During Passover, no leavened products are eaten. (4) Many say benediction of thanksgiving before meals and grace at the end of the meal. Time and a quiet environment should be provided for this.

Sabbath: Observed from sunset Friday until sunset Saturday. Orthodox law prohibits riding in a car, smoking, turning lights on and off, handling money, and using television and telephone during the Sabbath (also known as Shabbat). Health care providers need to be aware of this when caring for observant Jews at home and in the hospital. Medical or surgical treatments should not be scheduled for the Sabbath, if possible.

Death: Judaism defines death as occurring when respiration and circulation are irreversibly stopped and no movement is apparent. (1) Euthanasia is strictly forbidden by Orthodox Jews, who advocate the strict use of life-support measures. (2) Prior to death, the Jewish faith holds that visits by family and friends is a religious duty. The Torah and Psalms may be read and prayers recited. A witness needs to be present when a person prays for health so that if death occurs G-d will protect the family and the spirit will be committed to G-d. Extraneous talking and conversation about death are not encouraged, unless initiated by the patient or visitors. In Judaism, the belief is that people should have someone with them when the soul leaves the body, so family and/or friends should be allowed to stay with patients, even after a person passes on. After death, the body should not be left alone until it is buried, usually within twenty-four hours of death. (3) When death occurs, the body should be untouched for eight to thirty minutes. Medical personnel should not touch or wash the body, but allow only an Orthodox person or the Jewish Burial Society to care for the body. Handling of a corpse on the Sabbath is prohibited for Jewish people. If need be, the nursing staff may provide routine care of the body, wearing gloves. Water in the room should be emptied, and the family may request that mirrors be covered to symbolize that a death has occurred. (4) Orthodox Jews and some Conservative Jews do not approve of autopsies. If an autopsy must be done, all body parts must remain with the body. (5) For Orthodox Jews, the body must be buried within twenty-four hours. No flowers are permitted. A fetus must be buried as well. (6) A seven-day mourning period, called a shiva, is required by the immediate family. They must stay at home except for

(table continues)

(Table 3–1 continued)

Religious Group	Beliefs and Practices
(Observant Jews, continued)	Sabbath worship. Among some Conservative and Reconstructionist Jews, the shiva is sometimes held for three days or even one day. (7) Organs or other body parts, such as amputated limbs, must be made available for burial for Orthodox Jews, since they believe that all of the body must be returned to earth.
	Birth control and abortion: Artificial methods of birth control are not encouraged. Vasectomy is not allowed. Abortion may be performed only to save the mother's life. Conservative and Reconstructionist branches do not prohibit birth control or vasectomy; abortion is generally considered a matter of personal choice.
	Organ transplant: Recent rabbinical rulings allow for organ donation, based on the belief that life (that is, the life of the prospective organ recipient) must be preserved whenever possible.
	Shaving: The beard is regarded as a mark of piety among observant Jews. For the very Orthodox, shaving should not be done with a razor but with scissors or an electric razor, since a blade should not contact the skin.
	Head covering: Orthodox men wear skullcaps (called yarmulkes or kippot) at all times, and women cover their hair after marriage. Some Orthodox women wear wigs as a mark of piety. Conservative Jews cover their heads only during acts of worship and prayer.
	Prayer: Pray three times daily; pray directly to G-d, including a prayer of confession, which is required for Orthodox Jews. Health care personnel should provide quiet time for prayer.
Reform Jews	**Birth:** Reform Jews may or may not adhere to the practices referred to for observant Jews. They favor ritual circumcision, but it is not imperative.
	Care of women: Do not observe the rules against touching.
	Dietary rules: Usually do not observe kosher dietary restrictions.
	Sabbath: Usually worship in temples on Friday evenings.
	Death: Advocate use of life support without heroic measures. Allow for cremation, but suggest that ashes be buried in a Jewish cemetery.
	Organ transplants: Recent rabbinical rulings allow for organ donation, based on the belief that life (that is, the life of the prospective organ recipient) must be preserved whenever possible.
	Head coverings: Generally pray without wearing skullcaps.

(From Gershan 1985; Greenberg, Chir, & Wiesner 2004; Monk et al., 2003; Judaism 2006; Sinclair, D. 2003; Ultra-Orthodox Judaism 2003; Union of American Hebrew Congregations 2002; Wintz & Cooper 2003.)

Christianity

Roman Catholicism

IMPACT OF BELIEFS AND PRACTICES ON HEALTH CARE

In caring for the Roman Catholic patient, the health care provider must be aware of the importance of the sacraments, especially baptism, the Eucharist (the presence of Christ under the appearances of bread and wine), penance, and the anointing of the sick. Dietary habits may also be a concern to the patient, as well as the issue of birth control. Private devotions often play a role in the healing process. Religious practices and beliefs are very important to many and may affect the outcome of a patient's illness. Roman Catholics believe in the trinitarian nature of God: God the Father; Jesus Christ, the Son of God; and the Holy Spirit. See Table 3–2 for more detailed information.

Eastern Orthodox

IMPACT OF BELIEFS AND PRACTICES ON HEALTH CARE

Christians were united as one church from the time of Jesus' death and resurrection until the time when Constantine established Constantinople and made it the capital of the Holy Roman Empire in 330 CE. When Rome was invaded, the popes turned to the Franks instead of the Eastern leadership for help. This, along with the theological differences over the wording of the Nicene Creed regarding the Holy Spirit, the use of pictures and statues in churches, the sacraments, the marriage of priests, and the use of Greek or Latin in worship services, created a widening gap between the Eastern and Western churches. The official split came in 1054 CE when the pope in Rome excommunicated the Constantine patriarch and, in turn, the patriarch of the East excommunicated the pope (Papadakis 2003).

Nurses, along with the entire health care team, need to be aware that administration of the sacraments is important to Roman Catholics. Dietary practices of fasting from meat and dairy products on certain days, rituals regarding death, and calendar differences should also be noted. See Table 3–2 for specific information.

Table 3–2   Roman Catholic and Eastern Orthodox Beliefs and Practices
Affecting Health Care

Religious Group	Beliefs and Practices
Roman Catholic	**Birth:** Since Roman Catholics believe that unbaptized children are cut off from heaven, infant baptism is mandatory. For newborns with a grave prognosis, stillborns, and all aborted fetuses (unless evidence of tissue necrosis and prolonged death are present), emergency baptism is required. The health care provider calls a priest to perform the baptism unless death might occur before the priest arrives. In that case, anyone can perform the baptism by pouring warm water on the infant's head and saying, "I baptize you in the name of the Father, of the Son, and of the Holy Spirit." All information about the baptism is recorded on the chart, and the priest and family are notified.

Holy Eucharist: For patients and health care providers who are to receive communion, abstinence from solid food and alcohol is required for fifteen minutes (if possible) prior to reception of the consecrated wafer. Medicine, water, and nonalcoholic drinks are permitted at any time. If a patient is in danger of death, the fast is waived since the reception of the Eucharist at this time is very important.

Anointing of the sick: The priest uses sacred oil to anoint the forehead and hands and, if desired, the affected area. The rite may be performed on any who are ill and desire it. Persons receiving the sacrament seek complete healing, and the strength to endure suffering. Prior to 1963, this sacrament was only given to those facing imminent death, so the health care provider must be sensitive to the meaning this has for the patient. If possible, the health care provider calls a priest before the patient is unconscious, but may also call when there is sudden death, since the sacrament may also be given shortly after death. The health care provider records in the patient's record that this sacrament has been administered.

Dietary habits: Obligatory fasting is excused during hospitalization. However, if there are no health restrictions, some Catholics may still observe the following guidelines: (1) Anyone fourteen years of age or older must abstain from eating meat on Ash Wednesday and all Fridays during Lent. Some older Catholics may still abstain from meat on all Fridays of the year. (2) In addition to abstinence from meat, persons twenty-one to fifty-nine years of age must limit themselves to one full meal and two light meals on Ash Wednesday and Good Friday.

Death: Catholics believe in life after death. Each Roman Catholic should participate in the anointing of the sick as well as the Eucharist and penance before death. The body should not be shrouded until after these sacraments are performed. All body parts that retain human quality must be appropriately buried or cremated. |

(table continues)

(Table 3–2 continued)

Religious Group	Beliefs and Practices

(Roman Catholic, continued)

Birth control: Prohibited except for abstinence or natural family planning. Referral to a priest for questions about this can be of great help. Health care providers can teach the techniques of natural family planning if they are familiar with them; otherwise, this should be referred to the physician or to a support group of the church that instructs couples in this method of birth control. Sterilization is prohibited unless there is an overriding medical reason for it.

Organ donation: Donation and transplantation of organs are acceptable as long as the donor is not harmed and is not deprived of life.

Religious objects: Rosary prayers are said using rosary beads. Medals bearing the images of saints, relics, statues, and scapulars are important objects that may be pinned to a hospital gown or pillow or be at the bedside. Extreme care should be taken not to lose these objects, since they have special meaning to the patient.

Rituals/Ceremonies: Attending mass on Sundays and holy days is required; observance of sacraments important; use of sacramentals, including holy water, rosary beads (for prayer), lighting of candles, use of blessed oil during certain sacraments; reverence of the name of Jesus and the crucifix; use of statues and pictures depicting Jesus, Mary, the mother of Jesus, the apostles and saints.

Eastern Orthodox

Birth: The child must be baptized within forty days after birth. If sprinkling or immersion into water is not possible, baptism is performed by moving the baby in the air in the sign of the cross. An ordained priest or a deacon must be notified for this.

Holy Eucharist: The priest is notified if the patient desires this sacrament.

Anointing of the sick: The priest conducts this in the hospital room.

Dietary habits: Fasting from meat and dairy products is required on Wednesdays and Fridays during Lent and on other holy days. Hospital patients are exempt if fasting is considered detrimental to their health.

Special days: Christmas is celebrated on January 7 and New Year's Day on January 14. This is important to the care of a patient who is hospitalized on these days.

Death: Last rites are obligatory. This is handled by an ordained priest who is notified by the health care provider while the patient is conscious. The Russian Orthodox Church does not encourage autopsy or organ donation. Euthanasia, even for the terminally ill, is discouraged, as is cremation.

Birth control: This, as well as abortion, is not permitted.

(From Papadakis 2003; Wintz & Cooper 2003; Monk et al. 2003.)

Protestant Faiths

IMPACT OF BELIEFS AND PRACTICES ON HEALTH CARE

The Protestant churches began doctrinally, as did the Roman Catholic and Eastern Orthodox churches, with the belief in the death and resurrection of Jesus. However, the early leaders used the Bible as the basic source of authority, and not tradition. This basic difference led to conflict within the Roman church, since the universal authority of the pope was questioned.

Because of the many different denominations within Protestantism, health care providers need to be especially aware of what is important to each individual patient. This information could be obtained from a spiritual needs assessment and added to the plan of care. Table 3–3 outlines the beliefs and practices of fourteen selected Protestant groups. These beliefs and practices might impact on the health care program needed for such patients.

Table 3–3   Various Protestant Beliefs and Practices Affecting Health Care

Religious Group	Beliefs and Practices
Assemblies of God (Pentecostal)	**Baptism:** Baptism by complete immersion in water is practiced when an individual has received Jesus Christ as his Savior and Lord, based on Acts 2:38.
	Holy Communion: Notify clergy if the patient desires.
	Anointing of the sick: Members believe in divine healing through prayer and the laying on of hands. Clergy is notified if patient or family desires this.
	Dietary habits: Abstinence from alcohol, tobacco, and all illegal drugs is strongly encouraged.
	Death: No special practices.
	Other practices: Faith in God and in the health care providers is encouraged. Members pray for divine intervention in health matters. Health care providers should encourage and allow time for prayer. Members may speak in "tongues" during prayer.
Baptist (over 27 different groups in the United States)	**Baptism:** Do not practice infant baptism.
	Holy Communion: Clergy should be notified if the patient desires.

(table continues)

(Table 3–3 continued)

Religious Group	Beliefs and Practices
(Baptist, continued)	**Dietary habits:** Total abstinence from alcohol is expected.
	Death: No general service is provided, but the clergy does minister through counseling, prayer, and scripture as requested by the patient or family, and the patient is encouraged to believe in Jesus Christ as Savior and Lord.
	Other practices: The Bible is held to be the word of God, so the health care provider should either allow quiet time for scripture reading or offer to read to the patient.
Christian Church (Disciples of Christ)	**Baptism:** Do not practice infant baptism but have dedication service. Believers are baptized by immersion.
	Holy Communion: Open communion is celebrated each Sunday and is a central part of worship services. The health care provider notifies the clergy if the patient desires it, or the clergy may suggest it.
	Death: No special practices.
	Other practices: Church elders as well as clergy may be notified to assist with meeting the patient's spiritual needs.
Church of the Brethren	**Baptism:** Do not practice infant baptism but have dedication service.
	Holy Communion: Usually received within church, but clergy will give it in the hospital when requested.
	Anointing of the sick: Practiced for physical healing as well as spiritual uplift and held in high regard by the church. The clergy is notified if the patient or family desire.
	Death: The clergy is notified for counsel and prayer.
Church of the Nazarene	**Baptism:** Parents have the choice of baptism or dedication for their infant. Emphasis is on the believer's baptism, which is regarded as a symbol of the New Covenant in Jesus Christ.
	Holy Communion: Pastor will administer if the patient wishes.
	Dietary habits: The use of alcohol and tobacco is forbidden.
	Death: Cremation is permitted, and stillborn infants are buried.
	Other practices: Believe in divine healing but not to the exclusion of medical treatment. Patients may desire quiet time for prayer.
Episcopal (Anglican)	**Baptism:** Infant baptism is practiced and is considered urgent if the infant is critically ill. The priest is notified to administer the sacrament. Laypersons may baptize in an emergency.
	Holy Communion: The priest is notified if the patient wishes to receive this sacrament.

(table continues)

(Table 3–3 continued)

Religious Group	Beliefs and Practices
(Episcopal, continued)	**Anointing of the sick:** Priest may administer this rite when death is imminent, but it is not considered mandatory. **Dietary habits:** Some patients may abstain from meat on Fridays. Others may fast before receiving the Eucharist, but fasting is not mandatory. **Death:** No special practices. **Other practices:** Confession of sins to a priest is optional; if the patient desires this, the clergyperson should be notified.
Lutheran (10 different branches)	**Baptism:** Baptize only living infants anytime, but usually six to eight weeks after birth. Adults are also baptized, and modes of baptism, as appropriate, include sprinkling, pouring, or immersion. **Holy Communion:** Notify the clergyperson if the patient desires this sacrament. Clergy may also inquire about the patient's desire. **Anointing of the sick:** The patient may request an anointing and blessing from the minister. **Death:** A service of Commendation of the Dying is used at the patient's or family's request.
Mennonite (12 different groups)	**Baptism:** No infant baptism, but the child may be dedicated if requested by the parents. **Holy Communion:** Offered twice a year, with foot washing as part of ceremony. **Dietary habits:** Abstinence from alcohol is urged for all. **Death:** Prayer is important at time of crisis, so contacting a minister is important. **Other practices:** Women may wear head coverings during hospitalization. Anointing with oil is administered in accordance with James 5:14, when requested.
Methodist (over 20 different groups)	**Baptism:** Notify the clergy if the parent desires baptism for a sick infant. **Holy Communion:** Notify the clergy if a patient requests it prior to surgery or another health crisis. **Anointing of the sick:** If requested, the clergy will come to pray and sprinkle the patient with olive oil. **Death:** Scripture reading and prayer are important at this time. **Other practices:** Donation of one's body or part of the body at death is encouraged.

(table continues)

(Table 3–3 continued)

Religious Group	Beliefs and Practices
Presbyterian (10 different groups)	**Baptism:** Infant baptism is practiced by pouring or sprinkling. Immersion is also practiced at times for adults.
	Holy Communion: Given when appropriate and convenient, at the hospitalized patient's request.
	Death: Notify a local pastor or elder for prayer and scripture reading if desired by the family or patient.
Quaker (Society of Friends)	**Baptism and Holy Communion:** Since Friends have no creed per se, there is a diversity of personal beliefs, one of which is that outward sacraments are usually not necessary since there is the ministry of the Spirit inwardly in such areas as baptism and communion. A few Friends groups baptize with water.
	Death: Believe that the present life is part of God's kingdom and generally have no ceremony as a rite of passage from this life to the next. Personal beliefs and wishes need to be ascertained, and the health care provider can then act on the patient's and/or family's wishes.
	Other practices: The name of the Quaker infant is recorded in official record books at the local meeting.
Salvation Army	**Baptism:** No particular ceremony, but they do have an Infant Dedication ceremony.
	Holy Communion: No particular ceremony.
	Death: Notify the local officer in charge of the Army Corps for any soldier (member) who needs assistance.
	Other practices: The Bible is seen as the only rule for one's faith, so the scriptures should be made available to a patient. The Army has many of its own social welfare centers, with hospitals and homes where unwed mothers are cared for and outpatient services provided. No medical or surgical procedures are opposed, except for abortion on demand.
Seventh-day Adventist	**Baptism:** No infant baptism is practiced, but dedication services are performed.
	Holy Communion: Although this is not required of hospitalized patients, the clergy is notified if the patient desires.
	Anointing of the sick: The clergy are contacted for prayer and anointing with oil.
	Dietary habits: Since the body is viewed as the temple of the Holy Spirit, healthy living is essential. Therefore, it is prohibited to consume alcohol, tobacco, coffee, and tea, and to use drugs. Some are vegetarians, and most avoid pork.

(table continues)

(Table 3–3 continued)

Religious Group	Beliefs and Practices
(Seventh-day Adventist, continued)	**Special days:** The Sabbath is observed on Saturday. **Death:** No special procedures. **Other related practices:** Use of hypnotism is opposed by some. Persons of homosexual or lesbian orientation are ministered to in the hope of correction of these practices, which are believed to be wrong. A Bible should always be available for scripture reading.
United Church of Christ	**Baptism:** Practice infant and adult baptism. Three modes are used as appropriate: pouring, sprinkling, and immersion. **Holy Communion:** Clergy is notified if the patient desires to receive this sacrament. **Death:** If the patient desires counsel or prayer, notify the clergy.

(From American Baptist Churches USA, http://www.abc-usa.org; Christian Church Disciples of Christ: http://www.disciples.org; Church of the Brethren: http://www.brethren.org; Episcopal Church, http:// www.episcopalchurch.org; Episcopal Church of the United States: http://www.ecusa.anglican.org; Evangelical Lutheran Church in America: http://www.elca.org; General Council of the Assemblies of God: http://ag.org/2006; The Lutheran Church Missouri Synod, http://www.lcms.org; Mennonites USA: http://www.mennonitesusa.org; Monk et al., 2003; Official Site of the International Church of the Nazarene: http://www.nazarene.org; Southern Baptist Convention: http://www.sbc.net-Southern Baptist Convention)

Islam

IMPACT OF BELIEFS AND PRACTICES ON HEALTH CARE

Caring for the Muslim patient requires knowledge of the importance of Qur'anic law and customs. Muslims profess belief in one God, called Allah, who was revealed to them by the Prophet Muhammad. The Holy Qur'an is their scripture. They believe in a judgment day and life after death. Islam has set rituals and requirements to be followed in the areas of birth, diet, prayer time, care of women, and death (Abu-Allaban 2004). See Table 3–4 for specific information on providing health care for Muslims.

Table 3–4 Muslim Beliefs and Practices Affecting Health Care

Religious Group	Beliefs and Practices
Islam	**Birth:** A baby is bathed immediately after birth, before giving it to the mother. The father (or the mother, if the father is not available) then whispers the call to prayer in the child's ears so that the first sounds she hears are about the Muslim faith. Circumcision is culturally recommended before puberty. A baby born prematurely, but of at least 130 days' gestation, is given the same treatment as any other infant. Male infants are circumcised.
	Dietary habits: No pork is allowed, nor alcoholic beverages; some shellfish is prohibited as well; it is important to ask about dietary habits. All halal (permissible) meat must be blessed and killed in a special way. This is called zabihah (meaning, "correctly slaughtered").
	Death: Prior to death, family members ask to be present so that they can read the Qur'an and pray with the patient. An imam may come, if requested by the patient or family, but is not required. Patients must face Mecca, confess their sins, and beg forgiveness in the presence of their family. If the family is unavailable, any practicing Muslim can provide support to the patient. After death, Muslims prefer that the family wash, prepare, and place the body in a position facing Mecca. If necessary, health care providers may perform these procedures as long as they wear gloves. Burial is performed as soon as possible. Cremation is forbidden. Autopsy is also prohibited, except for legal reasons, and then no body part is to be removed. Donation of body parts or organs is not allowed since, according to culturally developed law, persons do not own their body.
	Abortion and birth control: Abortion is forbidden, and many conservative Muslims do not encourage the use of contraceptives since this interferes with God's purpose. Others feel that a woman should only have as many children as her husband can afford. Contraception is permitted by Islamic law.
	Personal devotions: At prayer time, washing is required, even by those who are sick. A patient on bed rest may require assistance with this task before prayer. Provision of privacy is important during prayer.
	Religious objects: The Qur'an must not be touched by anyone who is ritually unclean, and nothing should be placed on top of it. Some Muslims wear taviz, a black string on which words of the Qur'an are attached. These should not be removed and must remain dry. Certain items of jewelry, such as bangles, may have religious significance and should not be removed unnecessarily.
	Care of women: Since women are not allowed to sign consent forms or make a decision regarding family planning, the husband needs to be present. Women are very modest and frequently wear clothes that cover the whole body. During a medical examination, the woman's modesty should be respected as much as possible. Muslim women prefer female doctors. For forty days after giving birth and also during menstruation, a woman is exempt from prayer, since this is a time of cleansing for her.

(From Abou-Allaban 2004; The Council on American-Islamic Relations–CAIR About Us, 2006; Religious Tolerance, 2006; Islam; The Islam Page, 2006; Monk et al., 2003.)

Other Theistic Faiths

Christian Science (Church of Christ, Scientist)

IMPACT OF BELIEFS AND PRACTICES ON HEALTH CARE

The Christian Science Church sees God as divine love, truth, life, mind—the source and substance of all true being—and emphasizes the motherhood as well as the fatherhood of God. Adherents believe that a person's true being is spiritual, whole, and perfect, since humans were created in God's own image. Evil, sin, sickness, and death are not of God, but are rooted in the mistaken conception of life as material and separated from God. They believe that prayer is essential to living in harmony with God. They teach that heaven and hell are considered present states of thought rather than eternal dwelling places after death (Church of Christ, Scientist 2006).

Health care for many Christian Science patients (but not all) will be limited, since they may prefer to follow their own church's healing method through use of God's power. Christian Scientists are likely to be seen at birth or in an emergency room for care of fractures. Christian Scientists do respect the dedication and accomplishments of medical personnel in relieving suffering. They are also meticulous in obeying the law, even when it is restrictive to them, in order to respect the rights of others. See Table 3–5 for further details.

Jehovah's Witnesses

IMPACT OF BELIEFS AND PRACTICES ON HEALTH CARE

The Jehovah's Witnesses trace their historical foundation to the Bible and the fact that in Isaiah 43:12 Jehovah said, "Ye are my witnesses . . . and I am God." Their leader is Jehovah, and members of the organization acknowledge Jesus as the son of Jehovah, witness to the power of Christ, and follow the principles set by the faithful followers throughout biblical history.

Jehovah's Witnesses respect the health care given by physicians but look to God and divine laws as the final authority for their decisions. Because of this, the health care provider must be familiar with their beliefs, especially with regard to use of blood. They believe that taking blood or blood products into the body is a violation of the laws of Jehovah, as written in Genesis 9:3–4, Leviticus 17:14, and Acts 15:28–29. See Table 3–5 for further information.

The Church of Jesus Christ of Latter-day Saints (Mormons)

IMPACT OF BELIEFS AND PRACTICES ON HEALTH CARE

The Latter-day Saints believe in God as our father, Jesus as the son of God and our Savior, and the Holy Spirit as the source of truth. They emphasize faith in Jesus Christ, repentance for sins, and the necessity of receiving the Gift of the Holy Spirit. They look to the Bible and the Book of Mormon as the source of God's word. They believe that families can live together through eternity; they practice baptism by immersion for children eight years of age and older; they receive the Lord's Supper every Sunday with bread and water (Church of Jesus Christ of Latter-Day Saints 2006).

The Latter-day Saints emphasize healthy living and also adhere to health care requirements. In order to better care for the Mormon patient, health care providers should be familiar with their practices regarding sacraments, diet, care of their dead, and personal hygiene. For more information about this group, see Table 3–5.

Unitarian Universalism

IMPACT OF BELIEFS AND PRACTICES ON HEALTH CARE

The Unitarian Universalist Association does not require any member to adhere to a given creed or set of religious beliefs. However, basic beliefs of those within the association include belief in the inherent worth and dignity of every person; justice, equity, and compassion in human relations; acceptance of one another; a free and responsible search for truth and meaning; the importance of personal conscience; and the responsibility of all to work toward peace, liberty, and justice (Unitarian Universalist 2006).

Unitarian Universalists are free to decide what they believe is best for their health. See Table 3–5 for specific information on health care.

Table 3–5 Christian Science, Jehovah's Witnesses, The Church of Jesus Christ of Latter-day Saints, and Unitarian Universalist Beliefs and Practices Affecting Health Care

Religious Group	Beliefs and Practices
Christian Science	**Birth:** Use physician or certified nurse-midwife during childbirth. No baptism ceremony. **Dietary habits:** Since alcohol and tobacco are considered drugs, they are not used. Coffee and tea are often declined. **Death:** Autopsy is usually declined unless required by law. Donation of organs is unlikely, but is an individual decision. **Other practices:** Depending on how strictly they follow the teachings of Christian Science, they do not normally seek medical care, since they approach health care from a different, primarily spiritual, framework. They commonly utilize the services of a surgeon to set a bone but decline drugs and, in general, other medical or surgical procedures. Hypnotism and psychotherapy are also declined. Family planning is left to the family. They seek exemption from vaccinations but obey legal requirements, reporting infectious diseases and obeying public health quarantines. Nonmedical care facilities are maintained for those needing nursing assistance in the course of a healing. The *Christian Science Journal* lists available Christian Science health care providers. When a Christian Science believer is in the hospital, the health care provider should allow and encourage time for prayer and study. Patients may request that a Christian Science practitioner be notified to come. (Christian Science practitioners are not licensed health care professionals.) Their training consists of deep, prayerful study of the Bible and of the textbook of Christian Science, *Science and Health with Key to the Scriptures*, by Mary Baker Eddy. Before Christian Science practitioners can be recognized and advertised in *The Christian Science Journal*, they must complete a course of intensive instruction on healing and improving humankind from an authorized teacher.
Jehovah's Witnesses	**Baptism:** No infant baptism is practiced. Baptism by complete immersion of adults is done as a symbol of dedication to Jehovah, since Jesus was baptized. **Dietary habits:** Use of alcohol and tobacco is discouraged, since these harm the physical body. **Death:** Autopsy is a private matter to be decided by the person and family involved. Burial and cremation are acceptable. **Birth control and abortion:** Use of birth control is a personal decision. Abortion is opposed, based on Exodus 21:22–23. **Organ transplants:** Use of organ transplant is a private decision and, if a transplanted organ is used, it must be cleansed with a nonblood solution. **Blood transfusions:** Blood transfusions violate God's laws and therefore are not allowed. Patients do respect physicians and will accept alternatives

(table continues)

(Table 3–5 continued)

Religious Group	Beliefs and Practices
(Jehovah's Witnesses, continued)	to blood transfusions. These might include use of nonblood plasma expanders, careful surgical techniques to decrease blood loss, use of autologous transfusions, and autotransfusion through use of a heart-lung machine. Health care providers should check unconscious patients for medic alert cards that state that the person does not want a transfusion. Since Jehovah's Witnesses are prepared to die rather than break God's law, health care providers need to be sensitive to the spiritual as well as the physical needs of the patient.
The Church of Jesus Christ of Latter-day Saints	**Baptism:** If a child over the age of eight is very ill, whether baptized or unbaptized, a member of the church's priesthood should be called. **Holy Communion:** A hospitalized patient may desire to have a member of the church priesthood administer this sacrament. **Anointing of the sick:** Mormons frequently are anointed and given a blessing before going to the hospital and after admission by laying on of hands. **Dietary habits:** Abstinence from the use of tobacco; beverages with caffeine, such as cola, coffee, and tea; alcohol and other substances considered injurious. Mormons eat meat but encourage the intake of fruits, grains, and herbs. **Death:** Prefer burial of the body. A church elder should be notified to assist the family. If need be, the elder will assist the funeral director in dressing the body in special clothes and will give other help as needed. **Birth control and abortion:** Abortion is opposed except when the life of the mother is in danger. Only natural means of birth control are recommended. Artificial means can be used when the health of the woman is at stake (including her emotional health). **Personal care:** Cleanliness is very important to Mormons. A sacred undergarment may be worn at all times by Mormons and should only be removed in emergency situations. **Other practices:** Allowing quiet time for prayer and the reading of the sacred writings is important. The church maintains a welfare system to assist those in need. Families are of great importance, so visiting should be encouraged.
Unitarian Universalist	**Baptism:** Infant baptism is unnecessary and if used at all is without trinitarian formula. Usually dedicate their children. **Death:** Cremation is often preferred to burial. **Other practices:** Use of birth control is advocated as part of responsible parenting. Strong support for a woman's right to choose regarding abortion is maintained. Unitarian Universalists advocate donation of body parts for research and transplants.

(From Church of Christ, Scientist 2006; Jehovah's Witnesses 2006; Church of Jesus Christ of Latter-day Saints 2006; Unitarian Universalist 2006.)

Summary

Keeping informed about the myriad of beliefs and practices of various religious groups creates quite a challenge for the nurse and the rest of the health care team. Each religion has its own unique history, developed from the interplay of people, geography, culture, and government. Many religions have adherents all over the world. Although theistic religions all profess belief in one God, each group differs in some respects. Differences exist in health-related practices relevant to birth, the practice of sacraments, prayer, diet, special religious days, death, birth control, abortion, organ transplants, euthanasia, and the use of drugs. Nurses might be involved in any of these aspects of a patient's care.

Since our religious beliefs are intricately woven into our lifestyle, they frequently influence our reaction to stressful situations and our coping abilities during times of personal crisis, such as the birth of a child, an illness requiring medical or surgical intervention or dietary changes, and a death of someone dear to us. Having knowledge about a patient's religious views allows the health care provider to offer spiritual assistance at such times. The health care provider can use information about various religious practices to better communicate with patients and minister to their spiritual needs.

Acknowledgments

Special thanks to each of the following individuals or groups who reviewed and gave input to the various sections of this chapter:

Rev. James M. Bank, AB, STB, AM, Boston University, former teacher of New Testament at Boston University, currently minister of The First Unitarian Church of Baltimore, Baltimore, Maryland.

Rev. Stewart F. Bingman, MDiv, United Theological Seminary, Protestant minister for forty-five years.

Christian Science Committee on Publication for Maryland.

Susan Harwick, RN, BSN, member of St. Mary's Ukrainian Orthodox Church, Allentown, Pennsylvania.

Jehovah's Witnesses Information Center, Baltimore, Maryland.

Rev. William J. O'Brien III, BA, Loyola College, St. Mary's Seminary, Roman Catholic chaplain, University of Maryland Hospital, Baltimore, Maryland.

Akil Rahim, president/imam, Muslim Charities Institute of Islamic Technology, Columbia, Maryland.

Rabbi Moshe Sauer, Jewish chaplain, University of Maryland Hospital, Baltimore, Maryland.

Bishop Gary B. Wixom, The Church of Jesus Christ of Latter-day Saints, Columbia, Maryland.

Reflective Activities

1. In a small group, share experiences you have had with people who hold religious beliefs different from your own. Do your experiences change depending on whether you are in the health care environment or not?

2. With a partner, share which of your own personal religious beliefs have been or would be affected if you were admitted to a hospital.

3. Discuss with a hospital dietitian how different religious dietary laws are met.

4. Within a small group, choose a specific religion and, after research about beliefs and practices relevant to health care, present a skit to illustrate how best to meet the religious needs of a patient and her family.

References

Abu-Allaban, Y. (2004). Muslims. In *Handbook of Spirituality and Worldview in Clinical Practice*, 111–24. Allan M. Josephson and John R. Peteet (eds.). Washington D.C.: American Psychiatric Publishing, Inc.

Assemblies of God (USA). (2007). http://ag.org/top/Beliefs/index.cfm; accessed February 10, 2007.

Catechism of the Catholic Church, 2nd ed. (2006). Washington D.C.

Church of the Brethren. (2006). http://www.brethren.org; accessed September 5, 2006.

Episcopal Church of the United States. (2006). http://www.ecusa.anglican.org; accessed September 2, 2006.

Church of Christ, Scientist. (2006). http://www.churchofchristscientist.org; accessed
    September 5, 2006.
Church of Jesus Christ of Latter-Day Saints. (2006). http://www.lds.org; accessed Sep-
    tember 5, 2006.
Council on American-Islamic Relations. (2006). http://www.cair.net.org/asp/aboutcair
    .asp; accessed September 3, 2006.
Gallup Poll. (2007). Religion. http://brain.gallup.com/content/?ci=1690.
General Council of the Assemblies of God. (2006). http://ag.org/2006; accessed Sep-
    tember 5, 2006.
Gershan, J. A. (1985). Judaic ethical beliefs and customs regarding death and dying.
    Critical Care Health Care Provider 5: 32–34.
Greenberg, D., Chir, B., & Wiesner, I. S. (2004). Jews. In Handbook of Spirituality and
    Worldview in Clinical Practice.
International Church of the Nazarene (2006). http://www.nazarene.org/; accessed Sep-
    tember 5, 2006.
Islam 101. (2006). http://www.islam101.com; accessed September 5, 2006.
Islam Page. (2006). http://www.islamworld.net; accessed September 5, 2006.
Jehovah's Witnesses. (2006). http://www.watchtower.org/; accessed September 5, 2006.
Josephson, A. M., & Peteet, J. R. (eds.). (2004). Handbook of Spirituality and Worldview in
    Clinical Practice.
Judaism. (2006). Infoplease. © 2000–2006 Pearson Education, publishing as Info-
    please. http://www.infoplease.com/ipa/A0001462.html; accessed September 5,
    2006.
Mennonites USA. (2006). http://www.mennonitesusa.org; accessed September 2, 2006.
Monk, R. C., et al. (2003). Exploring Religious Meaning, 6th ed. Upper Saddle River, N.J.:
    Prentice Hall.
Moss, T. (2006). The growth of Christianity worldwide. http://www.virtuemag.org/
    articles/204; accessed October 2, 2006.
Papadakis, A. (2003). History of the Orthodox Church, 1–20. Greek Orthodox Archdiocese
    of America; http://www.goarch.org/en/ourfaith/articles/article7053.asp; accessed
    September 4, 2006.
Religious Tolerance (2006a). A Brief Review of the Early History of the Orthodox Church.
    http://www.religoustolerance.org/chr_orthh.htm; accessed September 5, 2006.
Religious Tolerance (2006b). Religions of the World. http://religioustolerance.org/
    worldrel.htm; accessed August 8, 2006.
Religious Tolerance (2006c). Islam: The Second Largest World Religion . . . and Growing.
    http://www.religiostolerance.org/islam/htm; accessed September 1, 2006.
Religious Tolerance (2006c). Christianity: From All Points of View. http://www.religious-
    tolerance.org/christ.htm; accessed September 1, 2006.
Sinclair, D. (2003). Jewish BioMedical Law: Legal and Extra-Legal Dimensions. Oxford Univer-
    sity Press: New York.
Union of American Hebrew Congregations. (2002). What Is Reform Judaism? New York:
    Union of American Hebrew Congregations. http://rj.org/whatisrj.shtml; accessed
    August 15, 2006.
Unitarian Universalist. (2006). http://www.uua.org/; accessed September 5, 2006.
U.S. Christian Church Disciples of Christ. http://www.disciples.org/; accessed Septem-
    ber 5, 2006.
Wintz, S., & Cooper, E. (2003). Cultural and Spiritual Sensitivity. http://wwwprofessional-
    chaplains.org/index.aspx?id=207; accessed February 10, 2007.

4

EASTERN PANTHEISM AND HEALTH CARE

VERNA BENNER CARSON

> To be aware of inner harmony is to abide with reality. To abide with reality
> is to be enlightened.
>
> —Tao Te Ching

True to our caretaking role, each of us is called on to be aware of and responsive to our patients' cultural, philosophical, and spiritual beliefs, especially as these influence health-related attitudes and behaviors. Many of our patients hold to religious beliefs that stem from a pantheistic worldview, including Hinduism, Buddhism, Taoism, and Confucianism (refer to chapter 1 for a discussion on the pantheistic worldview). This chapter focuses on Hinduism, Buddhism, and Taoism because they represent the major pantheistic religions; Hinduism and Buddhism are, respectively, the third- and fourth-largest religions in the world after Christianity and Islam (Monk et al. 2003, Beverslius 2000, Willis 2004). Historically the pantheistic religions were associated with peoples living in Asia—India, China, Japan, and Korea. Today, however, the tenets of pantheism, as well as theism, are more widespread and making inroads into societies that were once more spiritually and religiously homogenous. Therefore, we can never presume to know an individual's belief system merely by identifying his nationality. An article in the *Washington Post* (Cody 2007) emphasizes this point by reporting on the results of a government-sponsored survey in China that found that the number of religious believers is far higher than generally believed and may be as high as 300 million. Sixty-seven percent of Chinese identify with one of the traditional Chinese religions, such as Buddhism, Taoism, and Islam. However, the study concluded that the number of Chinese who identify themselves with Christianity may reach 40 million. This study underscores the importance of a caveat expressed in chapter 3—that there is no substitute for asking the patient and/or family what they believe and how they practice those beliefs.

Hinduism

Overview

Hinduism is perhaps the oldest religion in the world, dating back to antiquity. Hinduism has no specific founder(s). Worldwide, it is the third-largest religion, with over 900 million adherents; approximately 1 million members reside in North America. Most of those who adhere to the Hindu religion live on the subcontinent of India, although there are Hindus in other parts of Asia, including Nepal, Sri Lanka, Pakistan, and Bangladesh (Jambunathan 2006).

General Beliefs and Practices

Hindus are not bound together by a common creed or doctrine. There is no institutional organization, although many of the sects of Hinduism are so organized. Hindu theology holds that Brahman is the principle and source of the universe, the Divine from which all things emanate and to which all things return; Brahman is impersonal. Everything is divine and one with Brahman; this is pantheism. Bear in mind, however, that this Hindu theology—espoused by monks and theological leaders—may not be the version of Hinduism that is practiced by many lay Hindus around the world. Hinduism is considered polytheistic because Hindus worship many, perhaps thousands, of deities. You may be wondering how a religion can be both pantheistic and polytheistic. The explanation is that the deities in Hinduism are merely expressions, or incarnations, of Brahman. These expressions of Brahman meet the needs of Hindus to attach a face and personality to the object of their worship. It is difficult to worship a divine essence that is impersonal, faceless, and formless. Hindus believe in the Atman that is the soul, or essence of all reality—human, animal, insect, rock, tree, and the like. Essentially, the soul is not a separate entity but is identical with the Universal Soul or Brahman that is absolute truth and bliss. The Atman, like the Brahman, is eternal and, most important, it is said to be one's true nature. The only true reality is Brahman. Everything that we see around us is maya, or illusion.

Hinduism is a very tolerant religion and willing to accept that there is truth in other belief systems (Monk et al. 2003). In fact, Hinduism acknowledges that any sincerely religious person, regardless of whether she is Jewish, Christian, Muslim, or a member of another faith, is also a devout Hindu by nature of her religious sincerity. It is noteworthy that Hinduism recognizes Jesus Christ and Gautama the Buddha as incarnations of the God Vishnu, who, of course, is a manifestation of Brahman. As a rule, Hindus do not seek converts.

Karma is a core concept of Hinduism. Karma, a law of cause and effect, holds that physical and spiritual actions carry consequences (karma). Therefore, depending on how a person lives, good or bad karma accumulates. The goal of life is to be released from the cycle of birth, death, and rebirth, and to return to Brahman. Good actions lead to release from the cycle of rebirth. Bad actions keep the individual soul, or Atman, trapped in the cycle and may lead to rebirth as a lesser life form (as an animal, for example) or as a human being in a lower caste. Release from the cycle is achieved through a variety of paths or disciplines, each called a yoga (meaning "yoke"). These yogas include the way of:

religious devotion to a particular deity, such as Vishnu or Shiva, called Bhakti-yoga;

the way of good works or action, called karma-yoga;

the way of self-discipline through meditation, called raja-yoga; and,

the way of intellectual enlightenment, called jnana-yoga (Monk et al. 2003, Toropov & Buckles 2004, Willis 2004).

It is important for health care professionals to be aware of Hindu beliefs and practices that may have an impact on a patient's medical treatment. Table 4–1 details these.

Table 4–1   Hindu Beliefs and Practices Affecting Health Care

Diet	Many, but not all, Hindus are vegetarians. This practice is based on the belief in reincarnation and holds that an animal could represent the reincarnation of a person. Cows are especially revered. Many of the Brahmin caste in northern India consider eating meat to be religiously sanctioned. Women generally serve the food and may eat separately from men. During their menstrual periods women are not allowed to cook or have contact with other members of the family. When a health care provider is teaching Hindus about medication regimens, it is essential to take into account food rituals in relation to mealtimes and food selection (Jambunathan 2006). Hindus use the right hand for eating and the left hand for toileting and hygiene. Fasting is a practice on special holy days (Wintz & Cooper 2003).
Beliefs regarding healing	Some Hindus believe in faith healing. Others believe that illness is the Divine's way of punishing people for their sins.
Medical and surgical procedures	Hindus accept the use of medications, blood, and blood components. People who lose a limb are not considered outcasts from society, but the loss of a limb is viewed as karma for the sins of a previous life. Organ transplants are acceptable for both donors and recipients.
Reproductive practices	Hindu women prefer examination and treatment by a female practitioner. The birth of a male child is preferred. Hindus accept all forms for birth control; amniocentesis and artificial insemination are acceptable, although not always available; Hindus do not take a position on either therapeutic abortions or abortion on demand. Pregnancy is considered a hot period, which means that the Hindu woman will avoid hot foods, such as animal products, chilies, spices, ginger, and gas-producing foods because they are believed to cause overexcitement, inflammatory reactions, sweating, and fatigue. If eaten too early in the pregnancy, hot foods are believed to cause miscarriage and fetal abnormalities. Cold foods, such as milk products, yogurt, cream and butter, most vegetables, and foods that taste sour are thought to strengthen and calm the pregnant woman (Turrell 1985). During pregnancy there are rituals that are thought to protect the pregnant mother and the unborn child from evil spirits. Morning sickness is believed to be caused by an increase in pitta, or bodily heat. Iron-deficiency anemia is one of the nutritional disorders affecting women of childbearing age. This may be related to a belief that eating leafy vegetables produces a dark-skinned baby; consequently, this food item may be eliminated from the woman's diet (Jambunathan 2006). Both mother and baby undergo purification rites on the eleventh day postpartum. The baby is officially named on the eleventh day during the "cradle ceremony," and several rituals are performed to protect the baby from evil spirits. During the postpartum period, hot foods, such as dried fish, drumsticks, and greens, are considered good for lactation, while cold foods, such as buttermilk and curds, gourds, squashes, tomatoes, and potatoes, are restricted because they are gas-producing.

(table continues)

(Table 4–1 continued)

Religious support for the sick	Religious representatives are called priests; however, there are no church or temple organizations to assist the sick. Care of the sick is provided by family and friends within the individual's caste.
Death and dying	Pain medication may be refused because the patient is preparing for a good death, which is characterized by being in full possession of mental and physical faculties and fully cognizant of what is to come—not being overtaken by death, but deliberately letting go of life. Family members will most likely remain at the bedside singing and praying to help the dying person fix his mind on the Divine. Family may also request that the patient be lifted from the bed and placed on a purified spot on the ground (Vatuk 1996). After death, the death rite called antyesti is performed, consisting of a ritual bath, followed by a sprinkling of holy river water over the body of the dying person. The body is then covered with new clothes and parts of the body are dabbed with ghee (clarified semisolid butter); these practices not only purify the deceased but also strengthen the soul for the postmortem journey. The Hindu priest pours water into the mouth of the deceased and blesses the body by tying a thread around the neck or wrist.
	There are no religions customs or restrictions related to the prolongation of life. Death is viewed as just one more step toward nirvana or oneness with Brahman. Euthanasia is not practiced. Autopsies are acceptable. The donation of body parts is also acceptable. Cremation is the most common form of body disposal. Ashes are collected and disposed of in holy rivers such as the Ganges. Hindus in America may save their family member's ashes to later scatter them in holy rivers when they return to their homeland. A dead fetus or newborn is sometimes buried. There are family rituals in response to death. The eldest son performs prayers for ancestral souls, called shradda rites, but these are performed by all male descendants, each of whom offers pindam (balls of rice) on behalf of the deceased. Females may respond to the death of a loved one with loud wailing, moaning, and beating their chests in front of the corpse. This behavior symbolizes their inability to bear the thought of being left behind to handle life situations by themselves. This is particularly significant for females because widowhood is considered inauspicious. Health care providers need to offer support and understanding of the Hindu culture's response to death and grief (Jambunathan 2006).
Culture-bound syndromes	Some Hindus from northern India believe in ghost illness or ghost possession, a belief that a ghost enters a victim and tries to seize its soul. If the ghost is successful, death results. One sign of ghost illness is a voice speaking through a delirious victim. This may occur in children as well as adults. Other signs are convulsions, body movements indicating pain, choking or difficulty breathing, and, in the case of an infant, incessant crying (Freed & Freed, 1991).
Temporal relationships	The Hindu concept of time is past-, present-, and future-oriented. Hindus may not adhere to North American parameters of time, so being punctual for scheduled appointments may not be considered important. The health care provider should not misconstrue this behavior as a sign of irresponsibility, noncompliance, or not valuing health.

(table continues)

(Table 4–1 continued)

Disease and health conditions	Asian Indians migrating to the United States from the tropical regions of India may be susceptible to malaria. Respiratory infections, such as tuberculosis and pneumonia, are widely prevalent among Indians living in the mid-latitudes. Indians have a high morbidity related to cardiovascular diseases. Rheumatic heart disease is a major cardiac problem, along with hypertension. Dental caries and periodontal disease affect 90 percent of the adult population. Sickle cell disease is also highly prevalent (Jambunathan 2006).
Variations in drug metabolism	Asians are known to require lower doses and experience side effects at lower doses than Caucasians for a variety of psychotropic drugs, such as lithium, antidepressants, and neuroleptics. They are also more sensitive to alcohol than their Caucasian counterparts.

Buddhism

Overview

Buddhism emerged in the sixth century BCE and began as a reform movement within Hinduism. The movement was founded by Siddhartha Gautama, also known as Gautama the Buddha, who lived in what is modern-day Nepal. Buddha sought to restore the core of Hinduism at a time when the religion had become static and ritualized. Buddhism was accepted by powerful political leaders who believed that it had relevance to all people. It quickly became a missionary religion, seeking converts. Over many centuries and into modern times, Buddhism spread throughout Asia, where it became an important, if not dominant, religion in China, Japan, Korea, Indochina, Nepal, Tibet, and Sri Lanka. Hinduism in India adapted to the criticism of Buddhists and eventually absorbed Buddhism so that today Buddhism is hardly represented in India at all. In the last century, with a resurgence of missionary zeal, Buddhism has spread throughout the world.

Main Teachings of Buddhism

Buddha's teachings centered around two basic truths: the fact of suffering and the possibility of escape from suffering. He taught that all suffering is caused by selfish patterns of thought and behavior. In order to eliminate suffering, individuals must learn to redirect selfish desires until these desires are extinguished, leaving individuals free to simply "be."

In order to achieve this release, a person needed to redirect her entire attitude toward reality, first, by accepting the Four Noble Truths, and second, by living according to the instructions contained in the fourth truth (which points to the Eightfold Path).

The Four Noble Truths are:

1. Life inevitably involves *dukkha* (suffering).
2. The cause of suffering is *tanha* (greed).
3. Suffering can be cured by overcoming selfish cravings.
4. The way to overcome selfish craving is to follow the Middle Path.

Buddha taught his followers not to worship him as a god. Instead, he taught them to take responsibility for their own lives and actions. He instructed them that the Middle Way or Path was the way to Nirvana. The Middle Way involved avoiding a life of luxury and indulgence but also avoiding too much fasting and hardship. He identified the Eightfold Path that provides the strategy for following the Middle Path as follows:

1. Right Understanding and Viewpoint: Awareness of the need to overcome selfish desire.
2. Right Values and Attitude: Display compassion rather than selfishness.
3. Right Speech: Abstention from lies and evil language.
4. Right Action: Help others, live honestly, avoid gossip and immoral conduct.
5. Right Mode of Livelihood: Do something useful and avoid jobs that harm living things.
6. Right Endeavor: Encourage good and helpful thoughts and discourage unwholesome and destructive thoughts.
7. Right Mindfulness: Gain self-knowledge and self-mastery.
8. Right Concentration: Maintain a calm mind by practicing meditation, which leads to Nirvana.

Although Buddha's insights were focused more on ethical patterns of living than on religious rites, rituals, and theology, his goal was more than teaching ethical behavior. He saw ethical actions as the method for moving toward Ultimate Existence. And what is the Ultimate Existence to which Buddha pointed his followers? It is insight into the very essence of life and the freedom to live on the basis of that insight. Gaining this insight is most often described as Nirvana or extinction of desire. Once an individual achieves Nirvana, he has no need for a continuing soul or self—he simply "is." Enlightenment ends the cycle of reincarnations because, according to Buddha, what is passed from one life to another life is the karma that is attached to a person's consciousness. Entering Nirvana negates the need for individual consciousness (Monk et al. 2003, Toropov & Buckles 2004, Andrews & Boyle 2007, United Religions Initiative 2002).

Again, as with Hinduism, the way that Buddhism is actually practiced around the world by Buddhist laypeople may be very different than the Buddhist philosophy described above and taught by Buddhist educators and monks. While Buddha discouraged people from worshiping him as a god, it is not unusual to have large Buddha statues at the center of temple worship, given the apparent intrinsic human need to worship something concrete, with a personality and a face. Let's examine common Buddhist health beliefs and practices that may impact on health care. Table 4–2 details these.

Table 4–2   Buddhist Beliefs and Practices Affecting Health Care

Diet	Dietary regulations vary within different branches of Buddhism, with some practicing strict vegetarianism. This is an area that requires assessment on the part of the health care practitioner.
Reproductive practices	Since Buddhists believe in reincarnation, they view birth as the beginning of a precious opportunity for the complete development of the mind and the practice of compassion. Birth control is acceptable. Although Buddhists do not condone the taking of a life, abortion may be allowed, depending on the condition of the mother. Mothers are regarded as more important than fathers because of their primary role in the birth of children and traditional child care. When a mother is sick, special kindness is shown to her.
Death	The time of death is very important to the Buddhist since this marks the transition to the next life. Buddhists devote considerable religious practice to preparing for death. Everything possible is done to provide peace and quiet to the dying person. For the Buddhist, dying occurs over a series of stages that involve disintegration of the physical aspects of life until finally the consciousness leaves the body. Buddhists believe that the more

(table continues)

(Table 4–2 continued)

(death continued)	peaceful, composed, and calm the mind is at death, the greater the chance for a better rebirth. Family as well as monks recite prayers for the dying person and also read sacred text. After consciousness has left the body and death has occurred, Buddhists believe that the consciousness enters a *bardo* or intermediary spirit body, which is the precursor to the next life. The consciousness may remain in the bardo for a very brief time or up to forty-nine days before a new life is born. Immediately after death, Buddhists believe it is best to keep the body in a peaceful state. Traditionally, the body is taken to the home for a period of three days. The body is not touched and prayers are said. This enables the consciousness to let go of its current body and life, and all its attachments, and more easily move onto the next life. Bereavement takes place at the time of death and for at least the first forty-nine days. During this time, prayers are said for the person to achieve a good rebirth. Buddhists believe it is good to continue living as long as possible, and to die in a natural and peaceful way is preferred. However, the use of life support machines are not believed to be helpful if the person's mind is no longer alert and the person is experiencing severe pain. Under these circumstances the Buddhist might decide to withhold extraordinary life-support measures. Generally a Buddhist death is followed by a three-day period during which the body is not disturbed.

Taoism

Taoism (usually pronounced "Dowism") is intertwined throughout Chinese life and culture and is practiced by approximately 20 million people, primarily in Taiwan (Religious Tolerance 2008). Tao means "the way" and refers both to a way of living in harmony with the universe as well as the Overall Governing Presence (or Power or Principle) that is manifested in the universe. To live according to Tao means that individuals avoid ambition, striving, self-seeking, or any other behavior that disrupts the natural harmony. The religious tradition of Taoism is traced to the writings of Lao-Tse who, as legend has it, lived in the first half of the sixth century BCE. Taoism grew out of his efforts to find a way to stop the constant feudal warfare and conflict of his day. Taoism draws from earlier Chinese tradition and also incorporates aspects of Buddhism. The goals of Taoism include:

Each believer is to work toward being in harmony with the Tao.

Taoists seek answers to life's problems through meditation; they do not pray to a "God" because they don't believe in a "God" who hears their prayers or acts on their behalf.

Taoists believe in reincarnation and that time is cyclical.

Each person is to develop the virtues of compassion, moderation, and humility.

Taoists believe it is important to let nature take its course and not to impede the natural flow of life (Religious Tolerance 2008, Monk et al. 2003).

Once again, as with Hinduism and Buddhism, the way Taoism is actually practiced by Taoist laypeople may be very different from the Taoist philosophy described above and taught by Taoist educators and monks. Many different religious and folk beliefs may be mixed together with the philosophy of Taoism, resulting in a unique and individual expression.

Let's examine Taoist health beliefs and practices that may impact on health care (see Table 4–3).

Table 4–3   Taoist Beliefs and Practices Affecting Health Care

Diet	An equilibrium must be maintained between "hot" and "cold"—whether this relates to food, herbs, or medicines. Foods are considered as either "hot" or "cold." Hot foods are generally high in protein, fat, and calories. Examples of hot foods include pork, chicken, organ meats, eggs, brown sugar, ginger, nuts, honey, onions, tea, coffee, and alcoholic beverages. Examples of cold foods include cereals, rice, wheat, potatoes, chickpeas, cold drinks, fruits, white sugar, milk, most vegetables, and soy products. Rice is a staple, which is eaten with a variety of meat, fish, and vegetable dishes (Chan et al. 2000, Liu & Moore 2000).
Health beliefs	Illness is caused by a blockage of chi (life energy), and is treated with acupuncture and the use of compounds such as herbal preparations. Heavy metals are also sometimes used and can lead to toxicity—most commonly lead and mercury poisoning (Ernst & Coon 2002).
Pregnancy and childbirth	Prenatal care is valued by Chinese women. They prefer female health care providers to males. Traditional Chinese medicine remedies may be used for nausea, fatigue, edema, and other conditions of pregnancy. Postpartum, many women practice *zuo yuezi* (sitting in for the first month) for thirty days. This includes not only staying in the house, but avoiding cold foods, drinks, wind, water, and any other cold substance or contact; a diet based on balance of yin (cold) and yang (hot) foods; abstinence from physical work as well as abstinence from excessively pleasurable activities. Bathing (especially washing the hair) is limited and may include a warm bath with ginger wine or another "hot" alcoholic beverage (Cheung 1997).

(table continues)

(Table 4–3 continued)

(pregnancy and childbirth cont.)	Contraception is acceptable; however, it should not be discussed in front of other family members or friends.
Death	End-of-life care centers around family and communications. Symptom management may be complicated by family and patient reluctance to voice complaints. Barriers to management of pain and other symptoms by patients and family members may be related to lack of knowledge about pain management, fatalism, fear of addiction, desire to be a good patient, and a fear of distracting the physician from treating the disease (Lin 2000, Tang 2001).
	Reluctance to discuss prognosis, and in some instances diagnosis. It is the norm for families to withhold information from the patient, to lie to the patient, or for the patient to pretend not to know what is really happening. Family is expected to prepare the body for burial. Traditionally, there is always an older relative or someone from the temple to instruct the oldest son or daughter on what to do regarding the washing and dressing of the body. Burial is preferred by most (Kagawa-Singer & Blackwell 2001).
Blood transfusions or organ transplantation	Generally no objection.

Chinese System of Medicine

Traditional Chinese medicine (TCM) is a complete medical system and is one that has been used by one-fourth of the world's population for the past three thousand years or more. TCM is a system that arose out of a particular philosophy and worldview. In this instance, the most relevant philosophy is Taoism. For the Taoist, health is a manifestation of the harmony in the universe, obtained through the proper balancing of internal and external forces. Underlying all phenomena and animating all life is a vital energy referred to as chi (pronounced "chee"). This is very similar to the Hindu concept of prana.

Chi is believed to be the foundation of life, birth, and change. Everything that exists in heaven and earth is enlivened by chi. Thus, chi in the periphery envelops heaven and earth; chi in the interior activates them. Chi is considered the source from which the sun, moon, and stars derive their light and thunder, rain, wind, and clouds derive their existence. Chi is responsible for the change in seasons, for all that we see, hear, feel, and sense in all other ways.

The chi manifests itself through the dual polar forces of yin and yang, defined as opposing energies, such as earth and heaven, winter and summer, and happiness and sadness. When yin and yang are in balance, individuals feel relaxed and energized; when they are out of balance, poor health results. The universal flow of yin and yang is reflected in the human body. Broadly speaking, the inside of the body is yin, while the surface is yang. The chest and the abdomen are yin, while the back is yang. All solid organs—such as the liver, heart, spleen, lungs, and kidneys—are yin, while the hollow organs, such as the gallbladder, small intestine, stomach, large intestine, and bladder, are yang.

In addition, Chinese medical philosophers have devised a five-element theory that is a more tangible expression of yin and yang. The five primordial elements are wood, fire, earth, metal, and water. All substances, including the organs of the body, are classified according to this scheme. For instance, the spleen and stomach are of the realm of earth, while the lungs and large intestines belong to metal. These categories are not static, but are cyclically and dynamically related. For example, fire animates earth, earth produces metal, metal enriches water, water produces wood, and wood gives rise to fire. The relationships can be both nurturing and destructive, indicating further the delicacy of interaction between yin and yang and the need for maintaining a balance between them. It is also important to note that in TCM, reference made to an organ does not carry the same meaning as in Western medicine. According to TCM, there are five organ systems—the kidney, heart, spleen, liver, and lungs. Despite their specific names, these five systems refer not to individual body parts but to complex networks. For instance, the kidney represents the entire urinary system, along with the adrenals. The heart represents both the heart and the brain (Traditional Chinese Medicine 2002).

In general, Chinese medicine addresses the mechanics of energy within the body. It employs a structural model of twelve pathways of chi, or meridians, and their branches. Illness is related to the blockage of energy along one or more of the meridians. However, through certain points on the body surface, one may gain access to internal organs and interior flows of energy. Today, there are as many as 722 points known, with about 40 to 50 in common use. Acupuncture, one of the procedures employed in TCM, uses needles to manipulate, disperse, or reactivate energy flow (Chow 1984, Traditional Chinese Medicine 2002).

Another technique employed by TCM is the less well-known procedure of moxibustion. Moxi, which derives from Artemesia vulgaris of the chrysanthemum family, is burned so as to produce heat over the energy points.

This penetrates the skin and alters the flow of chi. TCM also relies on the techniques of acupressure, the use of herbal medicines, nutrition, Chinese massage called tui na, and exercise such as tai chi and qi gong, which combine movement with meditation.

Diagnosis is an elaborate process. Interviewing, palpation, and pulse diagnosis are supplemented by the careful observation of body build, skin coloration, breath, body odors, nails, gestures, and mood, as well as inquiry into the practical and spiritual aspirations of the patient. The voice provides information about the patient's shen, or spirit. From this assessment, the TCM practitioner obtains a total health picture of the patient—physical, mental, emotional, and spiritual—and is able to make a more accurate diagnosis of illness. The TCM practitioner attempts to diagnose whether there is a blockage of chi affecting one or more of the patient's organ networks.

Another difference between the Chinese and the conventional allopathic approach to diagnosis is pulse diagnosis. Within the Chinese system, this is a real art, requiring years of practice and attention to corresponding symptoms. Six pulses are felt on each wrist, using both a light and a firmer touch. There are a number of pulse qualities, such as fast, slow, vast, weak, slippery, astringent, stretched, or tardy. Pulse reading in Western medicine is a quick measure of cardiovascular function, but pulse diagnosis in Chinese medicine can take up to one or two hours and can indicate to the TCM practitioner not just the patient's current state of health but also the past health history as well as the future health outlook.

TCM claims to be helpful in treating chronic conditions such as obesity, diabetes, complications of diabetes, high cholesterol, infertility problems, irritable bowel syndrome, and recurrent cystitis. There are other conditions where TCM may prove beneficial as well, including allergies, addictions, chronic pain, menopausal symptoms, arthritis, stress, sleep disorders, and constipation (Traditional Chinese Medicine 2002).

Summary

Every nurse should be sensitive to the patient's cultural background, religious beliefs and practices, and value system, and create an accepting atmosphere in which the patient feels free to express various concerns, from dietary needs to misgivings about the Western health care system. Ignorance and lack of exposure on both sides can be overcome to some extent by the nurse's willingness to ask, to listen, and to explain. Every patient understands the universal language of caring, openness, and warmth and of a respect for humanity that goes beyond color and creed. These are the best foundations for effective interpersonal communication and for the ability to provide spiritual care.

Reflective Activities

1. Reflect on what you believe are similarities between Western and Eastern spirituality.
2. Are there areas in Western and Eastern spiritual thought where there are irreconcilable differences? If so, what are they?
3. Reflect on the differences between a theistic and a pantheistic worldview. How would you bridge these differences in attempting to meet the spiritual needs of a patient and/or family who had a different worldview than your own?
4. How would you support the family of a dying Buddhist patient as they prepare for their loved one's death?
5. You are taking care of a patient who is diagnosed with cancer. His doctor recommends aggressive chemotherapy but the patient decides to forego all allopathic interventions and to rely solely on TCM. How would you support this patient?

References

Andrews, M. M., & Boyle, J. S. (2007). *Transcultural Concepts in Nursing Care*, 355–407. Philadelphia: Lippincott Williams & Wilkins.

Beverslius, J. (2000). *Sourcebook of the World's Religions*, 11–17 and 50–59. Novato, Calif.: New World Library.

Buddhist Beliefs and Practices Affecting Health Care. (2006). http://www.healthsystem .virginia.edu/internet/chaplaincy/Buddhism.cfm; accessed September 1, 2006.

Chan, S. M., Nelson, E. A. S., Leung, S. S. F., Cheung, P. C. K., & Li, C. Y. (2000). Special postpartum dietary practices of Hong Kong Chinese women. *European Journal of Clinical Nutrition* 54, no. 10: 797–802.

Chernin, D., & Manteuffel, G. (1984). *Health: A Wholistic Approach*. Diamond Bar, Calif.: Quest.

Cheung, N. F. (1997). Chinese zuo yeuzi (sitting in for the first month of the postnatal period) in Scotland. *Midwifery* 13, no. 2: 55–65.

Chow, E. P. Y. (1984). Traditional Chinese medicine: A wholistic system. In Salmon JW (ed.): *Alternative Medicines*. New York: Tavistock.

Cody, E. (2007). Poll Finds Surge of Religions among Chinese. *Washington Post* (February 8), A-15.

Ernst, E., & Coon, J. T. (2002). Heavy metals in traditional Chinese medicines: A systematic review. *Clinical Pharmacology & Therapeutics* 70, no. 6: 497–504.

Fenton, J. Y. (1988). *Transplanting Religious Traditions: Asian Indians in America*. New York: Praeger Publishers.

Freed, R. S., & Freed, S. A. (1991). Ghost illness of children in North India. *Medical Anthropology* 12: 401–17.

Handbook on cultural, spiritual, and religions beliefs. (2000). http://www.schl.nhs.uk/documents/cultural.html; accessed October 2, 2006.

Jambunathan, J. (2006). *Hindu-Americans*. http://www-unix.oit.umass.edu/~efhayes/hindu.htm; accessed September 6, 2006.

Kagawa-Singer, M., & Blackwell, L. J. (2001). Negotiating cross-cultural issues at the end of life. *Journal of the American Medical Association* 286, no. 23: 2993–3002.

Keown, D. (2003). *A Dictionary of Buddhism*. New York: Oxford University Press.

Lin, C. C. (2000). Barriers to the analgesic management of cancer pain: A comparison of attitudes of Taiwanese patients and family caregivers. *Pain* 88, no. 1: 7–14.

Liu, H. G., & Moore, J. F. (2000). Perinatal care: Cultural and technical differences between China and the United States. *Journal of Transcultural Nursing* 11, no. 1: 47–54.

Monk, R. C., et al. (2003). *Exploring Religious Meaning*, 6th ed., 21–25. Upper Saddle River, N.J.: Prentice Hall.

Nuernberger, P. (1981). *Freedom from Stress: A Wholistic Approach*. Honesdale, Pa.: Himalayan International Institute of Yoga Science and Philosophy.

Religious Tolerance. (2008). http://www.religioustolerance.org/taoism.htm; accessed March 30, 2008.

Tang, S. T. (2001). Taiwan. In B. R. Ferrell & N. Coyle (eds.), *Textbook of Palliative Nursing*, 747–56. New York: Oxford University Press.

Tigunait, R. (1983). *Seven Systems of Indian Philosophy*. Honesdale, Pa.: Himalayan International Institute of Yoga Science and Philosophy.

Toropov, B., & Buckles, Father Luke. (2004). *The Complete Idiot's Guide to World Religion*, 3rd ed., 165–93. New York: Beach Brook Productions.

Traditional Chinese Medicine (2002). http://www.umm.edu/altmed/ConsModalities/TraditionalChineseMedicinecm.html; accessed September 29, 2006.

Turrell, S. (1985). Asians' expectations: Customs surrounding pregnancy and childbirth. *Nursing Times* 81, no. 18: 44–49.

United Religions Initiative (2002). Buddhism: Basic Beliefs. http://www.uri.org/kids/world_budd_basi.htm; accessed September 6, 2006.

Vatuk, S. (1996). The art of dying in Hindu India. In H. M. Spiro, M. G. McCrea Curnen, & L. P. Wandel (eds.), *Facing Death*, 121–28. New Haven, Conn.: Yale University Press.

Willis, J. (2004). *The Religion Book*, 264–74. Detroit: Visible Ink Press.

Wintz, S., & Cooper, E. (2003). *Cultural and Spiritual Sensitivity*. http://wwwprofessional-chaplains.org/index.aspx?id=207; accessed February 10, 2007.

5

THE LEGAL ISSUES

RELIGION VERSUS HEALTH CARE

PATRICIA C. MCMULLEN AND
NAYNA D. C. PHILIPSEN

> *The First Amendment embraces two concepts—freedom to believe and freedom to act. The first is absolute but, in the nature of things, the second cannot be. Conduct remains subject to regulation for protection of society.*
> —Cantwell v. Connecticut[1]

The U.S. Constitution guarantees justice, liberty, and happiness, and protects religious freedom in a number of amendments. The First Amendment to the U.S. Constitution protects religion and the practice of religion in the Establishment Clause and in the Exercise Clause. The Fifth Amendment guarantees that "The right of the people to be secure in their persons ... shall not be violated." The Fourteenth Amendment guarantees liberty, due process, and equal protection. Religious belief may conflict with health care when individuals of goodwill (often a caregiver and patient) disagree, and when the conduct of the individual must be regulated to protect the welfare of society.

Selected Cases

Situation 1

An elderly Jehovah's Witness, unable to make decisions for himself, was admitted to the hospital with multiple organ dysfunction. The physician recommended a blood transfusion. His family refused for religious reasons. Later that night another physician, unaware of the refusal, ordered a transfusion. The next morning the nurse discovered the error.

Should the family be told about the error?

What should the caregiver do if a representative from the patient's church asks if he had a blood transfusion?

If the patient had been lucid and competent upon admission, had signed a consent form for the transfusion, and after he was scheduled for surgery his family refused to allow him to receive the transfusion for religious reasons, should he receive the transfusion?

Situation 2

A thirty-two-year-old Jehovah's Witness, the single mother of two young children, was admitted to the Emergency Department with internal bleeding after a car accident. The physician ordered an immediate blood transfusion and surgery, stating that with it she would most likely recover, but without it she would likely die. The patient, who was conscious and lucid, refused the transfusion on religious grounds.

Should her health care providers honor her request not to transfuse her, if they believe that she will die without the transfusion?

Should her health care providers perform the indicated surgery if it requires a blood transfusion?

What if the patient were correct, and receiving blood would result in her exile from heaven?

What should her health care professionals do if this patient's mother comes to the Emergency Department and demands that the transfusion be administered?

If the patient dies, but would have lived with the transfusion, may the negligent driver of the other car face manslaughter charges for her death?

Situation 3

A twenty-four-year-old woman is in her ninth month of pregnancy when her obstetrician determines that a stress test was abnormal, and that her baby should be delivered surgically by cesarean section as soon as possible to save its life. The woman states that, according to her religious belief, birth is normal, and she insists on waiting for labor to begin on its own and giving birth to her baby at home.

Should the state intervene to save the life of the fetus?

If her baby dies, is this woman guilty of child abuse, or of murder?

If she asks a certified nurse-midwife to assist her with a home birth, what should the midwife do?

Situation 4

Mr. and Mrs. Smock want to enroll their five-year-old son, Paul, in kindergarten. The school nurse advises them that Paul must receive all his immunizations before he can enroll in school. The parents tell her that immunizations are contrary to their religious beliefs, and that they cannot permit Paul to be immunized.

What should the school nurse do?

Can the state provide an exemption from the immunization requirement for religious refusals?

Must the state provide an exemption for religious refusal?

Does it make any difference if the Smocks have never taken Paul to a health care provider?

Does it matter if the Smocks have never taken Paul to church, and have no church affiliation?

Does it make any difference if there is an outbreak of rubella in the community?

Situation 5

A young woman enters a pharmacy with a prescription for four birth control pills, which the pharmacist recognizes as the "morning after" pill. He does not believe in abortion, and refuses to fill the prescription based on his religious belief that it is evil.

Should the state intervene and force him to fill the prescription?

Does it matter if the young woman is twenty-one years old?

Does it matter if she is married?

Does it matter if she is a rape victim?

Does it matter if the pharmacist refers her to another pharmacy that will fill her prescription?

Does it matter if the pharmacist refuses to transfer the prescription to another pharmacist?

These and similar situations may present spiritual dilemmas for individuals, their families, their health care providers, and their community. People who face a conflict between their religious beliefs and a medical option often experience spiritual distress. They may also feel stress from the conflict between their religious convictions and other strongly held values, such as liberty or beneficence.

Overview

Fortunately, in the vast majority of situations, an individual's religious beliefs, spirituality, and health care treatments present no conflicts—legal or otherwise. On the contrary, the best outcomes in health care result from "treating the whole patient," which means that the caregiver addresses the biological, psychological, sociological, and spiritual aspects of a patient, rather than just making a "diagnosis" or viewing the patient in terms of his "chief complaint." "Treating the whole patient" is consistent with what providers call "good bedside manner," which also correlates with decreased legal conflict.

Conflict between religious beliefs and health care arise in limited circumstances. First, the religious belief must lead to a religious-based act. Second, that act must be a health care choice on which an individual and the health care provider do not agree. The most common scenario is one in which the individual's treatment choice is different from the recommendation of a provider. No medical facility or caregiver has ever challenged a patient for agreeing with her doctor! These disagreements typically consist of a patient refusing care for religious reasons. Less frequently, conflicts occur because a caregiver refuses to provide particular services for religious reasons.

Conflict between religious-based decisions and health care practices increased in the late twentieth and the early twenty-first centuries. The rapid growth of technology led to the "medicalization" of life, and to practices that were inconceivable to our forebearers. The list of examples is long: antibiotics, routine lab tests, HIV testing, sonograms, magnetic resonance imaging (MRI), cardiopulmonary resuscitation (CPR), skin grafts, hip replacements, cosmetic surgery, early detection of pregnancy (at home), relatively safe and even optional cesarean delivery, birth control pills, artificial insemination, in vitro fertilization, genetic material donation, surrogate parenthood, safe termination of pregnancy, "medical management" of menopause, anesthesia/induced sedation and pain management, intravenous hydration, artificial feeding, artificial/assisted respiration, kidney dialysis, fetal diagnosis and therapy, immunizations, transfusion of blood or blood components, organ and bone marrow donation/transplants, genetic screening, genetic manipulation, cryopreservation of oocytes/spermatozoa and embryos, intravenous immunoglobulin therapy, the diagnosis and treatment of erectile dysfunction, the identification and treatment of many mental illnesses, most of our pharmaceutical products, and many, many others. Providers in each specialty could make a list of technological innovations to their practice area that exceeds the length of this one.

Cultural, ethical, and religious adaptation and assimilation have been slower than the evolution of technology in the health care environment. This has been dubbed "cultural lag". These changes present complex issues for our society, requiring a fresh application of religious principles. These applications involve not only responses from organized religion, but also responses from health care providers' professional organizations, legislators, and the courts. Questions of medical necessity and emergency, patient self-determination and autonomy, medical competency, substituted judgment, beneficence, paternalism, compelling state interests and the state's *parens patrie* (father of the people) interest, individual freedom, privacy rights, and fetal rights complicate decision making, sparking conflict between religion and health care.

Caregiver Refusals

A caregiver may refuse to provide requested or standard care when it conflicts with the provider's religious convictions. These conflicts have occasionally led to litigation. The scarcity of legal cases in this area may be partly a result of the imbalance of power and resources between care providers and care recipients. The most recent denials of care by providers leading to legal conflict have involved reproductive issues: pharmacists presenting religious-based objections to distributing birth control, or nurses and doctors refusing to participate in reproductive procedures for religious-based reasons. In these cases the courts must balance the rights of the caregiver with the rights of the individual and the welfare of society.

Courts have held that under some circumstances caregivers may be entitled to refuse to provide essential care to a patient on religious grounds without being guilty of patient abandonment, especially if they provide an appropriate referral to a provider who will honor that patient's wishes.[2] On a somewhat related issue, no constitutional provision guarantees an individual the right to demand special care based on religion, including payor reimbursement for an alternative therapy that is not provided to others. The law protects individuals from the imposition of unwanted care that may violate their autonomy, but does not guarantee special privileges based on religious beliefs.[3] Conflict also arises when caregivers impose non-health-related prerequisites for health care that conflict with religious beliefs. Recent examples of this include banning a particular head dressing (dreadlocks and yarmulkes) that the patients viewed as a religious practice and requiring a patient to wear an ID bracelet that he viewed as forbidden jewelry.[4] Courts have held that if the rule has a health benefit, and interference with religion was not the intent of the rule, it can be enforced.

Patient Refusals

Most policy statements, legislation, and court cases addressing conflict between religious belief and health care are in response to situations that involve refusal of a provider's recommended treatment. Typically the recommendation meets the appropriate treatment standard for prevention or cure. The problem arises when the standard is applied to an individual. No provider can tell whether, from that person's perspective, the standard is actually the best treatment in that particular case. That decision is always informed by the individual's spiritual resources, religious convictions, and values.

History and Legal Status of Religion-based Refusal of Care

Beneficence and Paternalism

Beneficence and paternalism took precedence in health care in the United States for many years. *Beneficence* meant the obligation of the health care provider to do what was "best for the patient," and was typically determined by the provider. *Paternalism* meant that the provider, usually the physician, had exclusive control of the health care decisions for patients, and did not even need to inform patients about their diagnoses or treatment options. In practice, this meant that providers often did not tell terminally ill patients that they were dying, or tell the mothers of infants born with severe malformations that their child was alive in the nursery next door, much less what treatment the baby was (or was not) receiving. Patients who disagreed with the treatment choice of a caregiver were not recognized as valid decision makers and were labeled as "noncompliant." To put on a hospital gown was to surrender the fundamental freedom of control over one's own body and life. Individuals continued to draw on their spiritual resources, but were often denied the opportunity to apply their religious convictions to the medical decision-making process. Under paternalism, it was more likely that the care was consistent with the religious convictions of the caregiver than those of the individual receiving the care. In a homogenous society, the religious convictions of patient and caregiver are often the same. With increasing diversity in our society, however, there is also wide diversity in religious convictions, and an increased likelihood of tension between patient and caregiver values.

The Establishment Clause

There are two portions of the U.S. Constitution that protect religion and the practice of religion. These two clauses are known as the "Establishment Clause" and the "Exercise Clause." In fact, the First Amendment's

Establishment Clause requires that all religious beliefs be treated equally. Therefore, courts have held that "organized religion" exemptions are unconstitutional. Religious freedom is an individual right, independent of belonging to an organized religion. However, membership and participation in religious activities are evidence that enhances the credibility of the individual's claim that his choices are religious-based.[5] A common example involves mandatory immunizations. States may create exceptions to the immunization requirement, but if the state allows religious-based refusals, it must allow individuals to claim religious-based objections to immunizations regardless of their membership in an organized religion.

Some religions have applied principles in ways that have led to more conflicts with medical technology than others. Jehovah's Witnesses elders announce policies about blood transfusions and blood products to members through their publication, *The Watchtower*. The U.S. Conference of Catholic Bishops in Washington, D.C., publishes the Ethical and Religious Directives for Catholic Health Care Services from its Committee on Doctrine.[6] Both of these organized religions have had high-profile objections to certain new health technologies as they work to apply a body of moral principles to medical matters. Jehovah's Witnesses have been the most vocal in opposing all blood transfusions, but have recently carved out exceptions for some blood-derivative products. The Catholic bishops have opposed artificial insemination and other artificial conception technologies, the morning-after pill/contraception (except in the case of rape), abortion at any point in pregnancy, and euthanasia (but not pain management that may incidentally shorten life). They have supported organ transplantation and treatment that takes into account the "well-being of the whole person."[7]

Self-Determination

Congress passed the Patient Self-Determination Act (PSDA) in 1991, thereby legislating, on a national level, that patients are the medical decision makers in their own care. Although alarming to some caregivers and institutions, the PSDA reflected public pressure for individual liberty and justice in health care, and the rising concern in society about the protection of individuals from the unchecked abuses of the imbalance of power inherent in the caregiver-patient relationship. It also opened the doors for individuals to receive health care consistent with their own religious values.[7]

Professional Ethics, Autonomy, and Justice

The PSDA appeared to turn medical ethics upside down. What had been "First, do no harm; second, do all the good you can" became "First, do what the patient wants; second, do no harm."

In fact, changes in the American Medical Association (AMA) Code of Ethics had already acknowledged the limits of beneficence, as well as the growing respect for patient autonomy (self-determination) and for justice (unbiased care) in health care. In 1847, Article II, section 6 of the 1847 AMA Code stated, "The obedience of a patient to the prescriptions of his physician should be prompt and implicit. He should never permit his own crude opinions as to their fitness, to influence his attention to them." By 1990, the AMA's Opinion of the Fundamental Elements of the Patient-Physician Relationship stated, "The patient has the right to make decisions regarding the health care that is recommended by his or her physician. Accordingly, patients may accept or refuse any recommended medical treatment."[8] In the Preamble adopted by the AMA House of Delegates on June 17, 2001, the first principle of medical ethics is "A physician shall be dedicated to providing competent medical care, with compassion and respect for human dignity and rights." Medical and nursing students in the twenty-first century learn to value patient autonomy, and to practice "patient-centered" care.

Institutional Policies and Informed Consent

In response to changes in the positions of professional associations, legislation, and a growing body of case law, institutions changed policies and procedures to specify the patient as the decision maker. These procedures guide providers in implementing the requirements of self-determination and provide that individuals give *informed consent* before treatment.

The legal basis for informed consent includes the First Amendment's Free Exercise Clause; the Fourteenth Amendment's right to privacy and self-determination and liberty interests; federal legislation, such as the PSDA; state legislation, including state professional practice acts (e.g., the Medical Practice Act and the Nurse Practice Act); regulation; policy; and federal and state common law (that is, case law). Courts in all states have made statements strongly supporting informed consent in a variety of cases, for example: "Basic to the informed consent doctrine is that a physician has a legal, ethical and moral duty to respect patient autonomy."[9]

Informed consent means that individuals are fully informed of their health status; of their treatment, testing, and procedure options; and of the consequences of these treatment options and of doing nothing. They are informed of any anticipated discomfort likely as a result of particular treatment options—or doing nothing. And they have the final choice as to whether to refuse or accept care. This includes the freedom to make decisions based on spiritual considerations. Issues have arisen around how much information is "usually significant" for a provider to disclose to qualify as informed consent and to allow for the patient's informed refusal of care.

Some clients have objected to the characterization of their medical choices as "refusals." According to Black's Law Dictionary (5th ed.), refusal is "The act of one who has, by law, a right and power . . . and declines it. Also, the declination of a right, or of a request or demand, or the omission to comply with some requirement of law, as the result of a positive intention to disobey . . . A rejection, a denial of what is asked." To many, refusal sounds more like a disguised echo of paternalism than like the promotion of patient autonomy. Some patients feel that providers continue to lack respect for their decisions. In their fight to promote the right to make their own health care decisions, they have formed patient advocacy groups, used civil and criminal law to enforce informed consent, and urged individuals to file complaints against caregivers with their licensure boards. Patient advocacy groups frequently arise as a consequence of issues with high religious controversy, such as euthanasia, abortion, and care options for pregnant women.

Competency and Substituted Judgment

What if an individual is not *medically competent*, that is, lacks the capacity to understand the information she needs to make a medical decision? Examples of individuals who are not medically competent include patients who are not conscious, those who have a serious mental handicap, and infants or children. In cases involving adults, the providers must determine whether the person made a decision while competent, using such tools as a Living Will or Durable Power of Attorney for Health Care, or by consulting with the next-of-kin. A person of strong religious beliefs should have a written and signed document stating related preferences and identifying the person who will make or support those choices on her behalf. If there is none, a court may have to determine who would best "stand in the shoes" of the individual to make medical decisions for her using *substituted judgment*.[10] In some cases involving Jehovah's Witnesses, representatives from the church have appeared in the clinical setting and begun to act in the role of decision maker.

In the case of younger individuals, a competent parent is the presumed decision maker. What if a parent makes a religious-based decision that appears to put the child at risk? Providers must then challenge the validity of this "legal presumption" and a court might override it. The law requires the surrogate decision maker to demonstrate beneficence. Nothing in the law requires the child to accept the religion of his parent(s) and, thus, decisions that arise from their religious beliefs.[11]

A pregnant woman is the decision maker for herself and therefore, indirectly, for her fetus. Fetal rights refer to the rights, if any, of a fetus or infant before it is born. What fetal rights exist, and when any such rights begin, is not clear, because before birth the fetus is completely dependent on the body of its mother. However, any fetal right may conflict with the rights of a woman, since any diagnosis or treatment of a fetus requires access to the mother's body. This raises issues of justice, because it is a violation of autonomy that only women would be required to suffer. In addition, individuals are not required to surrender bodily autonomy for other, more compelling treatment purposes, such as tissue donation to their own dying child, who is fully vested with all the rights of an individual, and clearly entitled to all parental duties of care. Issues surrounding possible duties and the appropriate application of moral principles to a fetus clearly challenge both organized religion and individuals of goodwill.[12]

Public Health "Police Powers"

The power to take action to enforce the public health is a police power. The Tenth Amendment generally reserves these powers to the state. Public health requirements, such as childhood immunizations, are therefore the responsibility of each state. Federal authority for public health is the exception. The exception includes international importation of disease, interstate spread of disease, certain Native American lands, and federal facilities and institutions (prisons, hospitals, the military). The federal government has authority to isolate and quarantine, concurrent with the state's authority. Federally quarantinable diseases are listed in Executive Order 13295 and include cholera, diphtheria, plague, tuberculosis, smallpox, yellow fever, and hemorrhagic fever. New diseases that pose similar threats (recent examples are SARS and avian flu) are added as they are identified. The federal government last used involuntary quarantine in 1963 in connection with a smallpox case. However, the U.S. Centers for Disease Control and Prevention (CDC) routinely use the Public Health Service Act to monitor and detain individuals at the U.S. borders. Actions such as quarantine and isolation make it clear that a public health interest can limit such fundamental and protected rights as an individual's freedom to move about at will and the freedom of religious expression.

Selected Cases

Return now to the situations at the beginning of this chapter. Reread them and use the above concepts as you draft your responses. Then compare your responses and reasoning to actual outcomes and the reasoning of the courts and to the discussion questions below.

Situation 1

Outcome: A nurse discovered blood infusing into an elderly Jehovah's Witness patient whose family had denied transfusion. She examined the chart and determined that it had been ordered overnight by a physician unaware of the refusal on the patient's behalf by his family. She notified the charge nurse, and hospital counsel advised that the blood transfusion must be discontinued immediately. The patient died soon after that. Staff argued about whether to tell the family about the blood error. No provider would tell the family about the error, and they were not told. The rationale given by caregivers was that it would distress the family, with no benefit. Caregivers assumed that the patient's religious belief—that receiving the transfusion would bar him from entry into heaven—was wrong. A caregiver on staff was very disturbed by the incident, and reported it to an outside party—the press![13]

Q1: Should the family be told about the error?

A: Providers should tell the next-of-kin, who represents the patient for health care purposes, about the error.

Q2: What should the caregiver do if a representative from the patient's church asks if he had a blood transfusion?

A: In some cases like this, church representatives had access to the patient's medical records, and the parties in court did not raise this fact as an issue, so the court did not address it. This would be a breach of patient confidentiality, unless the patient had requested that church representatives be told about the transfusion.

Q3: What if the patient himself had signed a consent form for blood transfusion upon admission?

A: In that case, the caregivers could give the blood. Substituted judgment by family members is only valid when the patient has no opportunity to make his own decision for his care. Each person has legal autonomy not just for medical decisions, but also in how to apply the teachings of his religion to his life decisions.

Situation 2

Outcome: When this patient refused the transfusion, the charge nurse and physician determined to notify hospital counsel immediately. The rationale was that she was the sole guardian for her two young children. Hospital counsel brought the case to court, and the court authorized the blood transfusion. The patient received the transfusion, and survived the accident.

Q1: Should her health care providers honor her request not to transfuse her, if they believe that she will die without it?

A: In general, care providers should honor the choice of the patient, even if she will die without the recommended care. In this case, however, the state had an interest in protecting the children from becoming orphans and wards of the state. That interest can outweigh the patient's interest in a religious practice. Providers should always refer a scenario like this one to hospital counsel.

Q2: Should her health care providers perform the indicated surgery if it requires a blood transfusion?

A: Providers should discuss the risk of the indicated surgery without blood with the patient, and they should make a determination together about the balance of risks and benefits of the procedure without blood. However, if the welfare of dependent children depends on the outcome, see Q1 above.

Q3: What if the patient were correct, and receiving blood would result in her exile from heaven?

A: If health care providers took action based on this kind of belief, rather than their own scientific knowledge, which other religious beliefs would be considered acceptable grounds for medical decisions?

Q4: What should her health care professionals do if this patient's mother comes to the Emergency Department and demands that the transfusion be administered?

A: If the patient's mother comes to the Emergency Department demanding that blood be transfused into her daughter, the mother can be advised to contact private counsel immediately. In general, the mother may be the next-of-kin for making a substitute judgment, but here the patient is a competent adult, and has clearly expressed her own wishes. Therefore, while her mother may try to change her decision, the patient's decision takes precedence over her parent's wishes.[14]

Q5: If the patient dies, but would have lived with the transfusion, may the negligent driver of the other car face manslaughter charges for her death?

A: If the client died, the negligent driver of the other car could be convicted of manslaughter. The fact that the victim was a Jehovah's Witness who refused a lifesaving blood transfusion is not a defense against manslaughter for the other driver, any more than the fact that a sick and elderly victim is more likely to die in an accident that a young and healthy person might survive constitutes a defense. People who behave negligently have to take their victims "as they find them."[15]

Situation 3

Outcome: The providers petitioned the court to order the woman to have a surgical cesarean delivery to save the life of her nine-month-old fetus. The judge granted the order. The woman escaped and went into hiding. She delivered a healthy baby at home without any further medical attention. These cases arise in the context of organized religious communities, such as the Amish, but can also arise from individual spiritual or religious convictions.[16]

Q1: Should the state intervene to save the life of the fetus?

A: Courts have been increasingly reluctant to order a pregnant woman to have a surgical delivery or to take any other steps to mandate procedures for pregnant women against their wishes. One reason is that the predictions of caregivers are frequently wrong and have been wrong in some well-publicized cases. In one such case, the court supported doctors at George Washington University Hospital and ordered a cesarean delivery for a twenty-four-year-old woman who was terminally ill and twenty-six weeks' pregnant, over the clear objections of the woman and her family. The deaths of both mother and baby were apparently hastened by the procedure. Later the ruling was overturned because it violated the mother's bodily integrity and autonomy.[17]

Q2: If her baby dies, is this woman guilty of child abuse, or of murder?

A: Some courts have held women responsible for the effect of acts (or in this case, omissions) during pregnancy that affect the child after birth. A Florida court even jailed a woman for delivery of an illegal drug to her child through the umbilical cord between birth and the clamping of the cord![18] These cases are in the minority, and not only because they violate autonomy or result in discrimination against women. Public policy and ethics suggest that a pregnant woman should consider the needs of her fetus. However, almost every pregnant woman has engaged in acts that may be harmful to the fetus. Should women be imprisoned for drinking alcohol during pregnancy? For failing to fasten their seat belt during pregnancy? For eating too much salt? For smoking? Public policy also suggests that each individual should engage in good health practices on her own behalf. For example, in many states drivers and passengers can be arrested for not fastening their seat belts. Finally, it is not in the interest of the state to engage in interventions that may worsen outcomes in the community. In Situation 3, one result of the court order was that the mother and baby received no further care. Some argue that if pregnancy resulted in loss of liberty, many more pregnant women would not seek prenatal care for fear of criminal prosecution or forced medical treatment.

Q3: If she asks a certified nurse-midwife to assist her with a home birth, what should the midwife do?

A: The nurse-midwife may provide services to this mother, following the same standards that she would follow for any mother, including careful documentation of professional recommendations and patient choices. Any information that the mother provides about her case should be treated as confidential, and be used to promote the health of the patient.

Situation 4

Outcome: The school nurse worked for a district that created an exemption for religious refusal of immunization. She asked the Smocks to fill out the standard form to request a religious exemption from immunization. However, other than the use of the word *religious* on the form, there was no indication that the Smocks had a religious basis for the exemption. In fact, little Paul had on occasion been removed from the Smocks' home because of neglect. The court ordered that Paul be removed from his parental home again, and receive medical care, including immunization.

Q1: What should the school nurse do?

A: The school nurse should gather information about the parents' claim of exemption, which she did. If the claim looks inconsistent and the nurse cannot verify the claim, the claim should be referred to the legal counsel for the school district, which this nurse also did.

Q2: Can the state provide an exemption from the immunization requirement for religious refusals?

A: Yes, a state may legislate an exemption from the immunization requirement for individuals who have a religious-based refusal. However, the exemption cannot target a particular religion, but must be available to all. The state intervened in this case because the claim of religious refusal and the actions of the claimant were inconsistent. If the parents had presented a credible claim that was consistent with overall behavior of caring for the child or of participation in other religious activities, the state would have been more likely to recognize the act as an expression of religious conviction. Even so, the state must weigh the competing interests in determining whether to create an exemption, or grant an exception to the immunization requirement.[19]

Q3: Must the state provide an exemption for religious refusal?

A: Where there is an overriding state interest, such as saving lives from communicable diseases, the state is not required to create exemptions. In spite of that, individuals can request an exception and, if their argument is strong and the state's interest relatively weak, it might be granted without the need for an exemption category.

Q4: Does it make any difference if the Smocks have never taken Paul to a health care provider?

A: If the parents have never provided medical care for their children, this is a fact that is more consistent with abuse and neglect than it is with religious conviction. Therefore, it makes a difference in determining the basis of the immunization refusal.

Q5: Does it matter if the Smocks have never taken Paul to church, and have no church affiliation?

A: Formal church affiliation may support credibility of a religious refusal, and never having taken the children to church may point up abuse and neglect in the overall analysis. However, engagement with a formal religion is not required for religious refusal.

Q6: Does it make any difference if there is an outbreak of rubella in the community?

A: An outbreak of rubella or any other serious communicable disease could create a public health emergency. In that situation, the state's need to protect the public health through immunization and possibly even quarantine would be much harder to overcome by any objector.

Situation 5

Outcome: The pharmacist in this case took the prescription and kept it. In taking the prescription, he accepted the duty of a pharmacist to this patient. The court found that the pharmacist could refuse to fill a prescription for religious reasons, if he also referred the woman to another pharmacy that could fill it. In this case, the pharmacist went further and attempted to block her access to emergency contraception based on his own convictions of evil (paternalism).

Q1: Should the state intervene and force him to fill the prescription?

A: The state weighed the interests of the professional and of the patient. It determined that the pharmacist has a right to religious refusal, but that right is limited because the patient cannot be refused care. The court balanced the two interests when it required a mechanism to ensure that another provider could meet the patient's health needs.

Q2: Does it matter if the young woman is twenty-one years old?

A: The age of the patient would not affect her rights to reproductive health care services. If this were a situation where the patient required substituted judgment, the pharmacist is not the presumed decision maker.

Q3: Does it matter if she is married?

A: The marital status of the patient is irrelevant to a determination of her rights, and is irrelevant in this scenario. If the patient were medically incompetent, the spouse might be the presumed decision maker.

Q4: Does it matter if she is a rape victim?

A: It might make a difference if this patient had been the victim of rape. If the pharmacist were Catholic, and claimed that the basis of his refusal was the teachings of his church, the fact of rape would present an inconsistency and undermine the credibility of his claim. The Catholic bishops permit the use of contraception in rape cases, because rape is not the moral way for life to be started.

Q5: Does it matter if the pharmacist refers her to another pharmacy that will fill her prescription?

A: If the pharmacist referred the patient to another pharmacy that would fill her prescription, that would meet the legal rights of all parties in most similar cases.

Q6: Does it matter if the pharmacist refuses to transfer the prescription to another pharmacist?

A: In taking the prescription and refusing to release or transfer it, the pharmacist affirmatively acted to violate the patient's access to care and her right to self-determination. This example reminds us that all rights, even those guaranteed by the Constitution, have limits. The religiously motivated acts of the pharmacist are protected until they interfere with other rights.

Recommendations for Providers

1. Inform patients of their diagnoses and all care or treatment options, including the outcomes with the option of no care or treatment.
2. Respect all patient choices, including those that seem very wrong to you as the provider, and document them in the health care records.
3. If a patient seems unable to understand his health care situation, identify the person who would exercise the right to make decisions for him.
4. Know the procedure to follow in a situation where the patient's choice or medical competency is not clear.

Summary

This chapter reviewed the constitutional guarantees and evolving law and policy that are the basis for contemporary state, client, and provider arguments in health care decision making and religious freedom. It also described key concepts and areas of significant conflict in religion and health care.

Reflective Activities

1. You are the nurse caring for a seriously ill man who refuses medical treatment for religious reasons. What measures can you institute to protect his religious rights? How can you reconcile these measures with state and hospital interests in maintaining his life?
2. Under what circumstances do you think parents should be allowed to discontinue medical treatment for their child?
3. You are the judge in a state court. By what means do you feel you should collect data to decide if a treatment should be ordered? Whose wishes should receive the highest priority? The client? The family? The hospital? State social services?
4. You are the obstetrician caring for a client who refuses treatment for religious reasons. If your client dies because of her refusal, what

effect would this have on your spirit? How would you deal with this situation?

5. Who do you think should be the primary decision maker for health care?

6. Do you think that the "right to accept or refuse" is a good way to describe the right to make your own decisions about your health care? Why or why not?

7. What are the limits of the average person's ability to give informed consent?

8. How much information about her preference for a treatment choice should a care provider give to a patient? (a) None, to assure that the patient is making a choice that is free from undue influence? (b) State a preference, but only when asked by the patient? (c) State a preference with your rationale, and try to get the patient to do what is best?

9. What do you think about the right of care providers to refuse to provide standard care, based on their own religious convictions? Recall the case of the pharmacist who refused to fill a prescription for birth control. Would his refusal have been better protected if there had been another pharmacist on duty who could have filled the prescription? Alternatively, should he have refused to accept the prescription at all, and simply advised the woman that he could not be her pharmacist? Does it matter that he was employed at a business that is a national chain, open to the public? What policies should the employer establish? How should this be communicated to clients?

10. What limits or court "tests" would you place on state and community interests, to ensure that they do not "swallow" the individual's right to make health care decisions or practice religious freedom, as medical paternalism once did?

11. Reflect on the following quotes. Do you agree? Why or why not?

• "Every human being of adult years and sound mind has a right to determine what shall be done with his own body." —*Schloendorff v. Society of New York Hosp.*, 105 N.E. 92, 93 (N.Y. 1914)

• "The judgment about which choice will best serve well-being properly belongs to the patient," and the physician must mention

all alternatives supported by "respectable medical opinion."
—*President's Commission for the Study of Ethical Problems in Medicine and Biomedical and Behavioral Research, 1982*

- "Informed consent requires a patient-based decision rather than the [paternalistic approach of the 1970s]." —*Culbertson v. Mernitz*, 602 N.E. 2d 98, 104 (Ind. 1992)

- "In some broad sense it might be said that a woman who fails to act before viability has consented to the state's intervention on behalf of the developing child." —*Planned Parenthood v. Casey*, 505 U.S. 833 (1992)

- New Jersey's "prudent patient" informed consent standard is "based primarily upon maturing concepts of patient autonomy and individual self determination." —*Schrieber v. Physicians Ins. Co. of Wis.*, 579 N.W. 730, 734 (Wis. Ct. App. 1998)

- "The Free Exercise Clause protects values distinct from those protected by the Equal Protection Clause." —*Employment Div., Ore. Dept. of Human Res. v. Smith*, 494 U.S. at 901 (1990).[20]

- "Ch. 2003-418, Laws of Fla., is unconstitutional on its face because it is an unconstitutional delegation of legislative power to the Governor and because it unjustifiably authorizes the Governor to summarily deprive Florida citizens of their constitutional right to privacy. . . . The Legislature assigned to the Governor the unfettered discretion to control the nutrition and hydration, indeed the life or death, of a limited class of Florida citizens. . . . The Court finds that the actions of the Legislature and of the Governor violated Mrs. Schiavo's right to privacy, due process, and the separation-of-powers doctrine." —*Michael Schiavo, as Guardian of the person of Theresa Marie Schiavo vs. Jeb Bush, Governor of the State of Florida, and Charlie Crist, Attorney General of the State of Florida*, Florida Circuit Court Civil Case No. 03-008212-CI-20 (2004)

- "The Board considers professional conduct to mandate that the physician makes certain that the patient is given the right to a reasonably informed participation in decisions involving his/her health care." Maryland Board of Physicians, Interpretation of Section 14-404 (A) (3) "unprofessional conduct in the practice of medicine."

Notes

1. *Cantwell v. Connecticut*, 310 U.DS 296, 303–04 (1940).

2. *Kong v. Scully*, No. 02-150 (Fed. 9th Cir., September 23, 2003). Four states permit pharmacists to refuse to fill a prescription for religious reasons, with certain conditions.

3. *Klassy v. Physicians Plus Insurance Co., et al.*, 276 Fed. supp. 2d 952 203 U.S. Dist Lexis 10956 (WI 2003); American Public Health Association (APHA). (2003). *Preservation of Reproductive Health Care in Medicaid Managed Care*. http://www.apha.org/private/2003_Proposed_Policies/12_Reproductive_Heath_Care.pdf. Accessed October 6, 2004.

4. *May v. Baldwin*, 109 F2d 301, 557 (C.A. 9 [Or.] 1997); *Jonathan Lee X v. Murray*, 976 F2d 726 (C.A. 4 [VA] 1992).

5. In the *Matter of Stratton*, 153 NC App 428, 571; SE 2d 234, Lexis 1183 (2002); *Walker v. Horn*, 385 F.3d 321 (3rd Cir., 2004).

6. For updated information, go to www.ascensionhealth.org.

7. See *Harvey v. Dr. Glen Strickland and Surgical Associates of South Carolina*, S.C. Supreme Court, July 1, 2002.

8. Council on Ethical and Judicial Affairs (CEJA), *Current Opinions* (Chicago: American Medical Association, 1990).

9. *Feeley v. Baer*, 679 NE 2d 180, 184 (MA 1997)

10. *Cruzan v. Director, Missouri Department of Health*, 497 U.S. 261, 280 (1990).

11. *Jehovah's Witnesses v. King County Hospital*, 390 U.S. 59 (1968).

12. American Academy of Pediatrics Committee on Bioethics, "Fetal therapy-ethical considerations," *Pediatrics* 103 (1999): 1061–63.

13. See Randy Cohen, "The Ethicist," *The New York Times Magazine* (June 18, 2006): http://www.nytimes.com/2006/06/18/magazine/18wwln_ethicist.1.html?_r=1&oref=.

14. See In re *Maria Isabel Duran*, 769 A.2d 497 (Pa. Super. 2001).

15. See *Klinger v. State of Florida*, 816 So2d 697; 2002 Fla. App. Lexis 4731 (2002).

16. *Jefferson v. Griffin Spalding County Hospital Authority*, 247 Ga 86, 274 SE2d 457 (1981); *Doe v. Doe*, 260 Ill. App. 3d 392, 198 Ill. Dec 267, 632 NE2d 326 (1994).

17. In re *Angela Carter*, 573 A2d 1235 (D.C. App. 1990); The American College of Obstetrics and Gynecology, "Patient choice in the maternal fetal relationship," *Ethics in Obstetrics and Gynecology* (2004): 34–37.

18. In re *Jennifer Johnson*, FL 5th Dist Ct. of Appeals (1991).

19. *McCarthy v. Ozark School Dist.*, 359 F3d 1029 (8th Cir., 2004).

20. Citing Justice O'Connor; see *Cantwell v. Connecticut*, 310 U.S. 296 (1940).

PART III

APPLICATION OF THEORY TO SPIRITUAL NEEDS

WHAT DOES SPIRITUAL CARE LOOK LIKE?

The next five chapters examine how nurses and other health care professionals actually respond to the spiritual dimensions of care. Chapter 6 discusses the process of identifying and meeting spiritual needs. Chapter 7 examines the spiritual needs of children and how to best meet those needs according to the child's or teen's developmental level. Chapter 8 spotlights the impact of spirituality in adults with chronic illness, with a special focus on mental illness and cancer. Chapter 9 addresses the importance of spirituality when aging impacts well seniors, frail elders, and their caregivers, as well as organizations and communities. Chapter 10 deals with the struggles of nurses and other health care providers as they grapple with the issue of death, as they provide care to dying patients, and as they meet the needs of grieving families.

6

SPIRITUALITY

IDENTIFYING AND MEETING SPIRITUAL NEEDS

VERNA BENNER CARSON

> Someday, after we have mastered the winds, the waves, the tides, and
> gravity, we shall harness for God the energies of love. Then, for the second
> time in the history of the world man will have discovered fire.
> —Teilhard de Chardin

If a physician sees a patient choking, the physician uses whatever measures are necessary to clear his airway and to restore breathing. If a patient
has an elevated temperature, the nurse administers the PRN order for an
antipyretic and wipes the patient's fevered brow with a cool cloth. When
a patient is recovering from a stroke and is learning to walk again and
manage the activities of daily living, the physical therapist and occupational therapist know exactly how to support the patient in her recovery.
If a patient needs support in accessing community resources, the social
worker can easily make those connections for him. However, if a patient
says that she is angry at God, feels abandoned, or cannot forgive, most
health care providers, including nurses, are tongue-tied, unsure about how
to respond. Of course, each of these situations—anger at God, a sense of
abandonment, or lack of forgiveness—is clearly the chaplain's domain.
However, patients do not always wait until the chaplain is present to raise
these issues—conversations happen when they happen—and nurses and
other health care professionals need to be able to respond with concern

and compassion. Unlike physical needs, which can be observed and quantified, spiritual needs must be inferred from patient behavior. In contrast to physical ministrations, which are often very concrete, spiritual ministry requires nurses and other health care providers to use only the tool of themselves—their compassion, their listening skills, their kindness, and all the things that make them unique and giving. This is no easy task, and it is one that health care providers avoid for a number of reasons. This chapter will first examine the reasons that the spiritual dimensions of patient care are neglected and then demonstrate how a systematic process can be effectively applied to spiritual aspects of care.

The following examples illustrate some of the ways in which patients express spiritual concerns.

Example 1

Mrs. Elliot, a thirty-two-year-old mother of three, is dying of cancer. While making rounds, the nurse finds Mrs. Elliot crying and in extreme pain. Mrs. Elliot is receiving high doses of morphine, with only slight reduction in her discomfort. Mrs. Elliot grabs the nurse's hand and cries out in anguish, "Why is God doing this to me? Why is he making me suffer so? Why is he taking me away from my children who need me so much?"

Example 2

Mr. Crone is scheduled for coronary bypass surgery in the morning. The nurse is reviewing the preoperative instructions with him when she notices that he is not paying attention to the instructions. "Mr. Crone, you seem as if you are a million miles away."

Mr. Crone replies, "You're wasting your time. I'm not going to make it tomorrow. I've brought this on myself, and I think God has had enough of me."

Example 3

Mrs. Johnson is waiting outside the operating room. She is scheduled for a cesarean section this morning. A chaplain notices that she is alone and is weeping softly. The chaplain asks what is wrong. Mrs. Johnson replies, "I want this baby so much. I'm diabetic, and I've already had two miscarriages. I'm so afraid. Will you pray for me?"

Example 4

Mrs. Santoz has been admitted because of an exacerbation of multiple sclerosis. She is confined to a bed and totally dependent on others for her basic care. A physical therapist is assisting the patient with range of motion exercises. Mrs. Santoz says angrily, "I hate this. I would rather be dead! I can't do anything for myself. I'm a total burden on my family, and they would be better off without me. My life is such a waste."

Example 5

Mr. Jackson, an avowed atheist, is recuperating from a severe myocardial infarction. He always seems angry and irritable toward whoever is caring for him. Mr. Katz, one of the evening nurses, notices that Mr. Jackson never has any visitors, although it is noted on the chart that he has a son. Mr. Katz asks Mr. Jackson about this and is told that he should mind his own business. Mr. Katz continues to interact with Mr. Jackson, and several days later he again brings up the topic of Mr. Jackson's lack of visitors. Mr. Jackson looks away and says with tears in his eyes, "I had a falling out with my son about a year ago. I miss him, but I'm not going to call him and tell him I'm in here. He'll think that I'm begging him to come back. He is going to have to contact me on his own."

Each of these examples, except the one involving the chaplain, would most likely cause discomfort and feelings of inadequacy in nurses as well as other health care providers. Let's take a look at the roots of this discomfort.

Societal Influences Regarding Spirituality

We are living in an increasingly secular society that is oriented toward the present and focused on material and tangible things. Concerns of the spirit, things that are sacred and eternal, receive far less attention in our world. Many of the resources at our disposal are used to make life easier, more fun, and less stressful. Energy is devoted to creating devices that make tasks less burdensome. Technology and technique are highly valued and in many ways have become gods to us.

Another societal influence on our perception of spirituality is the prevalence of a secular humanist philosophy, which is a distinctive worldview. Humanism is defined as a mode of action or an attitude that centers on distinctively human interests and ideals. This centering on human needs may turn us away from acknowledging a divine presence and influence in our lives (Sire 2004).

It is important to point out that humanism has had many positive effects on society. The humanist approach recognizes the worth of each individual, the importance of meeting the needs of each individual, and accepting and nurturing each human being. These ideas are also inherent in much traditional Judeo-Christian religious teaching and a theistic worldview. The critical difference between humanism and a theistic worldview is that in humanism human beings, rather than a Higher Power, are the center of the universe. Feelings, desires, and individual ambitions become the driving force, and life's meaning and purpose are derived from achievements and an awareness of our inner world. Humanists do not recognize the presence of a Higher Power nor do they ascribe to a Higher Power any influence on life's events. From a humanist perspective, all problems can be solved, all challenges overcome through the efforts of people, and that life's meaning is derived from personal achievements (Sire 2004).

Still another factor that affects our attitudes toward spirituality is the condition of the family. It is generally accepted that the family serves as a vehicle for individuals to initially experience religious concepts. The foundation for spiritual development probably has its roots in the first relationships that children develop with loving parents and siblings. This is where children receive the first images of what their particular religious faith tradition views as important. Divorce, disintegrated family units, and tremendous stress on the nuclear family make it increasingly difficult for the family to provide a solid foundation for spiritual growth.

Finally, the aura of mystery that surrounds the topic of spirituality is often felt to be too personal to explore. Many people, including nurses, believe that another's spiritual beliefs are private and are off-limits for discussion.

Impact on Nurses and Other Health Care Providers

Nurses along with other health care providers, are part of the society that they serve and are subject to the influences that shape the society as a whole. Although there is a trend in health care to provide whole person care, defined as encompassing the biological, psychological, social, and spiritual aspects of health, the area that is most likely to be ignored is the spiritual. The tendency to ignore the spiritual is related to two factors:

1. The health care provider's own spiritual development influences that provider's ability to recognize and to respond to spiritual needs in patients (see chapter 8). For instance, a patient's questioning of the existence and justice of the Divine may produce anxiety in a health care provider who has not resolved these questions for himself. Rather than deal with these uncomfortable feelings, the health care provider may find it easier to avoid discussing spiritual concerns altogether.

2. The lack of preparation in identifying and responding to religious and spiritual needs leaves health care providers feeling inadequate. Although the curriculum may include a course or two that focuses on religious and spiritual needs, the focus of health care training still remains on biopsychosocial content. The minimal preparation in the area of spiritual issues hardly qualifies the health care professional as an expert, and some health care providers have never received instruction in this area at all. Even though they may recognize its importance, they remain professionally uncomfortable in dealing with spiritual needs and therefore may ignore them (Carson & Koenig 2004).

Still another reason that nurses and other health care providers avoid discussing spirituality is that they believe that these needs fall solely within the chaplain's purview. The problem with this position is that many times patients express heartfelt spiritual needs when the chaplain is unavailable. It is inappropriate for the health care provider to delay or avoid responding to the patient's needs until a chaplain is on hand. There is no doubt that the chaplain is the spiritual expert, and fills an essential role on the health care team. Sometimes patients specifically request to speak with the hospital chaplain or a spiritual leader of their own faith. At other times patients need answers to theological questions that the health care provider is not qualified to answer. Patients may desire a specific religious service or rite. However, these situations do not preclude the health care provider's role in listening and responding with kindness and compassion to expressed spiritual needs, in addition to making a referral to the chaplain.

Application of a Systematic Process to Identify Spiritual Needs

Despite the many reasons for avoiding discussions of spirituality, meeting spiritual needs is and always has been part of the role of nurses and other health care providers (see chapter 1). Furthermore, it is not a choice, since a spiritual assessment is mandated by the Joint Commission on Accreditation of Healthcare Organizations (JCAHO) for all patients admitted to a general hospital, all psychiatric patients, patients in long-term care, hospice patients, and those receiving home care services (JCAHO 2004).

It is possible to approach spiritual needs in the same systematic manner in which health care providers approach biopsychosocial needs. Each of the disciplines within health care—medicine, nursing, social work, and the therapies—conducts a structured assessment to identify biopsychosocial needs that impact on care. Likewise, a structured approach is useful in identifying spiritual needs that may impact on care, and there are many examples of structured assessment tools that are used by chaplains, physicians, nurses, and social workers.

Chaplains generally distinguish between a comprehensive spiritual assessment (see Fitchett's 7 x 7 assessment in chapter 8), performed by a chaplain, and a required spiritual screening performed by other health care professionals. It is important to note that nursing, social work, and occupational therapy refer to the process of inquiry regarding spiritual issues as a spiritual assessment; however, this inquiry generally lacks the depth of the assessment completed by chaplains. However, before embarking on spiritual screening/assessment, there are some prerequisites. The first prerequisite is an acceptance that inquiring about spiritual issues is part of our professional responsibility. The second prerequisite is the skill of listening. A quick review of the five examples at the beginning of this chapter illustrates that, in each scenario, the patient openly identifies his or her spiritual need—the health care professional need only respond to what has been shared. Of course, not every patient will lay bare her spiritual concerns, so the third prerequisite is interviewing skills that identify and respond to less obvious spiritual cues given by the patient. A fourth prerequisite is excellent observational skills that allow the screener to pick up nonverbal behaviors indicative of stress.

Consider the following conversation between Nurse Bramer and his nursing supervisor, Nurse Smith. In this example Nurse Bramer believes he has assessed a patient's spiritual needs:

> NURSE SMITH: Were you able to gather any information about the patient's spiritual needs when you did the admission interview?
>
> NURSE BRAMER: Oh, sure. Mr. Johns is Catholic, and just recently started going to Mass again.
>
> NURSE SMITH: Does his return to church coincide with the onset of his illness?
>
> NURSE BRAMER: I don't know. I didn't think to ask about that. It seemed too personal.
>
> NURSE SMITH: Any more personal than asking about his bowel habits? I think we need more data about Mr. John's spiritual needs. With the surgery facing him, we want to help him draw on whatever support is available. I think you should call the chaplain about this patient—sounds to me as if his spiritual needs call for the expert.

It is common for health care providers to believe that they have assessed spiritual needs when, in reality, they have only inquired about a patient's religious affiliation. This information, though important, does not reveal the patient's deeper feelings about the meaning of life, love, hope, and forgiveness, which are the basis of spirituality. Nor does it determine whether membership in that faith community actually makes the patient feel like part of a caring community as opposed to being an outsider. A patient might belong to and be active in a particular religion and never have contemplated his spiritual nature. Conversely, just because a patient does not belong to a formal religion does not rule out his need for spiritual comfort nor the possibility of spiritual resources meaningful to him but not apparent to the staff. However, in many situations, such as the one cited above, the patient provides information that he recently started attending Mass again that suggests that a more comprehensive assessment is required; thus the referral to the hospital chaplain.

As illustrated in the previous vignette, the most important aspects of a spiritual assessment are a willingness on the part of the clinician (1) to really listen to what the patient is and is not saying about spirituality, and (2) to reflect on what has been said and to follow up with questions and observations to validate the patient's concerns. Signs of sadness, anger, agitation, or anxiety are behaviors that may reflect not only an emotional issue but a spiritual one as well. If the patient is hospitalized, it is also important for professional caregivers to observe whether the patient prays during the day or reads religious/inspirational material. Many of these observations are more easily made by nursing staff because they spend more time with hospitalized patients than other health care providers.

The content of a patient's verbalizations also gives the health care provider insights into the patient's feelings and needs. Review the examples at the beginning of the chapter. In each of these, the patients were virtually screaming out their spiritual needs—both through the words spoken as well as the emotions conveyed in their speech. Other areas that may hint at spiritual needs include issues such as a patient's response to pain. Does the patient seem to complain more than would be expected for the amount and type of pain being experienced? Is the patient restless and experiencing sleep difficulties? Of course, these behaviors could indicate physical needs, but they may also hint at spiritual distress as well. Does the patient refer to God in any way? Does the reference convey anger, fear, and awe, or is the reference made in a joking manner? Patients may also mention specific religious subjects, such as faith, hope, or prayer, or may discuss functions of their faith community that are a part of their lives. It is important to remember that all the factors that make health care professionals uneasy about conducting a spiritual assessment also impact on the patient's comfort in communicating spiritual needs (Carson & Koenig 2004, O'Brien 2003, Shelly 2000).

Also valuable is information about the quantity and quality of the patient's interpersonal relationships. Does the patient draw support from family and friends? Does the patient receive support from her faith community? If so, what form does that support take? How does the patient relate to health care providers? All these observations may point to whether or not the patient has a support system; whether or not there are people in her life who love her, show concern for her, and can be counted on to support her through her illness. If the patient is alone and lacks these supports, this may reflect a similar distance in relation to God. A concerned health care provider can make certain observations of a patient's environment. The presence of a Bible or other religious/inspirational reading material might indicate that the hospitalized patient is thinking about spiritual matters. Other things for the health care provider to observe would be whether the patient wears religious medals, pins, or articles of clothing. Prayer cloths are meaningful to certain religions. Whether the patient uses religious statues or other such items in observing religious rituals is also important (Carson & Koenig 2004, Shelly 2000). Table 6–1 summarizes these observations.

An adequate assessment also involves interviewing the patient to determine his specific spiritual concerns. These concerns can be ascertained through the use of the following five questions:

1. Do religious/spiritual beliefs provide comfort to you or cause you stress?
2. How might your religious/spiritual beliefs influence your health care decisions?
3. Are there any religious/spiritual beliefs you hold that might interfere or conflict with your medical treatment?
4. Are you a member of a religious/spiritual community, and, if so, is it supportive?
5. Are there any other spiritual needs that someone should address? (Koenig 2002)

It is important for clinicians to be aware that, just as spirituality may not be the easiest topic for them to explore with a patient, this is often a difficult area for the patient to discuss as well. The best approach avoids asking one question right after another, as if you're interrogating the patient;

Table 6–1   Observations to Be Made in a Spirituality Assessment

Nonverbal behavior	Observe affect. Does the patient's affect or attitude convey loneliness, depression, anger, agitation, or anxiety?
	Observe behavior. Does the patient pray during the day? Does the patient rely on religious/inspirational reading material or other literature for solace?
Verbal behavior	Does the patient seem to complain out of proportion to his illness?
	Does the patient complain of sleeping difficulties?
	Does the patient ask for unusually high doses of sedation or pain medication?
	Does the patient refer to God or a deity in any way?
	Does the patient talk about prayer, faith, hope, or anything of a religious/inspirational nature?
	Does the patient talk about a faith community that is part of her life?
	Does the patient express concern about the meaning and direction of her life? Does the patient express concern about the impact of the illness on the meaning of her life?
Interpersonal	Does the patient have visitors or does he spend visiting hours alone?
	Are the visitors supportive or do they seem to leave the patient feeling upset?
	Does the patient have visitors from his church, synagogue, mosque, or other faith community?
	Does the patient interact with the staff and other patients?
Environment	Does the patient have a Bible or other religious/inspirational reading material with her?
	Does the patient wear religious medals or pins?
	Does the patient use religious articles, such as statues, in observing religious practices?
	Has the patient received religious/inspirational get well cards?
	Does the patient use personal pictures, artwork, or music to keep his spirits up?

instead, questions are used to respond to verbal and nonverbal clues that indicate the presence of a spiritual need. The health care provider recognizes that not every patient will merit a complete spiritual assessment; however, it is important to identify the main areas of spiritual concern that will be affected by the patient's illness. In addition, the health care provider who is undertaking a spiritual assessment should approach the patient with acceptance, a gentle manner, and a sensitivity to timing and to the patient's feelings. Questions related to psychosocial and spiritual issues are generally left until the end of an interview, when the patient and the health care provider are feeling more at ease with each other. It is also helpful for health care providers to share with the patient their rationale for seeking information about spirituality. Patients should know that this information increases the health care provider's knowledge about their sources of strength and allows the health care provider to plan care more appropriately. In addition, the patient should know that this information will not be shared with anyone beyond the health care team.

Observations and an interview alone cannot form the basis for spiritual care. Each of the areas that the health care provider has observed—nonverbal and verbal behavior, interpersonal relationships, and the environment—all provide clues that require interpretation to be meaningful. It is essential for the health care provider to reflect on these observations and allow the patient either to validate or to correct the health care provider's perceptions. An incorrect interpretation of a patient's affect or attitude could lead to ineffective spiritual care. The following example illustrates the use of reflection to verify a health care provider's perceptions:

Let's return to Nurse Bramer to see how he validates his observations with Mr. Johns.

NURSE BRAMER: You seem sad this morning, Mr. Johns.

MR. JOHNS: No, not really. A bit reflective, but not sad. The surgery tomorrow is really making me think about my life—what I've done with it and what I'd like to do with it in the future—that is, if God allows me a future.

NURSE BRAMER: It sounds like this surgery has made you take stock of your life and how you want to continue.

Nurse Bramer has reflected back to the patient what he just said, to confirm it and to let the patient know that the nurse understood his concerns.

When evaluating the area of interpersonal relationships, the health care provider must look beyond mere numbers of visitors to the meaning of the visits and the effect the visits have on the patient. Is the patient alone because there is no one to visit, or is it because the family is experiencing transportation or financial problems? These observations must also be validated with the patient.

> NURSE BRAMER: I noticed that your son hasn't been in to see you in the last few days. Is there a problem?
>
> MR. JOHNS: He really wants to get in here, but he works the evening shift at the steel mill. Visiting hours conflict with his work schedule. He calls me at least once a day though. I wouldn't want him to take time off to come in here. He just returned to work after a long layoff. I did ask him to be here with me the day of the surgery, and he will be.

Although articles in the environment can also provide clues to a patient's concerns and beliefs, assumptions cannot be made as to the meaning of these articles. Items in the environment may indeed have deep religious significance, they may serve as good luck charms, or they may have no meaning at all to the patient. Again, these observations need to be validated with the patient. "I notice that you have several religious books on your bedside table. Do they have special meaning for you?" The patient is then free to express his feelings about these observations.

In considering an intervention for an expressed spiritual need, two principles must be kept in mind (Fish & Shelly 1985). First, a patient's relationship with a Higher Power is complex and individual. It is not possible to compile a list of standing spiritual orders appropriate for every patient who exhibits spiritual distress. Every patient must be approached in light of her unique needs. Second, nurses and other health care providers must be aware of their own spiritual beliefs. If providers feel uneasy with the issue of spirituality, they might tend to withdraw from a patient who is having a similar struggle. If providers themselves are angry with God, they might communicate these angry feelings in a manner that is harmful to the patient. If a provider doubts the existence of a Supreme Being, he might communicate this disbelief to a patient in a way that undermines the patient's beliefs, exacerbating the patient's spiritual distress.

It is possible, however, for a nurse or another health care provider to give spiritual care without having strong spiritual beliefs. Awareness of these feelings helps the clinician control these behaviors. A useful approach draws on communication skills and employs the ability to empathize with the patient through caring and concern. Although it is beyond the scope of practice for nurses and other providers to address specific spiritual or religious questions of their patients, they can provide spiritual care in a broader sense. Many health care providers believe that spiritual care entails only discussions pertaining to God or a Higher Power. However, the most effective spiritual intervention is the health care provider's offering of self. The tools to enhance the spiritual well-being of another include the willingness to listen, to empathize, to be available, to be vulnerable, and to be committed (Jourard 1964).

Spiritual Interventions

There are three broad categories of spiritual interventions available to the health care provider for meeting spiritual needs. The term ministry is used to describe these interventions, and it refers to the use of our gifts, talents, time, and energy in the service to another. Although the term ministry draws from a Christian perspective, the idea of providing loving service to another is certainly not limited to Christianity. Ministries fall into three broad categories:

Ministry of presence—involves a willingness to be an active listener, empathetic, vulnerable, humble, and committed.

Ministry of word—involves a willingness to conduct the spiritual screening/assessment, to talk about spiritual/religious concerns, to offer verbal support and encouragement regarding the patient's spiritual beliefs, to make a referral to the chaplain or, if the patient desires, to the patient's spiritual leader (minister, priest, rabbi, imam); to use scripture or other religious/inspirational literature as a means of alleviating the patient's spiritual distress; to advocate for the patient's spiritual/religious beliefs with the health care team; and to pray if this is what the patient asks for or initiates.

Ministry of action—involves a willingness to take action on behalf of a patient's spiritual needs. (Carson & Koenig 2004)

Ministry of Presence

Probably the greatest tool available to health care providers for meeting spiritual needs is their own presence and ability to touch another person both physically and spiritually. A health care provider does this through a personal relationship developed with the patient. This relationship allows the clinician and the patient to mutually experience the uniqueness of the other. It is in this relationship that the health care provider is able to learn about the patient's needs, wants, hurts, joys, and ambitions. It is through this relationship that the health care provider communicates personal spiritual strength and a willingness to care, listen, and be available to the patient. The health care provider's presence itself touches the patient's distressed spirit, just as a cool hand might soothe a fevered brow.

Being present so as to touch another's spirit requires five essential elements (Fish & Shelly 1985): listening, empathy, vulnerability, humility, and commitment.

LISTENING

The ability to listen is both an art and a learned skill. It requires the health care provider to completely attend to the patient with open ears, eyes, and mind. Listening is an active process that requires the health care provider's full concentration. It is essential for the listener to pay attention to both the auditory and the visual stimuli that she receives from the patient, and then analyze these stimuli to ascertain the patient's intent.

People often do not reveal their most intimate personal thoughts and feelings in a direct manner, but rather cloak them in obscure language. This masking of what represents the true self is a protective, or defensive, measure. If people reveal too much of themselves too soon, the listener may react in a hurtful way. The listener may scorn, criticize, or even scoff at the speaker. Rather than expose ourselves to the possibility of being hurt, we hide what we really feel and may only allude to it in a roundabout way. This places a burden on the listener to be attuned to and pursue clues that the speaker gives. Let's return to the example of Nurse Bramer and Mr. Johns.

NURSE BRAMER: Your surgery is tomorrow, Mr. Johns. How are you feeling about it?

MR. JOHNS: Oh, fine . . . I guess [tears in his eyes].

NURSE BRAMER: Your words say "fine," but your face is telling me something else. Why don't we talk for a while?

MR. JOHNS: I don't know what is wrong with me. I know that I need the surgery—it's the best thing for me. I can't go on living with this awful angina pain. I tell myself that I'm trusting in God, but still I feel—I don't know—I guess I'm afraid.

In this example, Nurse Bramer not only listens to Mr. Johns's words but also attends to the tears in his eyes. The nurse shares with Mr. Johns the discrepancy between his verbal and nonverbal messages. By taking the time to do this, Nurse Bramer communicates that he is indeed interested in Mr. Johns and cares about his feelings. This is the essence of listening. By listening to what Mr. Johns says, as well as to what he does not say, the nurse is making himself present to Mr. Johns.

Several barriers may interfere with the nurse's or another health care provider's ability to listen actively. Each of these barriers reflects the health care provider's inability to be totally present for the patient. First, the health care provider may be distracted by other things and may not be paying full attention to the patient. In the example of Mr. Johns, Nurse Bramer might have been thinking about other tasks that he needed to do and missed the tears in Mr. Johns's eyes when he said, "Oh, fine . . . I guess." Second, the health care provider may miss the meaning of the patient's message because of a failure to clarify the meaning of a word, a phrase, or a facial expression. Nurse Bramer validated Mr. Johns's nonverbal expression and this is essential to good communication. Not only does nonverbal expression make up most of what we communicate, but it is so easily misinterpreted by the listener. Third, the health care provider may interject personal feelings and reactions into the patient's situation rather than allowing the patient to explore and discuss his own feelings and reactions. The last barrier occurs when the health care provider is busy formulating a response while the patient is still talking. In this instance, the health care provider never hears the patient's message.

In the situation between Nurse Bramer and Mr. Johns, they both spoke English. This is not always the case. Sometimes the patient and the health care provider speak different languages; English may be a second language for one or both of them. Cultural differences also impact on the interpretation not only of what is said but what is communicated without words. The nurse must be sensitive to these potential communication barriers and be cautious about drawing erroneous conclusions about what the patient is and is not saying. For instance, a patient's diffidence might be interpreted by the nurse as arrogance, when in fact it masks a deep-rooted fear about being in the hospital and having "foreigners" give him care. The nurse must be willing to question conclusions that lead to irritation with, annoyance toward, or withdrawal from the patient. It is our responsibility as health care providers to find a way to communicate with the patients in our care. The use of family interpreters, volunteer interpreters, and attending to the whole message—verbal and nonverbal—allows us to more accurately assess a patient's spiritual needs.

EMPATHY

Empathy is the ability to vicariously experience the feelings of another. Empathetic clinicians are able to put those feelings into words and still remain objective in order to help the individual examine alternatives.

Empathy is different from sympathy. Sympathy allows the listener to share in the feelings of the other, but in the process of sharing, the listener loses her objectivity and is unable to differentiate between her feelings and those of the speaker.

Robert Kein, a sixteen-year-old with bilateral amputation below the knee as a result of a skiing accident, was assigned to Mrs. Johnson, a physical therapist. Mrs. Johnson, who had two teenage sons herself, found it very difficult to work with Robert. When she was in his room, she felt tearful, was unable to carry on a conversation with him, and experienced difficulty engaging him in rehabilitation for fear of causing him pain. She kept dwelling on how awful this must be for Robert and what it would be like if this happened to one of her sons. Mrs. Johnson was sympathetic to Robert and also ineffective because her close identification with his feelings interfered with her ability to focus on his needs.

One morning, Mrs. Johnson walked into Robert's room and found him crying. Her first response was to leave the room, thinking, "I can't handle this today." But she managed to stop herself, and she went over to Robert and touched his shoulder. He continued to sob and said, "What am I going to do? I wish I were dead. My whole life is sports. I would have qualified for an athletic scholarship if this hadn't happened. I feel like my life is over."

Mrs. Johnson recognized the feelings of despair that Robert was expressing and said to him, "It seems to you like your life is over. You are feeling that this is such an unfair thing to have happened to you. I agree with you, it is, but let's talk about it." Mrs. Johnson responded in an empathetic manner to Robert. She communicated to him that she was present for him, that she understood his feelings, and that she would be with him if he wanted to talk about his situation at greater length.

VULNERABILITY

Vulnerability seems to go hand in hand with empathy. As a nurse or another clinician allows herself to experience the feelings of the patient, she is allowing the patient to touch the core of her person. By entering into the patient's experiences, the health care clinician is open not only to pain and rejection, but also to joy and praise. The caregiver makes her own personal reserves of strength, faith, and courage available to another who is in need.

HUMILITY

When health care providers exhibit humility, they recognize that there are limitations to their personal knowledge and understanding, that they don't have all the answers, and that they should expect to learn from patients. Humility allows health care providers to accept both themselves and their patients as they are.

COMMITMENT

Commitment requires health care providers to make themselves available to patients as long as those patients need support. A committed health care provider shares in the loneliness, anxiety, and suffering experienced by a patient and does not to pull out of the relationship when it becomes uncomfortable. For instance, it is not uncommon for staff to avoid a patient who has a terminal disease. A real commitment to patients means being present for them both before and after they receive such a diagnosis. In fact, a real commitment involves being present for the patient and family throughout the dying process to assist them in dealing with the pain, fear, loneliness, sadness, and anger that follow such a diagnosis. A commitment like this hopefully helps patients deal with these feelings and achieve a peaceful acceptance of their death.

In summary, the act of being present for patients and touching their spirit is essentially a reflection of the health care provider's own spirit. The health care provider brings to the provider-patient relationship her own kindness, patience, love, gentleness, and honesty, and places these qualities at the disposal of someone in need. When health care providers share themselves in this manner, they can serve as a human bridge between the patient and the patient's perception of a divine power.

Ministry of Word

Great care and sensitivity are required to offer this aspect of spiritual care. As health care providers, we must choose our words carefully with full awareness of the power of words to heal as well as to inflict hurt. Health care clinicians frequently express a sense of inadequacy when faced with spiritual comments. Elizabeth Johnston Taylor (2007) discusses the use of restatements, open questions, reflection of feelings, and self-disclosure as communication strategies to respond to verbalized spiritual distress. Taylor (2007) uses the following example to illustrate these various responses.

The mother of a dying child says, "Why is this happening to my child? Why me? Is there a God?"

RESTATING generally uses fewer words than the patient has spoken but tries to capture the meaning of what the patient has said. Restating can be direct or tentative. It is important to avoid parroting what the patient has said, restating surface thoughts, or focusing on someone other than the patient. The usefulness of restating can be evaluated. If the patient clams up or keeps repeating herself, then the restatement has not helped the patient to gain understanding or to discuss additional dimensions of the situation. Using restatement, the health care provider might say:

"Watching your child die raises some very deep, disturbing questions."

"It seems that the unfairness of your child's dying is causing you to rethink what you believe about God."

"Because of this tragedy, you're wondering if God really does exist."

"You wonder why a lot, and if God is there." (Taylor 2007, 61–65)

USING OPEN QUESTIONS where the intent is to explore, and clarify thoughts and feelings, the health care provider might say:

"How does watching your child's death lead you to wonder about God's existence?"

"How does it make you feel when you wonder about the truth of your spiritual beliefs?"

"What kind of reaction do you have now to talking about these painful topics?"

"How do you feel about God not being there? How do you feel about asking why? What does your son think?" (Taylor 2007, 65–67)

USING REFLECTION OF FEELINGS to explore feelings more deeply and to gain insight, the health care provider might say:

Focus on a single word (for example, "Perhaps you're feeling sort of betrayed").

Use a phrase or metaphor to capture feeling (e.g., "You're feeling helpless in the face of this situation").

Use an experiential statement that implies a feeling (e.g., "Maybe you're feeling like the rug of your beliefs about God has been pulled out from under you").

Use a behavioral statement: "Maybe you feel like throwing in the towel." (Taylor 2007, 72)

THE USE OF SELF-DISCLOSURE requires the health care provider first to ask whether the needs of the patient or the health care provider will be met as a result of self-disclosure (Taylor 2007, 81–82). It is important for the health care provider to determine why the patient is seeking this kind of personal information. A response like, "Before I answer, could we take a look at what this means to you?" would allow the health care provider to assess the situation further. It is always important to follow up with an open question or reflection, such as "I wonder what is going on inside you now."

Willingness to Discuss Spiritual/Religious Issues

When health care providers conduct a spiritual assessment or screening, they are engaging in ministry of the word. By doing so, they are conveying to the patient and the family a willingness to discuss spiritual and religious issues. This willingness may indeed open the door to additional opportunities to talk about how spiritual beliefs and practices may impact on the current health situation. For instance, will spirituality or religion have any influence on the patient's ability to cope or on the patient's sense of purpose and meaning in life? Will spirituality and religion influence the patient's ability to adapt to his current health problem, or on choices that may face him and his family? As health care providers, we are not expected to provide answers to these questions, but facilitating the conversation is invaluable.

Supporting and Encouraging the Patient's Religious and Spiritual Views

The clinician's support of religious and spiritual views must always be centered on the beliefs and practices that provide comfort for the patient. This may present a challenge to health care providers, especially if the patient's religious and spiritual views derive from a different spiritual worldview than those held by the health care professional. As professionals, we must keep our focus on the patient and what is personally meaningful and comforting to her. Under no circumstances are we to proselytize. If the patient's beliefs and/or practices seem strange and unfamiliar to us, we need to ask for clarification and always be respectful.

Referral to Chaplain or Patient's Own Spiritual Leader

There are many reasons that a health care provider would make a referral either to the hospital chaplain or, if the patient or family requests it, to the patient's own spiritual leader. First of all, chaplains are not only spiritual experts, but are also members of the health care team. As members of the team, we do not need the patient's permission to make the referral. However, a referral to the patient's personal spiritual leader, including imams, ministers, priests, and rabbis, requires the patient's permission, due to Health Insurance Portability and Accountability Act (HIPAA) privacy regulations. Patients may raise theological concerns to the health care provider; such concerns are more appropriately dealt with by the spiritual and religious experts. The patient and/or the patient's family may request a specific religious rite or ritual that, again, is within the domain of the spiritual experts. The patient may request to speak to the chaplain or the representative from his own faith tradition. Sometimes the health care professional is not comfortable intervening in spiritual issues and may refer these issues to clergy. When a patient is in the hospital and a clergyperson is involved in her care, it is important that the clergyperson be greeted and treated with respect, made to feel that he is a vital part of the health care team, and offered assistance as needed as he ministers to the patient. The health care provider provides privacy during the cleric's visit and inquires if anything special is needed to conduct a specific religious ritual (for example, a table covered with a white cloth for the placement of a crucifix or a religious statue).

Use of Scripture or Other Religious Literature

The reading of scripture or other religious literature may provide comfort to a patient. However, the use of this intervention requires careful assessment, as well as a real sensitivity to the patient's expressed and unexpressed needs. If this intervention is used indiscriminately, the health care provider may be blocking the patient's true expression of feelings. Care is needed so as not to stifle feelings and avoid situations that either the health care provider is unable to handle or that require much reflection and dialogue.

It is certainly appropriate for the nurse or another health care provider to inquire if the patient has a special passage or reading and to ascertain why that passage holds special meaning to the patient. In this case, the caregiver is invoking something that already has personal meaning for the patient and may, indeed, serve as support for him.

Nurse Jenkins happened to go into Mrs. Lucas's room one last time before the end of the evening shift. Mrs. Lucas was having difficulty falling asleep. Nurse Jenkins asked Mrs. Lucas if there was a problem. Mrs. Lucas said, "Since I had the cataract surgery the other day, I haven't been able to read my Bible before I go to sleep. For years, I've been reading Psalm 23 right before I retire for the night. Reading those words seems to take away all my anxiety. Do you think you could read the passage to me?" Nurse Jenkins said, "I'll be happy to read it to you." Before the nurse finished, Mrs. Lucas had drifted off to sleep.

Prayer

The use of prayer as a spiritual intervention is very powerful. Prayer is described in many ways. The writings of the great spiritual leaders of all faith traditions acknowledge the centrality of prayer to a life in touch with a Higher Being. Prayer is an invitation to the Divine to enter into our existence in an active way. It is the bridge by which human beings engage in a personal relationship with the Almighty (Lewis 1985). Through this relationship, the individual communicates needs, feelings, fears, love, adoration, and awe to the Creator, and, in return, she feels the presence, comfort, and love of the Creator.

Illness can interfere with an individual's ability to pray. Feelings such as isolation, fear, guilt, grief, and anxiety often flow from the illness experience. These feelings can be barriers to relationships in general, and specifically to the relationship we have with God. Patients may find that prayers will not come, that they feel cut off from the Source of Life and unable to bridge the gap between themselves and their Creator. The nurse's or another health care provider's offer to pray with a patient can break through that sense of isolation and alienation and allow the patient to experience the comfort of God's love through the person of the health care provider.

There a few guidelines when using prayer. First, prayer or any spiritual intervention is never used out of intuition, but instead follows a careful assessment that has revealed the presence of a spiritual need. Second, prayer is never to be used as a substitute for the clinician's time and presence. Prayer is instead an adjunct to the health care provider's use of self to meet the patient's needs. Third, prayer is never used to meet the health care provider's needs but only to facilitate the patient's relationship with God. Finally, prayer is not used to communicate a magical view of God that conveys a false sense of hope and expectation.

Prayer can take a number of forms. For instance, the health care provider may choose to use a conversational type of prayer in which she reflects the patient's concerns and needs in the content of the prayer. Mrs. Pritchart was waiting outside the operating room. She was scheduled for a repeat cesarean section. Chaplain Owens noticed that Mrs. Pritchart had been crying.

CHAPLAIN OWENS: Mrs. Pritchart, you've been crying. What's wrong?

MRS. PRITCHART: I wanted to see my minister this morning, and he won't be able to get here before surgery. I wanted him to pray for me and the baby.

CHAPLAIN OWENS: Well, I'd be happy to pray for you and the baby. Would that be okay?

MRS. PRITCHART: Oh, yes. Would you please? This surgery really scares me.

CHAPLAIN OWENS: Dear God, please comfort Mrs. Pritchart as she enters surgery. Lift her fear and in its place give her peace and strength. Let her know that you are with her and the baby.

MRS. PRITCHART: Thanks so much. That really meant a lot to me.

Sometimes the health care provider is not comfortable praying out loud with a patient, or the patient is uncomfortable with the spoken prayer. In this instance, it is just as appropriate for the health care provider to tell the patient that he will remember her in private prayer.

Nurse Jones works in a medical-surgical unit. As part of her evening care, she always tells patients that she prays that God will grant them a peaceful and restful sleep. Her patients frequently make a prayer request of Nurse Jones.

Another approach with regard to prayer is to ask the patient if there is a special prayer that holds personal significance for him. It might provide a patient with great comfort to be able to recite such a prayer with the health care provider or in her presence.

Leslie Ann, a nine-year-old diagnosed with cystic fibrosis, was spending the night in the hospital without her mother. Leslie Ann's mother had to return home to take care of other family concerns. As bedtime approached, Leslie Ann started to cry.

LESLIE ANN: I want my mommy.

DOCTOR READ: Leslie, I can understand that it's very hard to be here without your mommy. Maybe I could do some of the things that she does for you when it's time to go to sleep.

LESLIE ANN: We always pray together and then Mom tucks me in and kisses me.

DOCTOR READ: I'd be happy to do that. How do you pray?

LESLIE ANN: We say a prayer that my mommy made up. Could you say it?

DOCTOR READ: Yes, why don't you say it and then I'll say it with you?

LESLIE ANN: While we say it, I'm going to close my eyes and pretend you're my mom.

DOCTOR READ: That's fine. Go ahead and tell me the words to the prayer.

LESLIE ANN: Guardian Angel, watch over my sleep. My worries and fears I give you to keep. Keep me through darkness of night. Wake me gently with God's morning light.

DOCTOR READ: That's a beautiful prayer. Let's say it together.

If the health care provider is of a religious faith different from that of the patient, it is important to ask the patient how he prays. For instance, a Buddhist patient might not want the health care provider to pray out loud, since his form of prayer is personal meditation. In this case, an offer to pray silently for the patient or to be with him while he spends time in meditation might be helpful. It is important to remember that the purpose of prayer is to support the patient in his relationship with God (however the patient perceives the Divine); therefore, the health care provider's approach should bring the patient peace and not create anxiety.

Advocating the Patient's Spiritual Beliefs with the Health Care Team

Sometimes it is necessary for the nurse or another member of the health care team to act as an advocate for the patient when the patient's spiritual beliefs are in conflict with the suggested treatment plan. Patients occasionally experience unnecessary turmoil because they are uninformed about religious exemptions that apply to those who are seriously ill or hospitalized. In this case, the clinician can contact the hospital chaplain to discuss this matter with the patient. Health care providers can bring in reading material that addresses this issue or can suggest that patients talk with members of their own faith community, or their own spiritual leader, for clarification of spiritual restrictions. Fasting is an example of a religious practice that is often exempted for the ill, for the elderly, and for pregnant women.

The patient is occasionally misinformed about the proposed treatment regimen. The health care provider ensures that patients receive the needed information about their health status and the proposed treatment plan. Patients are encouraged to discuss their perception of the nature and purpose of therapy so that misperceptions or misinformation can be corrected. The patient is informed of the possible consequences of refusing therapy, although health care providers should not to appear to be coercive or threatening.

When patients are experiencing true spiritual conflict and have been adequately informed about their health status, the health care clinician serves as an advocate by encouraging the other members of the team to consider alternate methods of therapy (e.g., use of nonblood circulatory volume expanders). The health care provider respects and supports the patient's decision, even if the decision conflicts with the health care provider's personal values. If this is impossible for the health care provider, the patient is assigned to another health care provider who is able to do this. Members of the health team are encouraged to discuss their feelings about situations like this so the patient is in no way avoided or treated with disrespect.

When parents have refused treatment for a child, the health care providers may suggest alternative methods of treatment that the parents can accept. If there are no alternative therapies available, the physician or the hospital administrator may seek a court order appointing a temporary guardian so that the child may be treated. This situation places the parents and the health care providers in an adversarial position. The health care provider's tasks are to provide spiritual support to the parents and their child through their own spiritual leader and to help the parents verbalize their anger. (See chapter 5 for a comprehensive discussion of situations in which religious beliefs conflict with necessary medical procedures.)

Ministry of Action

This is a broad spiritual intervention and applies to all the myriad of ways that nurses and other clinicians demonstrate compassion and concern for patients and their families. For instance, hospitalization can interfere with a patient's ability to practice important spiritual rituals and can produce feelings of anxiety, guilt, sadness, and grief, and a sense of loss. It is important for health care providers to reduce or eliminate as many factors as possible that contribute to this situation. The patient needs to know that his spiritual practices are acceptable and that the staff will do whatever they can to help the patient maintain these practices. For example, they may provide privacy and quiet for prayer, contemplation, or religious/inspirational reading by

Pulling the curtains or closing the door.
Planning care activities to allow the patient uninterrupted quiet time.
Turning off the television or radio.
If possible, holding telephone calls.

The nurse or another clinician can contact the hospital chaplain to clarify religious obligations when a patient is ill. In addition, certain religious services can be performed in the hospital. The health care provider can assist the patient in maintaining a diet consistent with religious practices as long as the diet does not interfere with the patient's health. This may require the health care provider to consult with both the dietitian and the patient's physician to determine if some fasting may be allowed or if a therapeutic diet can be modified in any way. The services of family and friends can also be used to supply the patient with special food unavailable in the hospital.

If the patient's health permits, the health care provider may arrange a visit to the hospital chapel or a quiet spot on the hospital grounds. In addition, the health care provider may arrange for the patient to have access to religious ceremonies conducted on the radio or television. In fact, some hospitals broadcast their own chapel services on closed-circuit television so that bedridden patients can feel that they are participating.

The clinician can encourage and enable the patient to perform a number of spiritual rituals not detrimental to her health. These include allowing time for prayer at bedtime or before meals and asking if the patient requires any assistance with these activities. A health care provider can help the patient deal with physical limitations that interfere with performing religious observances, such as turning the pages of a prayer book, holding the beads of a rosary, or lighting candles for the Sabbath. There may be habits of personal hygiene or attire that have special significance for the patient, and these need to be respected if at all possible (e.g., an Orthodox Jewish man's beard, or Orthodox Jewish woman's desire to keep her hair covered). The health care provider may—at the request of parents and when an emergency arises and a priest cannot be available— perform baptism for a critically ill infant born to Roman Catholic parents and make arrangements for other religious rituals (circumcision, anointing of the sick). Finally, in case of death, the health care provider should allow the family or the patient's spiritual leader to perform ritual care of the body.

Religious articles can hold great significance for a patient, providing a sense of comfort and security and a link to a time in life when things were better. Patients may feel that certain articles are essential to their religious practices, and without these items they may feel anxious. The health care team needs to be aware of the importance of such articles to the patient's overall spiritual and emotional well-being. These items should be treated with respect and protected from being lost or destroyed. For instance, a patient may wear a religious pin or medal, attached to a chain, or an article of clothing, such as a prayer shawl. Care needs to be taken so that such items are not lost in the laundry. Sometimes in an effort to tidy up a patient's bedside area, religious articles are inadvertently misplaced or tossed into the trash. If an item is lost, the health care provider should try to obtain replacements of the missing articles from either the hospital clergy, the patient's family, a personal spiritual leader, or members of the patient's faith community. A patient should be allowed to keep religious articles and books within reach or where these items are easily visible.

A ministry of action is a ministry of compassion, and this is the heart of spiritual care.

Summary

This chapter discusses the many reasons that the spiritual needs of patients are frequently neglected by nurses and other health care professionals. These reasons include the acceptance of a secular humanist worldview to the exclusion of a theistic worldview, the health care provider's own discomfort with the issue of spirituality, a belief that spiritual concerns are too private for the health care provider to assess, and a belief that spiritual concerns are the sole responsibility of the clergy. The reader is introduced to the concept that a structured process can be appropriately applied to the area of spirituality. Last, specific spiritual interventions are discussed.

Reflective Activities

1. Have you thought about your own spirituality? How does your belief system influence the care you provide to others?
2. If everyone has spiritual needs, how would you define these needs in an atheist? How would you meet such a patient's spiritual needs?
3. Have you ever identified a spiritual need in a patient? If so, what did you do about it? Why did you choose to do what you did?
4. What special gifts do you possess that you could put at another's disposal in responding to his spiritual concerns?
5. What are your feelings about prayer? Do you engage in prayer? What purpose does it serve for you? Could you offer to pray for someone else?
6. Consider performing a spiritual screening/assessment interview on a friend, a peer, or a family member. How do you feel when you inquire about spiritual matters? Do your feelings facilitate or impede the interview process?

References

Carson, V. B., & Koenig, H. G. (2004). *Spiritual Caregiving: Health Care as a Ministry.* Philadelphia: Templeton Foundation Press.

Fish, S., & Shelly, J. (1985). *Spiritual Care: The Health Care Provider's Role.* Downers Grove, Ill.: InterVarsity Press.

Joint Commission on the Accreditation of Healthcare Organizations. (2004). *2004 Comprehensive Accreditation Manual for Hospitals: The Official Handbook*. Chicago: JCAHO; www.jcaho.org.

Jourard, S. (1964). *Transparent Self*. Princeton, N.J.: Van Nostrand.

Koenig, H. G. (2002). Spiritual History. JAMA 288(4): 487–493 (July 26, 2002).

Lewis, C. S. (1985). Prayer. In J. Garvey (ed.), *Modern Spirituality: An Anthology*, 84–88. Springfield, Ill.: Templegate Publishers.

O'Brien, M. E. (2003). *Spirituality in Nursing: Standing on Holy Ground*, 2nd ed. Boston: Jones & Bartlett Publishers.

Shelly, J. A. (2000). *Spiritual Care: A Guide to Caregivers*. Downers Grove, Ill.: InterVarsity Press.

Sire, J. W. (2004). *The Universe Next Door*, 4th ed. Downers Grove, Ill.: InterVarsity Press.

Stoll, R. (1979). Guidelines for spiritual assessment. *American Journal of Nursing* 79: 1574–77.

Taylor, E. J. (2007). *What Do I Say? Talking with Patients about Spirituality*. Philadelphia: Templeton Foundation Press.

Travelbee, J. (1966). *Interpersonal Aspects of Nursing*. Philadelphia: FA Davis.

Vaughan, F. (1985). *The Inward Arc*. Boston: Shambhala Publications.

7

THE PSYCHOSPIRITUAL LIVES OF ILL OR
SUFFERING CHILDREN AND ADOLESCENTS

WHAT WE SHOULD KNOW, WHAT WE SHOULD DO

PAT FOSARELLI

> *If any of you put a stumbling block before one of these little ones who believe*
> *in me, it would be better for you if a great millstone were hung around your*
> *neck and you were thrown into the sea.*
>
> —Mark 9:42

Most adults are very fond of children, especially their own, and wish to shield them from "bad" things in life. Unfortunately, that cannot happen consistently. Devastating occurrences—such as illness, injuries, disasters, and death—happen every day, if not in a given child's immediate life, then certainly in friends' lives or in nature. Children see what is going on around them and respond to such events in a manner very much like that of important persons in their lives, especially their parents. The responses of older children and teens might also be influenced by the various media with which they come into contact.

Although this chapter is directed primarily at nurses, there are many health care professionals who enter the lives of children and teens experiencing loss or illness. So it is important for all those who work with children and teens to understand (1) normal development across childhood and adolescence; (2) how illness or loss affects developmental stages and common ways that children and teens respond to "bad" things in life; (3) the ways that coping strategies of significant adults and friends influence children's responses; (4) the role of the media in these responses; and (5) a summary of age-appropriate suggestions for psychospiritual care. The purpose of this chapter is to explore these five points by age for a variety of negative events that happen in young lives. The information for the fifth point is adapted from my own book, *Whatever You Do for the Least of These: Ministering to Ill and Dying Children and Their Families* (Fosarelli 2003). The reader who wishes more in-depth information on any age group is referred to that work.

This is a great deal of information. To keep it from becoming too unwieldy, each of the five points will be discussed by discrete age groups, starting with infants and toddlers and moving, sequentially, to older adolescents by the end of the chapter. Several theorists will be referenced, including Erik Erikson (1985), who was interested in how human beings formed relationships to others and to the world; Jean Piaget (Singer & Revenson 1978), who was fascinated by how children learned; and James Fowler (1995), who investigated faith development over a lifetime.

Like many adults, children and teens can experience the spiritual, not only in church or other houses of worship or in their private moments in prayer, but also as they interact with others, especially those who love them and those who have power over them. In children and teens, the spiritual is enmeshed within other domains of development, which is one of the reasons that a brief summary of development for each age is provided. By recognizing that children and teens experience the spiritual in the way in which they are treated, and by providing compassionate and sensitive care to them, we can meet their spiritual needs over and above the spiritual care given by representatives of their faith traditions.

Spiritual Care: General Principles

Children and Teens Themselves

Most of the spiritual care for young children is provided to them through their parents. Since very young children do not understand long sentences, many prayers might go over their heads, although many preschoolers want to say prayers themselves, and should be encouraged to do so. If parents agree, a representative of their faith tradition can be invited to pray with a child and his family, allowing a child who can do so to actually lead the prayer. Praying for an infant or toddler should be done in such a way that it does not frighten him, which means, for example, that any health care professional (or clergyperson) refrain from touching a young child who is experiencing stranger anxiety (see below). Praying for and with a pre-schooler must also be done gently, as young children feel vulnerable when they're ill, worried that God might be mad at them.

Spiritual care for elementary school–age children can be given to them directly or with their parents present. If parents and child agree, a representative of their faith tradition can be invited to pray with the child and her family. Many children will want their parents present if a minister or chaplain visits, or if someone prays with them. After checking with their parents to see how spiritual needs might be best addressed, a person addressing spiritual needs should always ask children of this age if they want to talk, let alone pray, and their wishes should be respected. Some children will not be at all interested in opening up to a stranger, while other children will be glad for any opportunity to talk about what's on their minds. Children should always be asked if they wish their parents to remain in the room with them in any case, as the vast majority of children will want their parents present for support. Many times, children will be so upset by unanswered prayers that they might express anger at God, which usually upsets parents or other caregivers. Elementary school–age children need to express their feelings, and they need to be reassured that nothing that they did caused the negative event (illness, death, loss) in their lives.

Spiritual care for teens can be given to them directly or with their parents present. If parents and teen agree, a health care professional or a representative of their faith tradition can be called to pray with the teen and his family. Many young teens still want their parents present if a minister or chaplain visits, or if someone prays with them, although some older teens prefer to be visited alone. After checking with their parents to see how spiritual needs might be best addressed, those addressing spiritual needs should always ask teens if they want to talk, let alone pray, and abide by their responses. If they wish to pray, they should also be asked if they would

like to lead the prayer. Some teens will not be at all interested in expos-
ing their innermost thoughts or praying aloud, while others will appreciate
the opportunity to offer a prayer in the company of others. Teens should
always be asked if they wish their parents to remain in the room with them
in any case, as many young teens and some older ones will want their parents present for support. Many times, teens will be so upset by their prayers
seemingly being ignored that they become angry with God or say that they
no longer believe in God. Like younger children, teens need to express such
feelings and receive reassurance that the illness, death, or loss is not a punishment for sin. In the Judeo-Christian tradition, the psalms can be used to
highlight that even the psalmist had strong, sometimes negative, feelings
about God, illness, trouble, and unanswered prayers.

Siblings

Siblings are often forgotten when another child is ill or experiencing a
loss. This is not acceptable, since siblings suffer, too. In general, the same
guidelines provided for children and teens apply to siblings as well, except
that two emotions are more common in siblings than in the affected child
or teen. The first is guilt. Although some children and teens who are ill or
who are experiencing a loss might feel some guilt over their circumstances,
believing that something they did (or failed to do) brought on their unfortunate circumstances, siblings are even more likely to feel guilt, especially
if their relationship with the affected sibling is conflicted. Even siblings
who love each other enormously have their spats from time to time, and
when one of them becomes ill or suffers a loss that the other sibling does
not also experience, the "spared" sibling might feel guilty over the times
that she was mean to her sibling. This is especially true if the "spared" sibling said things like, "I hate you"; "I wish you were dead"; "Why don't you
just go away?" or "God doesn't even like you."

The second emotion more common in "spared" siblings is jealousy.
An ill or grieving sibling usually receives more attention from parents and
other adults than other siblings do. This imbalance in attention received
might cause some otherwise healthy siblings to "become" ill (displaying
symptoms like the affected sibling or symptoms that will catch their parents' attention) or to engage in acting-out behaviors (such as temper tan-

trums, arguing, name calling, difficulties in school, and the like) in an attempt to get positive or negative attention. Obviously, the type of acting-out behavior depends on both the age of the child and his temperament. The best way to avoid having to deal with acting-out behaviors is to encourage parents to prevent them in the first place by giving all children in a family the attention and love they need and providing quality time with each one. If this can't be done for a particular period because of the needs of the affected child, then clear explanations as to why this is so should be provided to the other children. Also, if the parents can't provide such quality time, other relatives or trusted adults should be recruited to do so.

Parents and Other Caregivers

Much spiritual care might be needed by parents or other relatives of an ill or grieving young child or teen; these adults might believe that, somehow, they caused their current situation by real or perceived wrongs in their lives, or that God is punishing them through their child or teen. Many are angry at God because their prayers for healing have not been answered. *Always* ask whether overt spiritual care (by a religious professional, a health care professional, or anyone else) would be welcomed before initiating it. Some people, especially those who feel alienated from God or the church, will chafe at the idea of prayer or meeting with a representative of a faith tradition. *Never* force the spiritual (e.g., prayer or scripture) on anyone; doing so might only "prove" that religion is coercive, or that the professionals believe that the situation in question is, indeed, punishment for past misdeeds, which can only be rectified by prayers and acts of contrition. By all means, if young patients (children or teens), parents, or other caregivers show an interest, direct them to the chaplain's office and to the chapel. At difficult times, it is important for people of faith to know that God is there for them, especially through other people who demonstrate care and concern.

When speaking with parents or other caregivers, remember to inquire about any siblings and how they are doing. Inquire also about the parent(s) themselves and how they are coping. Ask if there is anything you can do, but don't make promises that you can't keep. Do not offer unsolicited advice. It is better to offer no advice than bad or wrong advice.

Even if a parent asks, do not speculate as to why this child is ill or if God is punishing the family for some reason. Never pry. "Well-intentioned but ill-conceived statements can not only hurt a parent (or child) emotionally but also spiritually" (Fosarelli 2003, 18). If a parent seems to want to pray with you or talk about God outside her child's earshot, give her an opportunity to do so by asking if you can speak to her for a moment out of her child's room or presence.

The best gifts you can give a parent (and the best evidence for a loving God) are simple presence and genuine listening.

Infants and Toddlers (Birth to 2½–3 Years)

Normal Development

PHYSICAL

A newborn child can do nothing on her own; her every need must be met by others. In the beginning, she has very little muscle control and an immature nervous system; her gaze seems bleary, and the slightest noise frightens her. Yet, by the end of the first year of life, this same infant will probably be able to see very well, sit alone, crawl, walk, say one or two words, and make lots of loud noises herself. What an amazing developmental progression in twelve short months! And the second twelve months are just as amazing because the toddler (so named because she "toddles" as she walks) not only walks but runs and climbs, "assists" in dressing herself and doing household chores, babbles constantly (every once in a while actually saying a few "real" words!), and is definitely her own person with her own wants, when *she* wants them. Physically, she is becoming stronger and more agile, which leads to her great desire to get her own way. In trying to get what she wants, her favorite word is often "No!" Toilet training might begin toward the end of the toddler years (roughly twenty-four to thirty months), with alternating successful and frustrating days common.

PSYCHOLOGICAL

The famous German psychologist Erik Erikson described psychological stages across the human life span. For each age, a person must successfully navigate the stage to be well prepared to move on to the next stage. His theory posits one characteristic versus another; this does not mean that development is an all-or-nothing proposition, but that development results in the achievement of one characteristic *predominantly* over the other. In Erikson's view, infants experience the stage called *trust versus mistrust*. Because those around them must do so much for them, infants will learn to gain trust in their world by trusting in those caring for them. As long as caregivers meet the infants' needs in trustworthy ways, infants will learn to trust. If caregivers do not provide care in a gentle or timely fashion, or if they completely fail to provide needed care, infants will learn not to trust.

SOCIAL

Young infants enjoy the company of anybody, even those whom they do not know. By six to nine months, they will avoid contact with unfamiliar people (so-called *stranger anxiety*) and will object with crying or screaming when a parent leaves the room or even their line of vision (so-called *separation anxiety*). These two anxieties are normal, even in infants who have forged healthy attachments to their parents, whom they trust.

Toddlers experience autonomy versus shame and doubt. Toddlers are eager to do things on their own; indeed, they must do so if they are ever to become independent. When their efforts fail, as they inevitably will, depending on the response of those around them, they might take such failures in stride or be ashamed of their inabilities, becoming fearful of trying again. This latter response is more likely to occur when significant adults ridicule or punish a toddler who has failed, for example, to eat neatly or use the toilet correctly.

Toddlers usually still avoid strangers and scream, cry, kick, and so on if such adults try to hold them. As the second year of life progresses, toddlers will become more comfortable with permitting parents to leave their sight—at least for a brief amount of time. These social stages might be more difficult if the toddler is in an environment in which he feels shame rather than affirmation (for example, being addressed as "You big baby" every time he cries).

COGNITIVE

The great Swiss psychologist Jean Piaget focused on how children learn. The details of his work are beyond the scope of this chapter, but his cognitive stages are useful to know. The stage for infants and toddlers is called *sensorimotor.* Infants and toddlers learn through their senses, especially by placing things in their mouths. By the end of the first year of life and certainly throughout the rest of a child's life, she can use her motor system (i.e., her arms and legs) to seek and retrieve objects of interest, unlike the situation when she was younger in which she had to wait for interesting objects to be brought to her. This is vitally important for continued learning to occur.

SPIRITUAL

James Fowler, a psychologist and an ordained minister, studied stages of faith development across the life span. For some age groups, his stages might act as proxies for spiritual development. Fowler called the period of infancy and toddlerhood a *prestage: undifferentiated faith.* This is akin to Erikson's stage of *trust versus mistrust.* If a young child is treated well, he will learn to have faith in those around him. If they, in turn, speak lovingly and reverently of "God," he will learn that "God" is someone special. Furthermore, if parents perform rituals while saying "God" (folding their hands, bowing their heads, closing their eyes, etc.), their child will learn to imitate those rituals himself. Although he would not be expected to have a full understanding of these rituals, he can understand that they are associated with "God." This will serve him well in the next stage of his faith or spiritual development. On the other hand, if a child hears the word *God* only when expressed in anger or cursing, or if the word is only said in connection with frustration, he might easily conclude that "God" is nothing special. If God's name doesn't come up at all, a young child will be thoroughly unfamiliar with it.

How Illness or Loss Affects Development

COMMON WAYS THAT INFANTS AND TODDLERS REACT
TO NEGATIVE EVENTS

Anything that curtails the infant's or toddler's ability to explore, to learn, or to form attachments interferes with developmental progression. An ill infant might not learn to sit until months after similarly aged infants do; a toddler might have difficulty developing a secure attachment to a parent who is absent a great deal because of illness. A seriously ill toddler might have marked stranger anxiety because she has been around so many strangers who have hurt her with needles and medical procedures in her young life. Furthermore, because infants and toddlers have not yet developed sophisticated coping mechanisms to handle stress, their responses to negative events are rather immediate and raw.

First of all, what is a negative or "bad" event in this age group? A "bad" (temporary or permanent) event for infants or toddlers is anything that disrupts the routine in their lives. Examples include personal illness or injury (especially if it is accompanied by pain), illness in a primary caregiver or the caregiver's absence for any reason, or removal from familiar surroundings.

What do infants and toddlers do when faced with such things? They cry and, if they are older, they might scream, kick, bite, or hit. Because their routines are thrown off, their sleep patterns might be disturbed, their appetites might be diminished, and their willingness to play or move around might be limited. Of course, sometimes when an infant or toddler is ill, the adults are the ones who prevent him from doing the things he loves; it is we who will not let him out of bed because he has an intravenous line; it is we who will not let him eat because he is NPO; it is we who awaken him to assess vital signs or draw blood. It must be clearly understood that all these activities exacerbate the loss of a young child's sense of normalcy, no matter how important the activities are by adult standards. After all, children of this age are sensorimotor by nature, and when that capability is disrupted, they will feel the loss. In addition, when we ask a parent to "step out of the room" while a procedure is to be done, not only is a young child experiencing pain but now he is terrified and experiencing suffering because of the (temporary) loss of his primary advocate. We can fully expect stranger anxiety and separation anxiety to be in full force. Someone who is calm and kind helps to comfort such a child.

Temperamentally, some infants and toddlers object noisily while others whimper quietly or even silently during a disruption of their routines. But make no mistake about it: Both groups of children are suffering. A person does not need to experience physical pain in order to suffer, although many people certainly suffer because of physical pain. A person can suffer because of any loss, and the loss of her daily activities or a loved one might, in some cases, be worse than suffering from physical pain.

What can be done for ill children? Obviously, certain procedures must be performed, and certain protocols must be followed. The best tactic is to try to provide as much normalcy as feasible, and to permit parents or other significant caregivers to be present as much as possible, even during certain procedures, as their presence might do more good than harm. Every situation is unique in this regard, because, obviously, the health care team doesn't want a parent becoming agitated in front of an already frightened child. Yet a parent or another familiar caregiver who can be a soothing presence should be considered part of the healing regimen. If a child can be held by a parent, let that happen; if a child loves a certain food and it's not prohibited, offer it; if a child has finally drifted off to sleep, try to postpone (within reason) the venipuncture, repeat abdominal exam, or vital sign assessment.

What can be done for children experiencing the loss of significant people or places in their lives? In these instances, the goal is to keep everything else as routine as possible. Admittedly, that is difficult when the adults are mourning themselves or are also displaced, but trying to preserve some semblance of normalcy for the young child is of paramount importance in terms of mental health, and might also benefit the adult in question, since doing so might distract him from some of his own suffering.

Saying prayers or singing hymns softly can be very reassuring to an infant or toddler, especially if she is already familiar with them, as doing so reminds her of her "normal" life. To avoid both frightening a child and the spread of germs, the touching of an infant or toddler during these sacred moments should be done only if (1) the young child does not have stranger anxiety, and (2) the person doing the touching has washed her hands thoroughly.

Helpful and Unhelpful Adult Coping Strategies

When adults are "out of control," many young children become very frightened. On some level, they recognize that their own inabilities or diminutive size mean that they lack the power to take care of themselves. As such, infants and toddlers look to parents or other trusted adults for care. The psychological stages of *trust versus mistrust* and *autonomy versus shame and doubt* are fully operative at this age, and young children need adults whom they can fully trust and who will genuinely affirm them.

So when an adult is highly emotional, an infant or toddler becomes afraid of the intensity of the reaction. Can this person still be trusted? Is the reaction the result of something that the child has done? As a result, an infant or toddler might try to cling to the adult, which might exacerbate the adult's reaction instead of calming it. Furthermore, if the adult, in turn, ignores the child, he might become even more distraught and clingy or might turn inward and ignore everyone around him, neither of which is helpful.

Yet the opposite reaction might also be unhelpful. Adults who speak to infants and toddlers in affected, high, syrupy voices do not always soothe. Young children need kind voices, spoken in normal tones. High, squeaky voices are too much like cartoon characters, and the child's situation does not warrant a cartoon atmosphere. In addition, adults who are overprotective might also engender fear in their children, because if the parent is frightened and hovering, maybe there's something scary for the child to fear as well.

The best adult reactions, whether the adult is the child's parent or his nurse, is kindness, gentleness, and warmth. The young child must feel affirmed and loved; he must not feel abandoned. A harsh or stern tone of voice has no place in situations in which a child is terribly frightened or in pain. If a child is experiencing pain, attempts to alleviate it must be prompt. If a child is suffering, attempts to address the suffering in a way that makes sense to a particular child must be initiated. This is an art because children of this age are preverbal, and adults must be able to read their nonverbal cues as well as to communicate their care in nonverbal ways. Nonverbal cues are important because adults can't adequately explain to a preverbal child what is happening and why it must be done, and a preverbal child can't express the reason behind his tears. A child who is more at ease will probably be more cooperative with medical interventions or with attempts to normalize his life in other ways.

Above all, the majority of infants and toddlers are best comforted by the people who care for them the most; ideally, those individuals should have unlimited access to the children. If the problem is that such a person is unavailable because of death, illness, or another situation, then the person to whom the child would bond most closely (after the primary caregiver) should be present, if at all possible. Although loving strangers are a blessing, if a child is experiencing separation or stranger anxiety, such strangers—even though kind and loving—might not be the answer. Adults who are "rejected" by infants and toddlers in these situations need to remember that it's not a personal rejection.

The Role of the Media in the Reactions of Infants and Toddlers

Because of their limited cognitive ability at this age and their limited ability to express themselves, the media plays less of a role at this age than at some of the other ages that will be discussed. Although the specific content of an image is beyond the grasp of infants and toddlers, the images themselves might be scary. Scary images will frighten infants and toddlers, so exposure to such images should be kept to a minimum. Practically speaking, that means no scary programs on television and no scary videos/DVDs when a young child is present. After all, who knows what she makes of the sights and sounds of many programs, even the evening news with its graphic depictions of war zones, crime scenes, and sites of natural and human-made disasters?

Specific Suggestions for Psychospiritual Care of Infants and Toddlers[1]

1. Enter the infant's or toddler's room quietly. Smiling and using a soft voice is best, but remember that coming too close might be frightening. Never try to hold or touch an infant or toddler who objects.

2. If the parent speaks about God, prayer, or a faith community in some way, consider asking her if she would like to pray. If she says yes, do so, and if not, don't. When praying aloud, try to use a familiar prayer like Psalm 23 ("The Lord is my shepherd"), or the Lord's Prayer. If possible, say a prayer that is familiar to the infant or toddler. Singing a hymn is appropriate if it is done quietly and especially if it is familiar to the young child whom you are visiting. If the parent would like to take the lead in the prayer or hymn, let him.

3. Always make sure that your hands are clean. If you must touch an infant or toddler, gently touch the top of the head and never touch his hands or face.

Preschoolers (3–5 Years Old)

Normal Development

PHYSICAL

The preschooler is in love with life and learning! Constantly moving and continuously talking, she explores her world through touching it and asking questions. She can now run, climb, and jump well, and she enjoys coloring and making things with clay, even if the objects don't always resemble what they are supposed to be. With a supportive adult or older sibling by her side, she might stretch her own limits in healthy, age-appropriate ways. She likes being able to dress herself (even if not perfectly) and feed herself, especially her favorite foods. Her appetite tends to be healthy, and with all her activity, she tends to sleep well at night. Her vocabulary grows by hundreds of words every few weeks, and she probably loves to sing, especially enchanted by rhymes.

PSYCHOLOGICAL

Erikson noted that this was the stage of *initiative versus guilt*. With their growing independence, preschoolers love to take the initiative in doing things. As long as their initiative leads to success, they are happy. When their initiative does not lead to success, and especially when it leads to more work for others, they might feel guilty, especially if that guilt is imposed on them by the adults in their lives or older siblings. Preschoolers express their guilt by acting out (e.g., hitting, throwing objects, etc.), tearfulness, or whininess. Some preschoolers who have not passed beyond the toddler tendency to temper tantrums might experience them as well. All these behaviors underscore how frustrated the preschooler feels in not being able to do what he wants to do when he wants to do it, a hard lesson for every human being.

SOCIAL

Preschoolers are usually very happy and very friendly with others. They enjoy playing with other children their age, although they still might have a problem sharing toys or a parent's attention with others. If they're over-indulged with material things, they might also become demanding or greedy.

COGNITIVE

Piaget called this stage *preoperational;* simply stated, it means that young children have a "logic" all their own, which is not at all how adults understand the term. Preschoolers do not understand and have no use for adult logic. For them, cause and effect can run forward or backward, and an association between two things means causation. Furthermore, they might attribute a causative relationship to things that actually have no relationship, let alone a causative one. Preschoolers have difficulty distinguishing reality from fantasy. It is difficult to say for certain whether most preschoolers are lying when they tell a "story," because they might really believe what they are saying. In addition, although they are learning words and songs at a brisk pace, they have difficulty ordering the sequence of events in a simple story.

SPIRITUAL

Fowler called the preschool stage *intuitive-projective.* Intuition is a sixth sense about something: we know about it even though no one taught us, and we didn't directly read about it. Projection is placing onto a unique person, place, situation, or thing one's experience from a similar person, place, situation, or thing from the past. In terms of God, preschoolers have insights about God that most logical adults simply don't have; because preschoolers think "outside the box," they are not constrained by thoughts that seem foolish. Their ideas about God are not necessarily wrong, but they are different from what adults would think and certainly express. Preschoolers tend to project onto God both the positive and negative attributes of those closest to them (i.e., their parents). If her father becomes angry when she doesn't eat her vegetables, God is angry also. If her mother tenderly rocks her to sleep when she's scared, God does, too. A child at this stage can be particularly harmed if she is abused by an adult who gives the impression that God wanted the adult to abuse her or that God will punish her if she tells on the abuser.

How Illness or Loss Affects Development

COMMON WAYS THAT PRESCHOOLERS REACT TO NEGATIVE EVENTS

Illness or loss can affect preschoolers' growing sense of independence. If a preschooler is ill, he might not be able to play outside or leave the hospital; if the family is facing some loss, he might be overprotected and not have the opportunities to develop like a normal child. In other words, such a child might not be permitted to take initiative. Consequently, he might regress to behavior more typical of younger children.

Because their coping skills are still rudimentary, most preschoolers react to negative events in their lives with tears or acting out in some way. Like their younger counterparts, serious negative events might interfere with appetite, activity, and sleep. Nightmares might follow in the wake of a negative event, thus disrupting sleep. Children need to be gently reassured when nightmares occur; it is terrifying to awaken in the dark after having a scary dream, especially if that child's life is different than it used to be.

Because they are trying to make sense of the world, preschoolers might ask endless questions about what has happened or is happening. These kinds of questions are good because, without them, children speculate as to causes of "bad" things, and in their prelogical stage, their explanations might not only be wrong but also terrifying. For example, a girl whose father has died believes that he did so because she wasn't nice to him. A boy who is ill believes that his illness is caused by something "bad" that he did. An actual example from my own experience follows. A four-year-old was warned by her mother not to leave the yard because a car might hit her if she wandered into the street. Chasing a ball, the girl ran into the street and was struck by a car. In the hospital, the child repeatedly stated that the car hit her because she was bad; in other words, the car was sent to hit her because she disobeyed her mother. No amount of explanation could change her mind.

Children of this age frequently believe that if something happens, they caused it. Such self-centered thinking is normal at this age, but not necessarily helpful. Furthermore, they frequently believe that whatever happened is some kind of punishment for what they did, and this is so even when a child does not have overly punitive parents. From the perspective of a preschooler, being ill does seem like punishment. He is confined to his hospital room, his room at home, or his house, and can't go out and play. He can't eat the foods he likes, and maybe he can't even eat at all. Grown-ups do things that hurt, like draw blood or administer shots, and these seem like punishments. Children might wonder what they did that was so bad that God is punishing them or won't listen to their prayers. It is useless to debate these points with a preschooler who is not thinking logically when the adult presumably is. It is better for an adult to ask what the preschooler's opinion is, and—unless it is completely wrong and needs to be corrected—to offer her (i.e., the adult's) opinion. This forms the foundation of good communication.

As an aside, even when human-made or natural disasters occur, preschoolers will assume that somebody did something to deserve it. Preschoolers will ask who was bad that a hurricane, tornado, or earthquake destroyed a certain town; they will ask what the United States did that made the Twin Towers fall in New York on 9/11. Furthermore, because of their limited capacity to understand distance or time, when they see an image of an event, they might think that it is very close to their homes or that it is happening now, even when neither might be the case. Preschoolers think in the present; to them, every event is happening in the present tense.

Sometimes, preschoolers will respond to negative events by pretending that they didn't happen and continuing to play. Although this behavior upsets many adults, it is the way that some children process and cope with negative events. Indeed, many children work through their anger, grief, loss, and fears precisely through play.

Fear is a strong emotion. Young children are afraid of being abandoned by loved ones when they need them most; they also fear pain. When children are ill, nurses or doctors might ask parents to leave at certain times while procedures are being performed, and this is agonizing for preschoolers, because they need Mommy or Daddy precisely at that time. Physical pain evokes much fear in young children, who will cry and scream (seemingly out of proportion to the pain experienced), either from a needle or from the illness/injury itself. It is usually not helpful to tell a preschooler to be a big boy or big girl and stop crying, because no preschooler is a "big" boy or girl; in such a situation, the preschooler might be petrified and tears are appropriate.

Helpful and Unhelpful Coping Strategies by Adults

Adults who trivialize a child's distress exacerbate a negative situation. Ridiculing, teasing, or shaming has no place in the care of a child who is truly suffering (regardless of the cause) or in pain. Although many adults might indicate that they are only saying or doing such things in order to distract a child, there are better ways of diverting a child's attention. All human beings—regardless of their age—need to have their fears, concerns, and questions taken seriously.

Similarly, overprotection or hovering over a child gives the impression that the situation is even worse than he imagines, which, in turn, makes him more fearful. Preschoolers have vivid imaginations, and when adults act frightened, children will conclude that something more is wrong than the parents (or medical team) are saying.

Adults who work with children who are ill, grieving, or fearful need to remain calm and gentle. There is no need to pretend to be stronger than one really is, but there is a need for the adult to say, unequivocally, that she is on the child's side and will be there for her, no matter what. The adult should support the child in whatever way seems best for that child. Some children might want to be held, while others will prefer playing a game or quiet conversation. More important, adults need to permit a child to ask whatever questions she has without judging those questions as unacceptable. And, perhaps most important, adults need to answer those questions as honestly as they can, without undue detail and without lies. Asking the child, "What do you think?" helps adults to dispel erroneous ideas that a child might have. This is especially true when God questions arise, such as "Why did God do this?" or "Why won't God do that?"

Furthermore, acknowledging a child's fears really does help him to work through them. When fears are ignored or trivialized, the child feels that he has nowhere to go with them. Engaging in conversation about these fears means that the adult is ready to hear the child's perspectives about the fears and then offer her own, ideally suggesting some strategies for working through them.

The Role of the Media in the Reactions of Preschoolers

Like their younger counterparts, preschoolers don't understand everything they see, but they are much better able to devise ideas about what is happening and why. Scary images will frighten preschoolers, no matter how much they try to be brave, so children undergoing negative situations in their lives might need their media exposure carefully monitored. Various forms of media should never be used to entertain a preschooler unless you are sure that there is not and will not be negative graphic images. Even a seemingly "innocent" image—for example, a little baby—might greatly upset a preschooler whose baby brother is very sick in the hospital or whose mother is pregnant and ill. A hospitalized child might be very frightened if a medical program is being broadcast on the TV in his room, especially if adults (or children) are portrayed as injured, angry, or afraid. Although preschoolers can talk about what they see and hear, they might not do so unless they trust those who ask them about the images and sounds. If they internalize frightening images and sounds, they are less able to rally the strength and resiliency they need in the face of difficult circumstances.

Suggestions for Psychospiritual Care for Preschoolers[2]

1. Approach a preschooler with a soft voice and a smile. If he looks at you with interest, say your name and interact with him from a distance initially. If he will not look at you, don't stare or demand that he look at you. Instead, give him space.
2. Introduce yourself to adults in the room, and ask how they are. Never speak *about* the preschooler as if she were not in the room.
3. Any conversation with a preschooler should be led by him. Although you can certainly ask a question, it's up to him to respond.
4. Preschoolers sometimes ask questions about why God doesn't make them better or happy again, if God is mad at them, or if God knows where they are. Ask such a child what she thinks is going on with God. Answer any question briefly, but do *not* argue with a child's point of view.
5. If children or their parents mention God, prayer, or a faith community in some way, consider asking if they would like to pray. If they say yes, do so, and if not, don't. If the child would like to pray, ask him what prayer he would like to say and if he would like to lead it. In these matters, follow his lead.

Early Elementary School–Age Children (5–10 Years Old)

Normal Development

PHYSICAL

Taller, heavier, stronger, and more agile, elementary school–age children enjoy their bodies' abilities. They like to play physical games like tag and softball; they like to stretch their abilities by running faster and jumping higher. Their fine motor skills are improving as well, so they like to color, draw, and make objects with their hands. Their vocabulary is impressive, and they seem to have boundless energy. Most elementary school–age children have excellent appetites, sleep well, and get a lot of exercise, although there is an increasing tendency for many children of this age to be sedentary.

PSYCHOLOGICAL

Erikson called the stage of elementary school–age children *industry versus inferiority*. Young elementary school–age children are learning many things in school and in life. The adults in their lives stress that if the children work hard, they will succeed. So children work hard and are pleased to see the results of their work, which encourages them to work even harder. Yet no matter how hard some children work, they never excel; many times, they can't even find a single area at which they can be solidly competent. This can lead to feelings of inferiority.

SOCIAL

Children of this age begin to have best friends, peers with whom they can play, talk on the phone, and sit with at lunch. Such friendships teach important lessons about fairness, give-and-take, and forgiveness. Although squabbles frequently occur, if adults steer clear of them, most children work them out themselves.

COGNITIVE

Children of this age are challenged by the many subjects that they must master in school. They must learn letters, words, spelling, reading, and writing. They must learn numbers and arithmetic functions. They must learn about the world at large through science, history, and geography. Unlike their younger counterparts, they can no longer count on an idiosyncratic "logic" to get them through, for all these fields are subject to adult logic. In order to learn what they need to know by heart, they first must learn through their hands. In other words, they need concrete objects to learn. For example, if a person takes two cookies from eight cookies, she will be left with six. Collecting leaves in the fall demonstrates that each tree's leaves are not only shaped differently than others, they're also different colors, even different hues of the same color. Flash cards help children of this age learn their spelling words for the test. Piaget called this stage *concrete operations.*

SPIRITUAL

Fowler noted that children of this age love myths—stories about good versus evil in which the heroes and heroines are larger than life. He also noted that children of this age are very literal in the way they think. That makes sense since they are rewarded in school for being very literal. Words have to be spelled in a certain way in order for them to be marked correct; numbers have to be added and subtracted just right to get the correct answer. A child doesn't get credit for a wrong answer. At this age, what children learn is very cut-and-dried, and that spills over into their faith lives as well. They love the stories in scripture; the more amazing the story, the better! That appeals to their "mythic" stage. But they are very literal in their knowledge. For children of this age, there are right answers about God, and there are wrong answers about God; there are no gray areas or areas of ambiguity. They are literalists when it comes to stories from scripture and the tenets of their faith traditions.

How Illness or Loss Affects Development

COMMON WAYS THAT YOUNG ELEMENTARY SCHOOL-AGE CHILDREN REACT TO NEGATIVE EVENTS

No child wants to feel left out or different from his peers. When an illness, loss, or family situation makes a child feel different, it might have an impact on his self-esteem. Illness or a family situation might mean that a child can't attend school, be on the team, or do his favorite things; it is not uncommon for such children to worry that no one will like them any longer or that the other kids will think they are dumb, since they are missing so much school. In addition, the physical pain or side effects associated with medical regimens might make them feel sick and grouchy all the time.

Young elementary school–age children have an increasing ability to make sense of their world, by asking questions and learning through reading or listening. When something "bad" happens, their first impulse is to try to explain it in the best ways they can. Since they are just learning adult logic, their ideas are not always on target. In addition, they are still a bit self-focused, so they continue (to some degree) to attribute fault to themselves if something goes bad. For example, an eight-year-old boy is convinced that he is responsible for his baby sister's illness, because he told her that he hated her. A seven-year-old believes that the reason her father left her and her mom is that she tore up a picture of her father when she was angry with him. A nine-year-old is convinced that he has a brain tumor because he once used a cell phone, and he heard a news story about cancer and cell phone usage. A six-year-old believes that her father was killed by a drunk driver because she forgot to pray for him before she went to bed on the night that he died. After 9/11 and several natural disasters, many children wondered whether people had done something wrong or whether God was angry with human beings as a whole.

Regardless of how children work out the details of why something bad happened, they are often left with anxiety. As with younger children, this anxiety can manifest itself in tearfulness or acting-out behaviors, such as arguing, cursing, or destroying property. Sometimes, it is all talk, full of raw bravado, especially among little boys, who declare that they will "zap" their cancer cells or "kill" the bad guys who create terror.

Although children of this age do usually have better coping skills than younger children, not all of them cope well, and such coping ability is a function of their pre-event personalities. Many children, when seriously ill, will regress to a younger age, when they were healthier. Other children, when faced with the impending death of a parent, try to re-create life the way it was before Mom was so ill. Even at this young age, some children turn to alcohol or drugs, especially if those around them do so and they can get a supply. Other children become addicted to food, video games, or television.

Children of this age might take their frustration out on those who love them the most in a kind of "You only hurt the ones you love" scenario. Some children are terrors at home or with relatives, but are still well-behaved in school or with friends because it is important for them to maintain control in some situations. Some of these children might be physically or verbally abusive with health care professionals, especially nurses, who are charged with their care. Other children, especially those in chronic pain, lash out at anyone who comes close. Children who suffer from a chronic illness might experience a double dose of suffering. They might have pain (which is bad enough), but they also might be limited in what they can do currently. At an age when it's important to play outside with friends, such children might be "stuck" in a hospital room or at home, unable to engage in normal activities, such as team sports or school. This increases their suffering, especially if their friends don't visit, call, or e-mail.

Because no child wants to feel "different" from others his age, if an illness (or its treatment) has caused changes in his body, he might refuse to see anybody. To prove that they're not "different," some of these children will "forget" to take needed medications, in an effort to see if they're really needed in the first place. Even a child who has lost a parent to death or lost a house to a tornado feels "different" and doesn't want others to look too hard at him. When such a child is around others, he might put on a brave face, saying outwardly that everything is alright or that it's "no big deal," all the while mourning inwardly.

Finally, the issue of God's role in a child's situation is an important, though potentially difficult, one to address. Many children raised in a particular faith tradition believe that God loves them, is their best friend, and will help them. In addition, they believe that they communicate with God through prayer. Imagine their distress when their prayers are not answered! It's hard enough for adults to understand unanswered prayers, but it's nearly impossible for many children because they take God so seriously. A human best friend will usually do anything for his friend. If God is the child's best friend and the child petitions God in prayer, then why is he still infected with HIV? Why did Mommy die? Why doesn't the family have a home to which to return? Why did terrorists blow up another building, killing more people? Because children of this age are so literal, they conclude that God isn't listening, is too busy, doesn't love them, or is angry at them when prayers for "important" things are not answered. It does not help to argue with such points of view.

Helpful and Unhelpful Coping Strategies by Adults

As stated previously, adults who themselves are out of control do not help children to maintain control. Adults in highly charged emotional states, such as wailing, yelling, or cursing, do not bring calm to a child. Attempts to make jokes or trivialize what the child is feeling are also usually not helpful, because they fail to take her situation seriously. Adults who refuse to engage children in conversation, refuse to answer their questions, or lie to children do more harm than good because children experiencing something "bad" need to talk, be listened to, and be affirmed. Adults should not project their feelings onto a child in an attempt to "toughen her up." A child is not a little adult; she is a child and should be treated as one.

What does a helpful adult do? He listens attentively, asking questions for clarification, but letting the child do most of the talking. He answers questions as honestly as he can, unafraid to say, "I don't know." He commiserates with the child whenever he can. He refrains from giving pat or glib answers to questions or concerns that mean a great deal to the child. If a child brings "God talk" up, a helpful adult is open, and, if he feels uncomfortable with the subject, he tries to find another person with whom the child can be relaxed enough to open up. He honors the child and takes the child's concerns seriously.

A helpful adult tries to alleviate the child's suffering in any way she can, including advocating appropriate pain medication if the child is in serious pain. She encourages the reestablishment of a routine to increase the chances that the child will feel "normal" again. She remembers his age and his circumstances. She is there on both the good and bad days and doesn't take the bad days personally. She permits the child to do what he can and does not expect him to do what he can't; she, too, does what she can and doesn't beat herself up for not doing what is not in her power to do.

Even though such persons sound like saints, they are just human beings trying their best to alleviate the suffering of children. In this way, children meet the love of God in and through other human beings.

The Role of Media in How Elementary School–Age Children React to "Bad" Events

Many elementary school–age children have a certain fascination with the macabre; in some cases, they have nightmares after viewing such images or can't get them out of their minds. If they view media that highlights the macabre or the violent, especially in relation to a natural or human-made disaster, murder, or car crash, they might dwell on it, becoming overwhelmed with fear and anxiety. On the other hand, some elementary school–age children, usually boys, actually enjoy the blood and gore and relate it to their own situations with gusto, almost trying to "weird out" adults who speak to them. As with younger children, it is probably best to minimize exposure to violent, bloody, or frightening images, especially when children have so many other negative events in their lives.

Suggestions for Psychospiritual Care for Elementary School–Age Children[3]

1. Approach an elementary school–age child quietly, with a soft voice and a smile. Acknowledge (with a smile) the parent or other adult(s) in the room, but speak to the child *first*. If she responds or looks at you with interest, introduce yourself and initiate a conversation. If she is in the middle of doing something—watching TV, for example—don't keep interrupting or demanding that she look at you. Instead, ask her if this is a good time to visit. If she asks you to leave, consider doing so. It might be a bad time for her.

2. Introduce yourself to the parent or other adult(s) in the room. Never speak *about* the elementary school–age child as if he were not in the room; that is rude. Also, try not to permit a parent to speak for her child; indicate that it's important for you to hear what the child himself wants to say.

3. Any conversation with a child of this age should be led by him. Although you can certainly initiate a question, it's up to him to respond. In addition, there might be topics that would be better left unexplored. Letting the child lead the conversation makes it more likely that such topics will not be broached.

4. Children of this age are sometimes rude in the way they express themselves, especially when they are ill, frustrated, or sad. Although adults need to ease up a bit when children are not at their best, the intentional hurting of another (either physically or verbally) cannot be permitted. If a child is really out of sorts, leave.

5. If a child cries, let her cry without trying hard to cheer her up or make her laugh. You can ask her if she would like a tissue or if she would like to talk about what is making her so sad. Never trivialize her concerns or questions.

6. Children of this age sometimes ask questions about why God doesn't make them better or happy again, if God is mad at them, or if God still knows where they are. Ask such a child what she thinks is going on with God, as that will provide insight into her way of thinking. Answer any question briefly, but do not argue with a child's point of view, and do not become personally offended if she expresses anger at or disappointment in God. After all, many people in scripture did the same thing! Instead, gently express your own ideas, never being afraid to say, "I don't know" (which will usually be the most honest answer to many questions). Above all, always assure such a child of God's love and care.

7. If children or their parents mention God, prayer, or a faith community in some way, consider asking if they would like to pray. If they say yes, do so, and if not, don't. Never force prayer. If he would like to pray, ask him what prayer he would like to say and if he will lead it. Keep prayers simple. Never "judge" a child's prayer for it is his way of speaking to God.

Preteens and Young Adolescents (10–14 Years Old)

Normal Development

PHYSICAL

The elementary school–age child is growing up fast. Now she looks like a young lady, instead of a little girl; he looks like a young man, instead of a little boy. Both girls and boys grow in height, and they gain weight. Girls tend to become curvaceous, while boys gain muscle mass. Sexual characteristics appear, as girls develop breasts and have the onset of their menstrual periods, while boys develop adult male sexual organs, have an increase of hair on the body, and experience voice changes. For the most part, both girls and boys like these bodily changes, although they might be self-conscious if they develop either much earlier or much later than their peers.

If these young teens are interested, they can develop their bodies to become quite proficient at some sport or large-muscle physical activity, or they can become better at a fine motor endeavor that requires skill and hand-eye coordination.

PSYCHOLOGICAL

Erikson described the adolescent stage as *identity versus role diffusion*, meaning that the young person needs to establish an identity separate from that of his parents or family. The question seems to be this: Who is he in his own right? To do this, the young person tries to do things differently than his parents might do them and tries to develop interests that they would not share. Those children at the younger end of this age group are just beginning this process, while those at the older end are well into it. Although this is a normal part of growing up, role diffusion can be negative if it includes hanging out with the wrong crowd, experimenting with alcohol or drugs, or engaging in illegal or immoral activities.

SOCIAL

The preteen and young adolescent is just beginning to get interested in the opposite sex and usually feels more comfortable with her best friend or with a small group of friends. Initially, interaction with the opposite sex is facilitated by group activities, where there is much moral support. Girls of this age can spend hours on the phone, talking to someone whom they've seen all day in school.

COGNITIVE

Piaget noted that as adolescence was approached and then reached, young people had a greater capacity for abstract thought. He called this the *formal operations* stage, which is the adult stage of thought. The young teen can imagine himself in situations in which he has never been and can reflect seriously upon his future. He can also imagine a number of possible answers to various questions. No longer does he need concrete objects to learn every skill; some of his learning can be entirely through thought or by reading about or seeing something of interest.

SPIRITUAL

In terms of spiritual development, the young person moves into the Fowlerian stage of *synthetic-conventional*. The conventional is the norm, while the synthetic is the bringing together of many parts. Young people still have a strong sense of the conventional because it wasn't so long ago that they were literal in their faith. In other words, they still identify with the faith tradition in which they've been raised. Yet, as they grow up and meet many people, some of whom have very different beliefs than they do, they try to put it all together. Surely, other religions have good people; what do those people believe, and why? How do their beliefs compare with those of the young person? It is at this age that many young people begin to ask serious questions of their faith tradition and even of God in terms of why there is so much natural and human-made evil in the world.

How Illness or Loss Affects Development

COMMON WAYS THAT PRETEENS AND YOUNG TEENS REACT TO NEGATIVE EVENTS

To young people approaching adulthood, an illness or loss can be devastating. Just when they should be more independent, they have to be dependent on their parents for the most basic of needs. Just when they should be forging their own identity, they continue to be someone's daughter or son because they cannot do anything on their own. Just when their bodies and minds should be at peak performance, they are limited—sometimes because of their illness and the side effects of the medications that they must take, and sometimes because of the craziness in their families or living situations. Many domains of development may grind to a halt, or actual regression in development may occur. Either of these can be fostered by parents or other caregivers who are (understandably) highly protective of their ill, grieving, or fearful teens.

Although young teens are able to understand that sometimes bad things just happen, that doesn't mean that they have to like them. Like younger children, they may react with anger and acting out, or with tears and sadness. Sometimes, children of this age will try to rationalize "bad" events in the hope that making cognitive sense of them will enable them to better accept them. Preteens and young teens have very definite opinions about things in general, and they are usually not shy about sharing these opinions. Other young people pretend that nothing has happened, or that they are invincible; in that regard, they might "forget" to take needed medications in an attempt to prove that they don't need them. Still other young teens act as if, even though an event happened, it doesn't matter to them. All these are efforts to try to cope with an unwanted situation. Obviously, the healthiest way of coping is to acknowledge that a loss is occurring or has occurred and work through it, with a trusted adult or friend. But for some young people, this is far easier said than done, especially if their own coping skills are poorly developed, and there is not much support for them at home or among their friends.

A complicating factor is the young person's increasing maturity. Why call this complicating? For the first time, an ill, dying, grieving, or petrified child can both easily remember what life was like in happier times (i.e., when she was normal or could do more) and can have a sense of what she will miss in the future because of her illness or loss. A child of this age who is dying knows that he will never be a doctor when he grows up because he will never grow up. A girl whose parent was killed in a robbery or by a drunk driver knows that the parent will never be there for her wedding day.

Like younger children, young teens might treat those who love them the most very badly. A girl might not want to see her friends because her appearance has changed, or because her friends will look at her "weird" because she has lost a body part, a parent, or a place to live. Although she might state that she doesn't care if anybody communicates with her, she is frequently quite wounded if no one calls or writes. Various thoughts may enter her mind: Am I that easy to forget? Don't I matter to anyone?

Young teens can also be extraordinarily rude to nurses who are trying to care for them. They don't like to think that they are "guinea pigs," with doctors or nurses "experimenting" on them. They might hate the taste of certain medications, the pain of certain injections, and the side effects of certain treatments. All these limit the amount of cooperation that a young person might be willing to give to the medical team. When we also consider that an ill young person might be confined to bed or to her home, might not be able to eat normally, might be in constant pain, or might fear that she will be "nothing" in a very short time, it is no wonder that her coping skills are stretched to the limit. At a time when she wants to grow up like all the other kids her age, she is forced to be treated like someone much younger, and, to add insult to injury, her plight might never get any better than it is at present. This might precipitate thoughts about killing herself. It is no wonder that many young people in such circumstances need and benefit from mental health services.

They might also need and benefit from spiritual care, but the person who offers such care must be chosen carefully, because young teens have radar for hypocrites. Young people who are suffering want and need someone who will not be afraid of their questions, opinions, and anger. They have every right to feel cheated, but they do not have the right to hurt others or themselves. And some young teens do hurt themselves with alcohol or drugs, especially if members of their family do so or friends do so, and they can get a supply of drugs or alcohol. Other teens become addicted to sex, food, video games, or television.

Helpful and Unhelpful Coping Strategies by Adults

Adults can try to be people who will listen and who do not pretend or presume to have all the answers. They can refrain from constantly chastising a young teen for "talking that way" when the young person is ranting and raving. They can resolve not to lie to the young teen or to trivialize his fears, no matter how unreasonable or unlikely they might be. The best adult is one who takes his lead from the teen in a spirit of humility, knowing that he has not experienced what the teen is going through.

As was the case for working with a younger child, a helpful adult tries to alleviate the teen's suffering in any way he can, including advocating for appropriate pain management. He encourages the reestablishment of as normal as possible routine. He encourages friends to visit, call, text-message, or e-mail. When working with a teen who is ill or experiencing loss, he gives her enough space to do what she can without expectations that she will do more than she is able to do.

Mature, helpful adults seek to do what can be done, without being guilty over what cannot be done; they are there for the long haul—on both good and bad days. When bad days occur, which they will, helpful adults don't take the bad days personally. The example of such adults helps the young person to meet the love of God in and through fellow human beings.

Who are unhelpful adults? Those who talk too much, know it all, do not permit a young person to have a bad day, judge too much and accept too little, lie to "protect" the young person or for their own advantage, pry, try too hard to cheer up the suffering teen, or trivialize what the teen is experiencing—all these behaviors are not only unhelpful, they might be deadly. Such adults seem determined to control the situation and the teen, and that can spell disaster and tragedy. Sometimes, such adults are related to the teen, while at other times, they are part of the medical team.

The Role of the Media in How Young Teens React to Negative Events

Young teens are highly influenced by various media, and certain media are quite harmful. These include TV shows, movies, and video games that suggest that violence can solve any problem; that suicide is an acceptable form of problem resolution; that everyone is doing alcohol or drugs; and that everyone is having sex without any lasting consequences. For example, if suicide is glamorized, a terminally ill teen might decide to end it all and bypass his suffering. If violence is glamorized, a grieving teen might decide to avenge his father's death. If extramarital sex is glorified, an unwanted pregnancy (or a sexually transmitted disease) might result from engaging in unprotected sex, and if drugs and alcohol seem to be the things to do, death might result from overdoses. Why do teens do these things? They do so either to demonstrate that they have control over their bodies, or to demonstrate that whatever they do doesn't matter in the long run.

Suggestions for Psychospiritual Care for Preteens and Young Adolescents[4]

1. When you enter the room, introduce yourself and ask if you might visit. If the patient refuses to speak to you or asks you to leave, don't remain. You are not there for yourself and your own ego needs.

2. Introduce yourself to any adults in the room. Never speak *about* the young teen as if he were not in the room; that is demeaning. Try not to permit a parent (or another adult) to speak for the teen, by emphasizing that it is important for you to hear from the teen directly.

3. Do not launch into a discussion of religious or spiritual issues; connect with the young person on some other topic first. Religious or spiritual issues are very personal, and many preteens and young teens have a suspicion about "church types" or those who seem "holier than thou."

4. Always respect the wishes of preteens and young teens, especially their need for privacy. Even if they wish to speak about spiritual issues, some will want to talk about such issues in the presence of their parents; others will not. Always ask a teen if she would like her parent to remain, and abide by her decision.

5. Any conversation with a young teen should be led by her. Although you can ask a question, it's up to her to respond and move the conversation along. Because there might be topics that would be better left alone, letting the teen lead the conversation makes it more likely that such topics will not be raised.

6. Young teens can be very emotional or rude when they are ill, frustrated, or sad. Although adults need to be understanding with such teens, the intentional hurting of another person (physically or verbally) cannot be permitted. If a young teen is really cranky, end the visit. If a young teen cries, remember that he is having a hard time. Don't try to cheer him up, make him laugh, or trivialize his concerns or questions by making jokes. You can certainly offer him your presence and concern by asking him if he wants a tissue or wants to talk about what is upsetting him.

7. Young teens frequently ask questions about why God doesn't make them or life better again, if God is angry at them, or if God is punishing them. They might express their own anger at God for being unfair or for permitting suffering in their lives or in the world. Listen quietly, but do not argue with the teen. Do not become personally offended if she expresses anger at or disappointment in God; after all, even the psalmist did that! Instead, quietly express

your own ideas. Answer questions as honestly as you can, never being afraid to say, "I don't know" (which will usually be the most honest answer) to many questions. Above all, assure her of God's love and care. Your calm, accepting presence is the best evidence of your own belief in God's love.

8. If the teen has mentioned God, prayer, or a faith community in some way, consider asking her if she would like to pray. If she says yes, do so, and if not, don't. If she would like to pray, ask her what prayer she would like to say and if she would lead it. Never "judge" the teen's prayer, for it is her way of communicating with God in the midst of her suffering.

Older Adolescents (15–19 Years Old)

Normal Development

PHYSICAL

Most older adolescents have achieved their adult height, and they look like young adult men and women. Muscle mass and fat distribution are appropriate for their gender; exercise might promote greater muscle mass, while a sedentary lifestyle promotes more fat deposits. Older adolescents are stronger than many adults, and if they take a keen interest in a skill, they frequently can master it without difficulty.

PSYCHOLOGICAL

Older adolescents are firmly in Erikson's *identity versus role diffusion* stage, although by the time that they are in the latter years of adolescence, only a few are truly diffuse in their roles or goals. Much of their "diffusiveness" depends on the "diffusiveness" of their peer group. For a discussion of this stage, see the "Psychological" subsection under "Preteen and Young Adolescents."

SOCIAL

Although most older adolescents have a best friend of their own gender, they are probably still part of a group of friends, male and female. In addition, most adolescents date, with a fair percentage becoming sexually active. Peer pressure might be strong in terms of dating, sexual activity (and the types thereof), and alcohol and drug use.

COGNITIVE

Piaget's *formal operations* stage continues. For a discussion of this stage, see the subsection titled "Cognitive" under "Preteens and Young Adolescents."

SPIRITUAL

Fowler's stage for older adolescents is called *individuative-reflective*. It is reflective in that it takes much interior work to sort out what a person believes and accepts and what he cannot believe or accept. It is individuative because no one can do the work for anyone else. Can the young person believe what her parents believe and accept those religious beliefs wholeheartedly, or must she find a different way? This stage can take many years and much reflection. Illness and loss of any kind make the search all the more difficult and poignant.

How Illness or Loss Affects Development

COMMON WAYS THAT OLDER ADOLESCENTS REACT TO NEGATIVE EVENTS

Much of what has been said in the corresponding subsection under "Preteens and Young Adolescents" applies to older adolescents as well. In addition to what was mentioned in that section, several other points should be highlighted.

Because older adolescents are closer to leaving home than they were when they were younger, they experience an enormous impact from an illness or condition that forces them to depend on their parents for some of their most basic of needs. After all, what normal eighteen-year-old needs his parents to help him use the toilet? What normal seventeen-year-old requires her mother's assistance in dressing? How can teens forge their own identities under such circumstances? Loving parents want to be helpful. Many are (understandably) protective of their ill, grieving, or fearful teen, so afraid of losing him that they do too much, keeping him in a perpetual state of childhood. Some development ceases; actual regression in development may occur. Although older teens are usually embarrassed by this, many parents welcome their teen's dependence as a chance to "take good care" of them.

Older adolescents are sophisticated enough to understand that sometimes bad things just happen, but that doesn't mean that they have to accept them. Like younger children, they can react with anger and acting out, or with tears and sadness. In fact, on some days, older adolescents may act like children, and on other days like mature adults. Some older adolescents try to rationalize "bad" events, act as if nothing has happened or that they don't care, or act as if they were invincible; in that regard, they might "forget" to take needed medications (e.g., a diabetic teen who "forgets" to take insulin) to prove that they really don't need them. All these are unhealthy strategies to cope with a difficult situation.

Obviously, the healthiest strategy is to acknowledge that a loss is occurring or has occurred and work through it, with the assistance of trusted adults or peers. For some young people, this is an enormous challenge, especially if their own coping skills are poorly developed or they lack the support of family or peers.

An older adolescent's ever-increasing maturity means that, whether she is ill, dying, grieving, or petrified, she can both easily remember the way her life was previously and can have a sense of what she will miss in the future because of her illness or loss. An older adolescent who is dying knows that she will not live to enter law school. A teen whose parent was killed in a random act of violence knows that his parent will never be there for his graduation.

Adolescents in crisis share the unfortunate human tendency to treat those who love them the most very badly. They might yell and curse at their parents or younger siblings. They might cut off all contact with their friends or might not want their friends to see them because their appearance has changed, or because their friends will look at them "weird." They might act as if they really don't care if their friends keep in touch, but they are usually very wounded when friends no long call, e-mail, text-message, or visit.

An older adolescent can be incredibly rude to nurses who are trying to care for him, and because he may be larger than his health care providers, he can be quite intimidating if he's angered. He might think that the medical team is somehow "experimenting" on him. This is especially true when medications or treatments cause even more discomfort or pain than he already has. Such associated side effects limit the amount of cooperation that teens might be willing to give to the medical team, especially if they think that members of the team are "losers" or "idiots." When an ill young person is confined to bed or to his home, is not able to eat normally, is in constant pain, knows that his situation is not likely to improve, or fears that he will become "nothing" very shortly, it is no wonder that his coping skills are stretched to the limit. As was the case with younger teens, many young people in these circumstances need and benefit from mental health services.

They might also need and benefit from spiritual care, but the person who offers such care must be chosen carefully, because older adolescents might be very skeptical of "religious freaks." Older adolescents want and need someone who will not be afraid of their crisis-related God questions, opinions, and anger. They have every right to feel cheated, and any adult providing spiritual care to such teens does well to acknowledge that.

Helpful and Unhelpful Coping Strategies by Adults

As has already been discussed in the corresponding subsection under "Preteens and Young Adolescents," the most helpful adults listen without interrupting, do not pretend to have all the answers, do not constantly berate a teen for her attitudes, judge little and accept a great deal, tell the truth, and never trivialize a teen's fears, no matter how unreasonable or unlikely they might be.

Unhelpful adults talk too much and listen too little, convey a sense of superiority, forbid the expression of normal emotions, lie to "protect" or for their own advantage, are nosy, try too hard to make jokes or be cheerful, or trivialize the teen's experience. Such adults need to be in control of the situation and the teen, and that can spell disaster and tragedy, because it is completely unrealistic. After all, who can control the progression of a disease? Who can control the length and depth of another's grief? Adults who need to exert control might be relatives or part of the medical team or the pastoral staff.

The Role of the Media in How Older Adolescents React to Negative Events

Older teens are still very much influenced by various media. Some media depictions are harmful, such as those suggesting that violence can solve any problem; those promoting violence against women, minorities, or children; those touting suicide as a "cool" form of problem resolution; those implying that smart people can do alcohol or drugs without getting burned; and those claiming that everyone is having lots of sex without any lasting consequences. For example, if suicide is glamorized, a troubled teen might decide to catch some glamour for herself. If violence is glamorized, a grieving teen might decide to avenge his best friend's death, and get some notoriety in the process. If premarital or extramarital sex is glorified, a teen might decide to "score" with many partners in an attempt to prove his worth and invincibility; if drugs and alcohol seem to be the things to do, a lifetime of regrets might result from actions committed while under the influence. Teens engage in such behaviors either to demonstrate that they have control, or to demonstrate that what they do doesn't matter in the long run.

Suggestions for Spiritual Care with Older Adolescents[5]

See the suggestions provided under "Preteens and Young Adolescents."

Compared with younger teens, older adolescents are more likely to (1) want to be visited alone (rather than have their parent[s] present), (2) be even more suspicious of "God talk" or "church talk," (3) express much anger at God, and (4) have even more piercing questions about God and God's ways. They might be much more belligerent than younger children and teens because their frustration is so great. They really can appreciate what life was like before and how different it will be in the future. For example, they might really understand that they are dying, and what that means. Platitudes are never useful in communicating with older adolescents who are ill, grieving, or suffering in any way, but a genuinely caring presence is nearly always of great benefit.

Summary

All health care professionals who work with children and teens who are ill, in crisis, or experiencing a loss do well to understand how illness or loss affects normal development. They should also recognize common ways that children and teens respond to "bad" things in life and the ways that coping strategies of significant adults and friends influence those responses. Because most children and many teens are more holistic in their approach to life than are most adults, offering age-appropriate psychospiritual care can help to relieve the suffering that ill, grieving, or dying children and teens experience, and perhaps the suffering experienced by their parents and siblings as well. This chapter has offered some general guidelines by age.

We adults do well to keep in mind how very hard it is to be young and to be dying or to have a very uncertain future because of a significant loss in life. When we seek to listen more than we speak, and to learn more than we instruct, we can be of greatest service to children, teens, and their parents. We then model the love to which all major religions refer—love of the Divine for the human and human love for one another.

PIAGET STAGES

Birth–2 years: Sensorimotor
Preschool years: Preoperational
Elementary school years: Concrete operations
Adolescence & older: Formal operations

ERIKSON STAGES

Birth–2 years: Trust vs. mistrust
2–3 years: Autonomy vs. shame & doubt
3–5 years: Initiative vs. guilt
5 to 10–12 years: Industry vs. inferiority
Adolescence & older: Identity vs. role diffusion

FOWLER STAGES

Birth to 2–3 years: Undifferentiated faith
Preschool years: Intuitive-projective
Elementary school years: Mythic-literal
Preteen & early adolescent years: Synthetic-conventional
Mid- to later adolescent years: Individuative-reflective

Reflective Activities

1. Did you experience serious illness, loss, or suffering of any kind as a child or teen? What were the circumstances? How long did it take you to adjust to what was happening? Who proved to be the most helpful to you and why? Who was the least helpful and why?

2. Which children or teens is it easier for you to provide care for— those who show their emotions readily or those who keep them hidden? Why do you think you have the preference that you do?

3. Can you be silent in the presence of a child or teen who is ill, grieving, or suffering, or do you need to fill the space with words? How do you react when you ask the child or teen a question and his parents do the responding?

4. What feelings do you have when a child or teen who is ill, grieving, or suffering cries? If you feel discomfort, how do you relieve that discomfort? When a child younger than ten years old cries, what is your immediate response? If a teen cries, what is your immediate response?

5. What reaction do you have when a child or teen who is ill, grieving, or suffering asks many questions? If you cannot answer the questions, how do you usually respond? Does your response to difficult questions or questions to which you do not have the answer vary by the age of the child or teen? By her emotional state? By whether her parents are present?

6. How do you respond to a child's or teen's "God questions" or complaints that God has not answered his prayers? Do you need to defend God or offer pat answers? Do you need to pretend that you didn't hear the questions or complaints in the first place?

Notes

1. Adapted from Fosarelli (2003, 17–19). Used with permission of Liguori Publications, Liguori, MO 63057. 1-800-325-9521. www.liguori.org.

2. Ibid., 26–31.

3. Ibid., 39–45.

4. Ibid., 52–57.

5. Ibid., 63–68.

References

Erikson, Erik. (1985). *Childhood and Society.* New York: W. W. Norton & Co.

Fosarelli, Pat. (2003). *Whatever You Do to the Least of These: Ministering to Ill and Dying Children and Their Families.* Liguori, Mo.: Liguori.

Fowler, James. (1995). *Stages of Faith: The Psychology of Human Development and the Quest for Meaning.* San Francisco: HarperSanFrancisco.

Singer, Dorothy, & Revenson, Tracey (1978). *A Piaget Primer: How a Child Thinks.* New York: New American Library.

8

ADULT SPIRITUALITY FOR
PERSONS WITH CHRONIC ILLNESS

PATRICIA E. MURPHY, GEORGE FITCHETT,
ANDREA L. CANADA

> The Serenity Prayer
> *God, give us grace to accept with serenity*
> *the things that cannot be changed,*
> *Courage to change the things*
> *which should be changed,*
> *and the Wisdom to distinguish*
> *the one from the other.*
> —Reinhold Niebuhr

Introduction

Religion or spirituality (R/S) is an important way for many people with ill-nesses to understand themselves and the events that happen to them. A brief encounter with illness often makes people more aware of their vulnerabilities. A chronic illness has a far more profound impact on well-being, including possible job loss, shift in status in the family, and, perhaps, a premature death. Because chronic illness is persistent and, at times, progressive, those caught in its midst need to draw frequently on coping skills, including R/S. For some this leads to growth and for others to frustration. Research is increasingly able to provide models for the association of R/S and health outcomes. Interventions guided by this research are apt to make the best use of the resources of caregivers as well as of the patients themselves. This chapter will look at a model for religious or spiritual coping that will then be applied to mental disorders and cancer. There is a wealth of research on the relation of R/S to other chronic conditions (Koenig, McCullough, & Larson 2001). We hope this introduction of research-based spiritual interventions will lead the reader to explore this topic further.

Conceptual Model

We have placed our discussion of clinical practice in the context of a theoretical framework as well as research. This section of the chapter elaborates on our theoretical model. R/S provides a worldview beyond the individual. (For a treatment of a variety of worldviews related to spirituality, including various religions, agnosticism, and atheism, see Josephson & Peteet 2004.) A major function of religion is to help us learn to live with life's limitations and tragedies—not only to learn to live with them, but to find meaning in life in the face of them. Some people who consider themselves spiritual, but not religious, develop such a framework outside the teachings of a faith group. Our theoretical model focuses on this process; that is, on how people use R/S to cope with difficult life situations such as serious illness. This model is based on the stress and coping model of Lazarus and Folkman (1984), as well as Kenneth Pargament's (1997) rich description of religious coping.

Figure 8–1 summarizes the model. The model emphasizes four important elements in using R/S to cope with serious illness. The first element is the process of appraisal. You have probably observed that the same situation—recurrence of a serious illness, such as cancer, for example—can evoke very different reactions in different people. One explanation is that people make different judgments or appraisals of the situation. When we are faced with a stressful event, we make two types of appraisals. The first, called a primary appraisal, is a judgment about how dangerous the situation is. Does it look like it will be harmful, possibly threatening, or perhaps, just challenging? Our second judgment or appraisal is about the resources we feel are available to us as we begin to cope with the situation.

Figure 8–1   Conceptual Model of R/S Coping

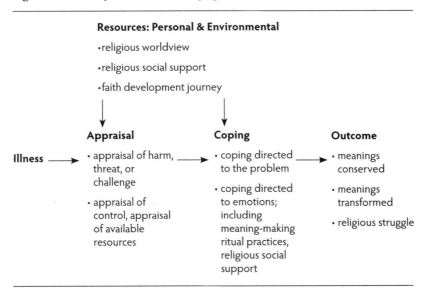

Does the situation appear to be within or beyond our control? Do we feel that we have the resources to help us cope with the situation right now, or are our resources stretched pretty thin?

The second element in our model of R/S coping is the personal and environmental resources that are available to us. You can see that awareness of these resources is part of the process of appraisal. Personal R/S resources include my R/S beliefs, formation, and practices. Environmental resources include support from members of my religious congregation or clergy, or a sense of connection that is part of spirituality. We want to emphasize the importance of three factors in the resources people bring to R/S coping. The first factor is a person's specific religious beliefs, such as belief in a loving God, belief in the power of demonic forces, or belief in a reality greater than oneself. The second factor is whether the person is connected to a congregation or group of people who share her beliefs. The third factor is where a person is in her journey of spiritual development. Where religious people are in the journey can be strongly shaped by their faith community, which, in turn, shapes their specific religious beliefs.

There are many theories of spiritual growth or faith development (Fowler 1981, Maitri 2000). About 86 percent of Americans identify themselves as religious (Hout & Fisher 2002), so we will look in greater detail at religious faith development. The model described by John Westerhoff (1976) sees the pilgrimage of faith proceeding through four styles. The first style is experienced faith, which refers to the nonverbal experience of the trustworthiness of existence, formed in infancy and childhood by our interactions with primary caregivers. The second style is affiliative faith, referring to the beliefs and practices we develop through participation in the religious life of our family. The third style is searching faith, the period when we question the faith of our family. This is a time of experimenting with alternative beliefs and practices, and, perhaps, a time of recognition of our own experiences of the holy. The fourth style is owned faith, referring to a time when, through the process of searching, we have formed a faith in which our beliefs are rooted in our experiences, and our rituals and practices give expression to those beliefs and experiences.

It is easy to see the importance of religious community in the stage of affiliative faith. In this stage, the family and/or the primary faith community communicates foundational beliefs and morals, and introduces the rituals that teach and reinforce them. Religious community also plays an important role in the stages of searching and owned faith. For many people, times of searching faith are experienced as a time of unfaith. Oftentimes, our exemplars in the affiliative period were, by contrast, people of steadfast faith. Religious communities that value and tolerate people in the midst of searching faith are not common. Such communities, when they are found, are often the communities that also welcome people with owned faith. They find themselves enriched, not threatened, by the diversity of beliefs and practices of a group of people with owned faith.

The third main element in our model is R/S coping activities. Some coping activities may be intended to directly address the problem. Other coping activities primarily help with the feelings associated with the problem. Sometimes the same coping activity may help in both ways. Common R/S coping activities include prayer, meditation, and devotional activities. One important aspect of R/S coping with serious illness is finding a balance between doing things that are within one's control and turning the rest over to God or a Higher Power. Another major feature of R/S coping is meaning-making. This is the process of attempting to integrate the meaning of the illness or another crisis into our preexisting beliefs (Park 2005).

The fourth component of our model is the outcomes of R/S coping. Pargament (1997) describes how people will, when possible, conserve key beliefs in the face of stress. However, there are times when illness or other life situations cause a crisis in belief; such times may be followed by transformation of beliefs. There are also times when a crisis in beliefs is not followed by transformation of beliefs, but by a prolonged religious struggle.

A considerable body of research, some of which will be described later in this chapter, has examined different elements of the process of R/S coping with illness. One interesting study has linked several elements of the model we have just described. In that study, Jacobson and colleagues (2006) conducted in-depth interviews with nineteen men and women with HIV/AIDS. They found that the study participants fell into one of four groups:

1. Men and women who had strong religious training, reported no time of searching faith, were able to conserve essential religious beliefs in coming to terms with their illness, and were not experiencing stress.
2. Individuals who had little exposure to religion in childhood, did not find their illness creating a religious crisis, and were not experiencing stress.
3. People who had religious training in childhood, had been through a journey of searching and owned faith, had experienced a religious crisis when they learned of their diagnosis, but were able to further transform meaning, and were not experiencing stress.
4. Patients who were like those in the third group, except that the process of transformation of meaning had not occurred for them. They were in a prolonged period of religious struggle and were experiencing stress.

As we can see from the model, and also from this study, the process of religious coping is a reciprocal process. That is, R/S resources affect how we cope with stressful situations, but the stress of a serious illness, can also affect religion or spirituality.

Spiritual Assessment

Our model of clinical practice is shaped by the model of R/S coping that we have just described. It is grounded in research that supports this model. As you can see from the model, clinical practice must be based on a careful assessment of a patient's personal and environmental R/S resources, as well as his faith/spiritual journey, and R/S coping process. A number of models have been proposed for in-depth spiritual assessment (Lucas 2001, Pruyser 1976), as well as for religious or spiritual history taking (Anandarajah & Hight 2001, Puchalski & Romer 2000), and screening for religious struggle (Fitchett 1999a, Fitchett 1999b, Fitchett et al. 2004, Fitchett & Risk, in press). One popular model for spiritual assessment, developed by a team of chaplains and nurses, is the 7 x 7 model (see Table 8–1; Fitchett 2002). This model places assessment of the R/S dimension of life in the context of a holistic assessment, including the patient's medical, psychological, family, psychosocial, and cultural background. The model focuses on seven specific dimensions for assessing the patient's R/S life. These include:

R/S beliefs
R/S sources of meaning
Moral obligations, based on R/S
R/S experiences
R/S rituals and practices
R/S community
Sources of R/S authority

The model employs a broad conceptualization of R/S, making it useful with those who identify with diverse religious beliefs as well as those who describe themselves as spiritual, but not religious. The model encourages both the patient and the caregiver to identify R/S resources as well as R/S needs.

Although spiritual screening and spiritual history taking by the health professional provide some information about a patient's R/S needs and resources, a spiritual assessment by a chaplain is indicated when more depth is desired. Unlike spiritual screening or spiritual history taking, spiritual assessment is usually based on listening to the patient's story as they need to tell it, and not on an interview with predetermined questions. The

Table 8–1   The 7 x 7 Model for Spiritual Assessment.

Holistic Assessment	Spiritual Assessment
Biological (Medical) Dimension	Belief and Meaning
Psychological Dimension	Vocation and Obligations
Family Systems Dimension	Experience and Emotions
Psychosocial Dimension	Courage and Growth
Ethnic, Racial, Cultural Dimension	Ritual and Practice
Social Issues Dimension	Community
Spiritual Dimension	Authority and Guidance

categories in the 7 x 7 model provide a framework for organizing, inter-preting, and summarizing the story the patient has told about his or her R/S needs and resources. A plan for spiritual care can be developed from this information. Case examples using the 7 x 7 model, including assess-ments and care plans, have been published elsewhere (Fitchett 2002; Fitch-ett & Roberts 2003)

Religious and Spiritual Coping in People with Chronic Mental Illness

This section will highlight the application of our conceptual model of R/S coping and will include some interventions. The section on coping with cancer will present, in detail, interventions for dealing with cancer that might be adapted for other chronic illnesses.

In the past, religious content was seen as a symptom in people with chronic mental illness (Turner et al. 1995). Contemporary emphasis on respecting diverse cultures, as well as ongoing research, show that R/S can be an important resource the person brings to coping with illness and the possible stressors that provoked an escalation of symptoms (Koenig 2001; Koenig, McCullough, & Larson 2001; Levin & Chatters 1998; McCullough & Larson 1999; Mickley, Carson, & Soeken 1995; Smith, McCullough, & Poll 2003; Ventis 1995).

The Importance of Childhood Religion for Coping

"Slowly the darkness began to weave its way into my mind, and before long, I was hopelessly out of control. I could not follow the path of my own thoughts. Sentences flew around my head and fragmented first into phrases and then into words . . ." (Jamison 1995, 79). This insider's view of the symptoms of bipolar disorder points to the interference with thought, feelings, and behavior that are part of the suffering individual's experience. The thoughts of a person with schizophrenia or schizoaffective disorder are apt to be even more fragmented. Although the thoughts of a person with depression appear to be more intact, a focus on worthlessness and guilt, along with a sense of hopelessness, caused by depression can be equally disturbing. This interference could impact appraisal and coping skills just described.

The first episode of a mental disorder usually does not occur until young adulthood (American Psychiatric Association 1994, Kessler et al. 2005, Kirkbride et al. 2006). There is evidence that the onset of schizophrenia is accompanied by a loss of brain cells with consequent cognitive deficits (Vidal et al. 2006). It is plausible that education and training in childhood prior to this change could be particularly important to those who suffer from schizophrenia. They may be much better able to recognize an R/S worldview established in childhood, than to develop a new framework for appraisal and coping as adults (for information about memory in schizophrenia, see Aleman and colleagues 1999). For the person experiencing mania, the structure of beliefs and ritual, along with calming practices from early life, might provide important resources. The person with depressive symptoms might have cognitions from beliefs and holy texts or from spiritual experiences as a child that could offset some of the negative thoughts associated with depression.

It is likely that persons with mental illness will be similar to other Americans surveyed in 1998, 93 percent of whom were raised in some religious denomination and 69 percent of whom attended religious services at least several times a month when they were twelve years old (General Social Survey 2007). Although some may have changed denominations or completely left organized religion as adults, they have probably retained some of the attitudes about the world, about themselves, and about others that religion teaches. Their religious worldview will impact their journey through illness. For patients whose thought processes are very disorganized, to have a framework at all in their otherwise chaotic experience is probably very valuable.

Resources and Coping

APPRAISAL

Early religious participation will have provided images of the Divine. For example, a patient diagnosed with schizophrenia as an adult believes that God loves him because his Sunday school during childhood had a wonderful playground. Ana-Maria Rizutto (1979) and others from a psychodynamic background theorize that early images of God come from parental figures. There is ongoing, though limited, research exploring religion both as compensation for or as related to attachment to maternal figures in early childhood (Kirkpatrick & Shaver 1990). For some, God is like a parent and makes up for a lack of a safe and consistent caregiver. For example, a group of patients discussing the image of God as father explained that because they kept moving from one foster home to another as children, God was the only father they really had. However, there are those who experience God as an abusive parent, particularly those who are sexually abused in childhood (Fallot & Heckman 2005). "He wasn't listening to me when I prayed for it to stop. He betrayed me" (Murray-Swank & Pargament 2005). In listening to the person who is suffering, it is important to be attentive to who God is for him or her. Often the image of God is not a simple question of helpful or harmful, but more often it is a mixture of these.

Fallot and Heckman (2005) found that women who had been sexually abused used more negative religious coping than those not abused in early childhood, but they also used positive images of God in their coping to the same degree as the general population. In some cases, images can be healed; in others, to use God language with a patient can be retraumatizing. For those with mental disorders, a world in the hands of a benevolent and/or powerful Deity may present a helpful backdrop for evaluating the threat of the onset of symptoms or the experience of the stressor that exacerbated them. Those engaged in religious struggle might need support in examining their understanding of God.

Secondary appraisals about the ability to cope with the threat are likely to have been learned by children who participated in religion in some way. At worship, during home rituals, and in some cultures through Bible reading at home, children will have heard repeatedly the sacred stories of creation and of protection in difficult situations with a sense of God's being in control of the world. Their congregation will have provided norms for leading a good life. Depending on the emphasis of the local congregation and denomination, they will also have heard of a demanding God with rules and possible punishment. The stressors in life—for example, death, illness, and frightening world events—will have been talked about, prayed about, and ritualized in a faith community. The child will have sung or heard the music of his congregation, often within the context of extended family. A piece of the child's identity will be the denomination to which he belongs. Because symptoms of mental illness interfere with thought, mood, and behavior, it might be important for adults to recall these resources, which include ideas, experience, and actions for coping.

WORLDVIEW

When appraising events, the beliefs, stories, and experiences of religion will provide a worldview with explanations for negative experiences, such as, "My voices tell me to kill myself, but I know God loved Job and tested him. I know God is testing me and loves me" or "I got this illness because I did something wrong." A patient with schizophrenia who had also been a victim of incest knew that he would be safe in heaven because the Bible says, "In my Father's house there are many mansions." He felt secure that the perpetrator would be safely locked away in a different house. Although some explanations are more beneficial than others, to have an explanation is better than facing the chaos of events where no one is in control.

RELIGIOUS SOCIAL SUPPORT

In appraising the ability to deal with events, religious training will have shown children what to do when someone dies, how people in their culture mourn, and what stories and songs carry the emotion of distress and offer hope. They will also have learned that the community is there for support. For example, an adolescent boy with cancer who had been physically abused by his mother's boyfriends was sent to church at age four as punishment. Until he died he drew on the love and care he had received from this experience, which helped offset the abuse and neglect he had suffered at home. He had the social support of a loving faith community. He also had the individual social support that religion contributes to well-being (Maton 1989, Pollner 1995). This boy knew Jesus was with him all along the way, even in the most difficult times.

A Sense of Self

Part of what individuals bring to adverse events is their sense of self, which begins to develop from infancy in interaction with their body, with others who offer a sense of connection, and in communication with the environment (Stern 1985). Throughout life, people are working at developing a sense of self that is good enough, safe enough, and connected with others (Kohut 1987). In his later years, Kohut spoke about how religion meets some of these human needs (Strozier 2001). The suffering of mental illness strikes precisely at this core of a sense of self. In the negative thoughts of depression or the paranoid thoughts of psychotic disorders, a person does not feel good enough or safe enough. Connections seem lost or broken because relatives and friends often find the person's manic or depressed behavior difficult to tolerate, so that there is less support from others temporarily and often long term. The person with schizophrenia might lose the ability or desire to communicate effectively. Behaviors of personality disorders can make it even more difficult for the friend or relative to stick by the person when symptoms are acute. The person with a chemical dependency is more connected to the chemical than to other people.

The pain of mental illness does not focus on pain in the back, or the leg, or some specific part of the body. The person's whole self is in pain. For some, this pain leads to suicide (Bauemeister 1990). For example, a young man newly diagnosed with schizophrenia complained that someone had stolen his soul. This is an eloquent description of what it must be like to be separated from the usual patterns of feeling and thinking that help reinforce a consistent sense of who you are. The language of religion, learned prior to the first incident of a mental illness, might take a person to a place where she has a greater sense of self and control. For example, a patient with disorganized speech was able to sing along with a familiar song at the beginning of a spirituality group. When asked what the song was like for him, he responded, "My words came out straight." He had some sense of control in dealing with his symptoms. Briefly, his mind worked well enough for him to utter a response with an organized structure.

The first step in interventions for mental illness is to establish a therapeutic alliance. For people whose symptoms often seem more obvious than the self behind them, it is good for the therapist to remember, in religious language, that this is someone made in the image of God, or, in spiritual language, that this is someone with whom I share a deep, spiritual connection. It might be easy to do this with some people. It will be harder to do this with someone who is in pain and suicidal or someone who is delusional. To acknowledge inwardly this connection is not the same as crossing boundaries. It is simply a place to be, which the client is apt to notice at some level. For example, a patient with schizophrenia who might have been frightening to some other patients because of his size was afraid to leave his room, but wanted the chaplain to visit. His first words were, "You're not afraid of me, are you?" He could pick up right away that the chaplain was meeting him and not just his symptoms and that made him feel less anxious.

Faith/Spiritual Development

A patient with a recurring depression who had attended church as a child, but had not attended church as an adult, joined a church and the choir. The patient was bright enough to know which personal beliefs would be welcomed by all the church members and which beliefs needed to be shared more cautiously. The patient's smile when talking about singing in the choir and receiving support from the church communicated how much this had contributed to her quality of life. This exemplifies the model for religious coping presented earlier. The patient's worldview stemmed, in part, from early childhood training about a demanding God and abuse as a young teenager. At times the sense of guilt that accompanies depression pulled the patient back to a negative worldview. The patient had been faithful to a journey of spiritual growth, working with her psychiatrist and the chaplain over several years, and had found a loving and concerned God. She was able to question earlier beliefs from her family and to develop an alternative set of beliefs. She could also identify with her current church community, and, at the same time, hold to her own beliefs and experiences. This development reflects both the patient's internal resources and the work of caregivers who helped her work through some of her negative religious thoughts. Although the patient's emotions were impacted by early childhood images, the patient was able to draw on newer cognitions to help counter a negative view of herself.

Awareness of a person's level of faith development facilitates meeting the patient at the level of the patient's needs. Some people have fairly simple religious schema from childhood that serve them well. Some have questioned their faith and have come through this questioning phase on solid footing. Others experience stress because of their questioning of earlier beliefs. Knowing this, the caregiver can help each individual rely on the strength of his religion or walk with him through a difficult time of transition.

SPIRITUAL AND NOT RELIGIOUS

Some people were never exposed to religion in their family, and some have chosen to abandon religion. The varied definitions of spirituality and problems with measures limit research on the impact of spirituality for these individuals. Oftentimes, patients are seeking to develop or expand their sense of spirituality in order to cope with their illness. Inviting these people to describe experiences they have had of a sense of connection or being in touch with a transcendent reality can help them deepen their spiritual awareness. Some will focus on nature or art. Sometimes they recall experiences at camp as a child. Telling the story can serve as a reminder of a reality greater than their symptoms. Even though they have a hard time feeling peaceful in the midst of symptoms, recalling the event can soothe and calm them, at least temporarily. Talking about meaning in life may help a person claim an inner self that has coped and journeyed through joy and suffering up to that point. Even though his illness would prevent his return to his life's work, for example, a patient who could claim how good he had been at his job and who could describe his altruistic motives for his work was able to discover that he was, indeed, a spiritual person. He had a long way to go in terms of grieving for the work he could no longer do. However, he had discovered a spiritual side to himself to help go through that journey.

Use of Religious or Spiritual Coping by People with Persistent Mental Illness

Along with the individual examples given above, there is growing information about the use of R/S coping reported by people with mental illness. Surveys show a high level of belief in patients with psychiatric symptoms that is comparable to the level found in the general population (Fitchett, Burton, & Sivan 1997; Kirov et al. 1998; Kroll & Sheehan 1989; Neelman & Lewis 1994; Reger & Rogers 2002).

Tepper and colleagues (2001) found a high level of religious coping (80 percent) in patients with serious mental illness. Of these individuals 30 percent claimed their religious beliefs and practices were their most important way to cope. When their symptoms became worse, 48 percent reported increasing their use of religious coping strategies. Those with the highest use of religion had fewer hospitalizations. The number of years of religious coping was related to fewer symptoms of psychosis, depression, and phobic anxiety. Most used a private form of religious activity, and 35 percent indicated that they regularly attended worship services, which is similar to results (35 percent) in Fitchett et al. (1997), but less than findings (50 percent) by Kroll and Sheehan (1989). A survey of a general population in 1998 (General Social Survey 2007) showed 33 percent of respondents attended worship services almost weekly or more.

An open-ended survey (Russinova, Wewiorski, & Cash 2002) asked people with schizophrenia, bipolar disorder, and major depression what alternative health care practices they used and then explored the respondents' perceived benefits. The most frequent responses were religious or spiritual activities (schizophrenia, 58 percent; bipolar, 41 percent; major depression, 56 percent) and meditation (schizophrenia, 28 percent; bipolar, 54 percent; major depression, 41 percent). When asked about the benefits of these practices, respondents were allowed to use their own words, which the authors then grouped by theme. Respondents reported "increased emotional calmness (40 percent) as a benefit from R/S activities. R/S activities also gave them "greater meaning and purpose in life" (36 percent) and "connectedness to nature or a higher power" (39 percent). Social benefits from R/S activities were "improved interpersonal relationships" (24 percent) and decreased social isolation (26 percent). As benefits of meditation, respondents claimed emotional calmness (77 percent), "improved concentration" (24 percent), "improved health" (27 percent), "feeling centered/grounded" (25 percent), and increased "capacity to cope" (22 percent).

Outcomes of Religious or Spiritual Coping for Mental Health

What evidence supports the experience of these people? Recent reviews of research in religion and mental health, based primarily on general populations of adults, students, or the elderly, show mostly positive associations of religion with psychological well-being, hope and optimism, purpose and meaning, lower levels of anxiety and depression, greater social support, and less substance abuse (Koenig 2001; Koenig, McCullough, & Larson 2001; McCullough & Larson 1999; Levin & Chatters 1998; Mickley, Carson, & Soeken 1995; Smith, McCullough, & Poll 2003; Ventis 1995). Koenig (2001) names some of the reasons religion might promote better mental health. Religion offers a positive worldview for life events. On the level of emotions, prayer or worship as well as beliefs may "evoke positive emotions—joy, wonder, awe, thankfulness. Religion provides rituals for important moments in life, like the death of a loved one. Religious beliefs also prescribe support and care for others, encouraging character traits such as altruism, kindness, generosity, forgiveness, and love for neighbor . . ." (Koenig 2001, 105). Finally, religion provides norms of behavior that can decrease negative stressful events (Koenig 2001).

These reviews also cite a few studies showing either a harmful relationship or no relationship at all. Some potentially harmful aspects of religion described include creating unusual thoughts through cults, causing guilt or shame, promoting regulations that might add stress, avoiding facing stressors realistically, and holding deviant beliefs by some groups (Mickley, Carson, & Soeken 1995). In many of the studies, the relationship might be complex in terms of which comes first, religion or outcome. Newer, better-designed studies try to address the question of causality.

Religious or spiritual care does not lend itself to evidence-based practice to the same degree that other clinical endeavors permit. However, there is value in looking to the research on relationships to help the caregiver focus interventions based on our information to date. Spiritual care for patients with mental disorders might address three frequently studied aspects of religion: attendance at worship services, private prayer or meditation, and the importance of religion and beliefs to the individual.

Attendance at Worship Services

Attendance at worship services is one of the most commonly used measures of religiosity in studies looking at mental health outcomes. One study (Strawbridge et al. 2001) looked at frequency of attendance in a general population that included people with symptoms of depression. Twenty-nine years after collecting the initial information, the researchers found that those who attended worship services frequently were more likely to stop being depressed and to increase the number of social relationships they had. These effects were particularly strong among women in the sample, who also indicated they were more likely to stop heavy drinking. There is some evidence that male veterans who were sexually abused attended worship services less frequently than those who were not abused (Chang et al. 2003). Those who attended worship services more frequently had better mental health. However, in a group of veterans who were sexually abused and in treatment for chemical dependency, there was no difference (Lawson et al. 1998). Another study showed that patients, hospitalized for depression, who attended worship services frequently had shorter lengths of stay, lower levels on the Beck Depression Inventory, and lower levels of current and lifetime alcohol abuse than their hospitalized counterparts with lower rates of worship attendance (Baetz et al. 2002). In a study of the elderly that looked at depression over a period of six years, people who attended worship services more often were consistently less depressed (Braam et al. 2004). On a less positive note, those who attended worship services occasionally or decreased their attendance became more depressed over time.

What does this mean for the depressed person? Clearly, some people derive benefits from regular attendance at worship services. For the less frequent attenders, it is intriguing to wonder what is happening. Seriously depressed people might have decreased attendance because of their symptoms and experience a sense of guilt and isolation. Still others might be holding on to a negative experience with their denomination. A simple question about participation in worship services earlier in life and a question about whether that pattern has changed lets the patient tell his story.

For example, a patient being treated for depression who spoke about what religious music did for him as well as the sense of support he received, described himself as feeling more peaceful and stronger after talking about worship services. When the experience of worship is positive, allowing individuals to tell you about it helps put them in touch with their own resources and focuses them on positive aspects of their life, rather than ruminating on the negative. Sometimes people who cut back on their attendance at worship services describe a sense of guilt. Giving them space to talk about it can help relieve the pressure. Some patients with chronic mental illness have insight into the fact that their symptoms are interfering with their ordinary behavior. Asking them how they would judge a friend with depression who had skipped worship services for a while can help give them a perspective on themselves. For patients who place authority in the leadership of their congregation, it might take having their pastor, rabbi, priest, imam, or a chaplain process their change in attendance with a plan for rejoining the congregation when they feel better or offering them a choice of finding another way of religious coping.

Of those who no longer attend worship services, some have drifted away because they never found worship services meaningful and some have walked away because they left behind a negative experience. Describing this exodus can increase the person's sense of self-efficacy. It is worth letting her claim she had the freedom to leave the congregation of her youth. Listening to the patient's story of departure might also reveal an experience, real or perceived, of some sort of harm at the hands of God, a religious leader, or the community. The individual could be using depressive thinking that includes overgeneralizing or expecting either/or answers. Talking about a perceived slight could promote overall growth. This could be an area that calls for a process of healing—always keeping in mind what will serve the patient's mental health. If worship services had been a source of strength, then finding a way back to worship service attendance could give the person with chronic mental illness an important source for coping.

For example, a patient with manic symptoms who was not allowed off the floor to attend worship services set up a small altar in her room. When asked about her altar, she explained that attending worship services helped her focus and feel more organized. This is a fairly common comment of patients with bipolar disorder. In finding that patients with this disorder who had been more unwell in the past five years attended worship services more frequently, Mitchell and Romans (2003) suggested that organizational ways of practicing religion might be more accessible to people at a time when symptoms lead to difficulty concentrating. In their survey Russinova and colleagues (2002) found that 41 percent of people with bipolar disorder, 58 percent of people with schizophrenia, and 56 percent of people with major depression ranked religious or spiritual activities as one of their most frequent ways of coping.

Although church members are not always welcoming of people with schizophrenia, religious congregations and attendance at worship services can be a readily accessible form of social support. In a group of people with schizophrenia who agreed to participate in spirituality classes, 65 percent attended worship services frequently for social reasons and because they enjoyed the music (Lindgren & Coursey 1995). As one person receiving help for recovery from symptoms of schizophrenia reported about his congregation, "They support you and always ask for prayer requests and things like that . . . and they know about my mental illness" (Sullivan 1998, 29).

Private Prayer and Meditation

A common method of coping is prayer. Several well-designed studies show no association of prayer with less depression (Baetz et al. 2002; Bosworth et al. 2003; Koenig, George, & Peterson 1998). A study by Ellison and his colleagues (2001) indicated that people who prayed more were more depressed. The authors suggested that stressors might lead to both greater depression and an increased use of prayer to cope. Studies rarely look at the kind of prayer a person is using. An exception is research by Poloma and Pendleton (1991). In that study, the kind of prayer a person used appeared related to his psychological outcome. Those who used colloquial prayer and meditation had greater life satisfaction, existential well-being, and happiness. People with higher levels of petitionary and ritualistic prayer indicated more negative affect and less happiness. Ritualistic prayer was still associated with negative affect when demographic variables were taken into account. The authors suggested that other types of prayer might be more difficult when symptoms were active so that the distressed person had to rely on ritual prayers.

For the person with mental illness, the area of prayer requires particular attention. Oftentimes, the symptoms of mental illness lead to a sense of isolation. Sometimes individuals feel guilty and abandoned by God. Their medication does not offer a quick relief of symptoms; neither does their request for God to take away their illness. It can be extremely valuable for patients to talk about their experience. If the experience is related temporarily to symptoms, verbalizing a sense of abandonment, particularly in a group, can be very helpful. It is important for the caregiver to acknowledge the pain the person is experiencing. It can be helpful for others in the group to let the person know that they have had a similar experience. A cognitive approach of reminding them about the difference between feeling God's presence and believing in God's presence at a time when their feelings are not working offers a path past blaming themselves for not being able to pray well. Asking how long that experience lasted in the past can offer a reminder that their experience will not last forever. Patients who have dealt with mental illness over many years often come to a sense of faith that gives them support and helps them cope. For example, a patient with schizophrenia shared that he had begged God to cure him of his illness. Eventually, he had an experience in which he knew God had answered his prayer. God did not take away the illness; rather, God promised to always be with him.

Some people also speak of using prayer or meditation as self-soothing or a way to find calm (Fallot 1998b). Some have found that formal prayers or religious songs work as a way to focus their attention away from hallucinations. A patient once explained that her mother had taught her to say the rosary when her thoughts were too confused. This gave her some control over her symptoms. Prayers in the Bible can also offer comfort, according to one patient, who said, "Sometimes you are so depressed you can't pray. Then you read the Psalms and it's like telling God how you feel." People who have coped with mental illness themselves are often the best experts when it comes to knowing what form of meditation or prayer helps. Often, however, health care providers don't even ask.

Importance of Religion and Beliefs

Well-designed longitudinal studies report the benefits of religion in the face of depressive symptoms. Internalized beliefs and salience of religion for elderly adults has been associated with fewer symptoms of depression (Idler & Kasl 1992), lack of chronic course of depression that remitted (or went away) over time (Braam et al. 2004), shorter time for remission from depression (Koenig et al. 1998), and lower levels of depression after six months (Bosworth et al. 2003).

Clinically depressed persons who had beliefs in a concerned and caring God were less hopeless and, therefore, less depressed (Murphy et al. 2000). In fact, in this same sample, belief in a concerned God was the only predictor of response to treatment for depression after eight weeks, when demographic variables and initial levels of hopelessness were considered (Murphy & Fitchett 2006). The hopelessness theory of depression (Abramson, Metalsky, & Alloy 1989) suggests that, in the presence of an adverse event, the person who attributes the event to stable, internal, and global causes is likely to become hopeless and, therefore, depressed. For example, if I believe that I have been and will always be (stable) worthless (internal), then I can't change (hopeless) the reason why I always have bad things happen to me. If I believe that this worthlessness leads to bad outcomes in all areas of life (global), I am trapped and can never change things for the better. There is evidence that this hopeless attitude leads to depression (Metalsky and Joiner 1992, Reno and Halarais 1989). Religious beliefs may offset these negative cognitions. For example, in a sample of people whose illness might lead to depression, religious people who were HIV positive had lower levels of hopelessness than nonreligious individuals (Carson et al. 1990).

Religion presents a God who listens (Bennett 2001). The God of the Psalms is willing to listen to hopeless, distressed people. For caregivers, the first step is to listen and to acknowledge how painful this sense of hopelessness is, rather than offering solutions or nice quotes from the Bible. The next step toward diminishing the pain of hopelessness is to help the person connect with his religious resources, whether it is a favorite Bible story, a psalm, or a song that contradicts the hopeless thoughts. In a study of the relationship of hope to spiritual well-being, Carson, Soeken, and Grimm (1988) found that the younger participants in the study had less religious well-being. The authors cited a passage from Thomas Merton that suggests that it is only after touching despair that a person truly needs to turn to God (81). Many patients who have coped with chronic mental illness have often stood at this place of despair. The caregiver need not fear it. Rather, it is the path by which many patients have moved to a deeper level of faith and a higher level of mature faith. Spirituality groups provide a wonderful context for older patients to model this capacity to cope with the darkness for those newer to the impact of a chronic mental disorder.

International research into the role of religion in the lives of people with schizophrenia (Kirov et al. 1998, Mohr & Huguelet 2004) has described generally beneficial aspects of religion and religious beliefs as well as the importance of religion and using religion to cope. "The nun always told me that the gospel is the world upside down and I didn't understand and one day, I saw all my life. I was so ashamed of myself, I had done so many silly things, I was a wreck and I told myself 'I have a dignity in God, I am a person, even if I am schizophrenic, on welfare, I am a person'" (Mohr & Huguelet 2004, 174). The authors also noted harmful aspects of religion for patients when they were delusional, such as taking literally a biblical directive to pluck out your eye if it offends you. While patients are experiencing psychotic symptoms, it might be particularly important to listen to the religious content of their words to help them focus on positive religious messages.

For example, a patient with schizoaffective disorder with manic symptoms claimed to be God's wife. This placed her above everyone else on the inpatient unit with her own conviction that she did not need medication. Many images from religion are well suited to giving a patient experiencing a manic episode an "understanding" of her experience. Whereas the non-religious person might claim to be the president or to receive directions only from him as part of her experience of grandiosity, the religious person is apt to identify with the Divine. For some patients, these delusional thoughts can interfere with compliance with medication. Further exploration with the above patient about the advantages of being related to God yielded the response that it gave her unconditional love and meant she would never die. Although religion was interfering with treatment, it was giving the patient a way to cope with the stress of the recent death of her brother in a car accident.

Once delusions are active, they are unlikely to change without medication. It could be the content of the delusion is serving a purpose for the patient. It was difficult for this patient to grieve the loss of her brother because of her illness. An empathic response to the reason the patient is using given images might create a better relationship with the caregiver. This could lead to compliance with treatment. Cognitive theory is being used for treatment of both schizophrenia and bipolar disorders (Rector & Beck 2001, Scott et al. 2006). For religious people, perhaps early cognitive interventions consistent with the patient's beliefs could offset beliefs supporting noncompliance.

Pardini and colleagues (2000) examined the mental health benefits of religion and spirituality of people in recovery from substance abuse. Religion contributed to social support and resistance to stress. These individuals preferred the term *spirituality* to *religion*, although the two were highly correlated. Spirituality was associated with greater optimism and lower stress in this sample. The author acknowledged the difficulty in defining the term *spirituality*, which means different things to different people (Cook 2004). Laudet (2003) cited articles suggesting that the component of spirituality that is a part of twelve-step programs might be an important obstacle to participation. When examining the attitudes of people in treatment for substance abuse of whom less than half were in twelve-step programs, none of the respondents reported this as a problem. The major obstacle was lack of motivation. Drug users receiving methadone or involved in a needle-exchange program reported religious healing most frequently (20 percent) as a form of alternative therapy (Manheimer, Anderson, & Stein 2003). Almost half of those who remained in recovery for addiction to opioids considered religion or spirituality an important support in their maintenance (Flynn et al. 2003).

The co-morbidity of chemical dependence with other mental disorders is high—about 66 percent in one study (Kessler et al. 1996). The causal relationship and mechanism are complex, although one theory is related to stress level (see Goeders 2003). Religion is a protective factor against chemical dependency, possibly due to religious prohibitions against substance abuse (Kendler, Gardner, & Prescott 1997). Those who have broken these restrictions might experience guilt and alienation from religious congregations. Perhaps the role of religion for those already addicted is related to the protection against some stressors that religion provides (Ellison et al. 2001; Krause & Van Tran 1989; Maton 1989; Smith, McCullough, & Poll 2003; Strawbridge et al. 1998). Some patients with a dual diagnosis say they find it helpful to have an image of a demanding God who can put order in their lives when they have fallen back into substance abuse. This image of a powerful Other who has expectations about behavior offers them a sense of hope. For those who are able to use the twelve-step program, their need for a Higher Power can lead to spiritual maturity (Miller 1998). Along with growth in acceptance and humility that are part of this process, forgiveness might be an important piece of the spiritual development that leads to recovery.

Adaptation of Spiritual Assessment for People with Mental Illness

Religion can play a mixed role for patients. Learning about the individual patient's experience is crucial. Fallot (1998a) described an adaptation of Fitchett's (2002) 7 x 7 model of spiritual assessment that is used at a community mental health center. He focused on letting the client describe *beliefs and meaning, experience and emotion, rituals and practice,* and *community,* paying attention in each of these categories to the use of explicit religious language, the role of the client's R/S experience in overall well-being, and the connection of religious material with psychotic symptoms. This information was used to create a care plan that took spirituality into account. Nurses in a study exploring how they distinguished psychotic from religious experiences found the same endpoint of overall well-being important. Aware that they brought their own beliefs and biases to the assessment, the nurses acknowledged the importance of looking at the patient holistically and accepting a sense of ambiguity in a field that, in the past, considered religiosity pathological (Eeles, Lowe, & Wellman 2003).

Because of past biases about religion in the content of delusions, it is particularly important to determine whether or not beliefs are consistent with the patient's culture. For example, a woman with a psychotic depression explained that her symptoms were due to a Voodoo curse. A staff person from her country of origin shared with us that Voodoo is a common belief in her village. That aspect of her experience deserved respect and was not delusional.

Interventions

There is a growing body of literature describing interventions for the religious or spiritual person. Earlier we noted that religious beliefs of the patient may contain both helpful and harmful components. Cognitive therapy is often used to help people examine and alter their beliefs in order to change their feelings and behaviors. Nielsen and colleagues (2000) explored this approach and provided a dialogue in which the caregiver used a story from the Bible to dispute a patient's beliefs about being a bad person. Not all caregivers will be familiar with the stories from a given religious tradition. Sometimes the patient will be able to recall a story that is helpful. Trained pastoral counselors or professional chaplains from various faith traditions who are familiar with the literature of their religion might be called in to assist with treatment.

Propst and her colleagues (1992) developed a protocol using religious cognitive-behavioral therapy (RCT) for treating depression. In a clinical trial involving participants for whom religion was important, those who received RCT lowered their depression scores more quickly than those receiving standard cognitive therapy, regardless of the religious beliefs of the counselors. Some individuals with chronic mental illness have viewed their illness as God's punishment or God as the source of their suffering (Lindgren & Coursey 1995). For them, religion causes pain, rather than offering solace. These patients might need an intervention that addresses such conclusions, without taking away patients' sense of meaning for their illness. Cognitive interventions to shift patients' religious beliefs could improve their quality of life.

Noting that drug addicts perceive themselves negatively with descriptors such as selfish and manipulative, a team developed a Buddhist-based meditation training to help addicts create a "spiritual self schema" (Avants, Bettel, & Margolin 2005). Participants in this eight-week training, which included contact with a therapist and guided daily exercises, increased their religiousness or sense of spirituality and decreased their use of drugs. Clients described themselves as feeling calmer and as having more control. Meditation exercises have also been effective in treating anxiety (Kabat-Zinn et al. 1992).

A group intervention for women with HIV (Pargament et al. 2004) includes components that might be useful in group therapy for people with persistent mental illness. Components of the program, "Lighting the Way: A Spiritual Journey to Wholeness," were based on the most recent information about the role R/S plays in coping. It incorporated cognitive and behavioral techniques as well as drawing on interpersonal experience and affect. Both R/S resources and religious struggles, such as anger at God, being branded with a stigma by religious communities, and feeling punished by God, were addressed. One session focused on hopes and dreams, allowing participants to name the dreams that were no longer possible because of their illness. People with chronic mental illness can benefit from learning to grieve the loss their symptoms bring. At the same time, they are able to choose realistic dreams for themselves and to claim meaning in their lives.

As Fallot (1998b) pointed out, true recovery is a long-term and often difficult journey. Hope is an essential ingredient for continuing the efforts needed to manage symptoms and grow in skills that promote quality of life and increase wellness. In providing case studies from "Solace for the Soul: A Journey Towards Wholeness," a treatment program for people who have experienced sexual abuse, Murray-Swank and Pargament (2005) provided a poignant example of this. After four weeks of treatment, a client who had been abused was able to shift her anger away from God toward the perpetrator. She still had a long way to go to recover from the abuse, but articulated hope: "I am getting there actually. I have moved from Hate down one step. I don't hate God quite as much. . . . I am on my way. After I started this program, at least there is a light. I have taken a few steps forward" (197).

Conclusions Concerning Chronic Mental Illness

We have seen that people with mental illness are likely to turn to religion or spirituality to cope with the ongoing effects of their symptoms. There is evidence that forms of religious coping can lead to greater well-being. Allowing people to talk about their use of religious or spiritual coping can help them draw on their own resources, giving them a sense of control. In listening, the caregiver might become aware of the need to address thoughts that are interfering with improvement or to refer the patient to a trained chaplain or pastoral counselor who can provide this service. When possible, groups can be a helpful setting for people to articulate ways their religion or spirituality helps them or gets in the way. Because psychiatry has historically equated religious content with pathology, it might be particularly important for caregivers to remember the importance R/S can hold for patients. There is no reason to fear inquiring about religion or spirituality in patients' lives. In fact, such an inquiry might lead to a better understanding, even of the delusional patient.

Dalmida (2006) offered some important reflections on the ethics of using spirituality in patient care. It is not the role of the caregiver to give advice. Rather, the person working with the patient should facilitate the patient's getting in touch with and utilizing the patient's own spiritual or religious resources. Care should be offered in the context of the patient's spirituality or religion and should not promote any specific religion. The health care provider is not likely to be trained to address specific spiritual needs and should not hesitate to refer a patient for pastoral care when there is a need.

Religious and Spiritual Coping in Persons with Cancer

We have looked specifically at an application of our conceptual model for religious coping in the section on people with chronic mental illness. In this section we will look more generally at R/S coping in people with cancer. We will highlight details of interventions for people with cancer that might be easily adapted for those with other chronic illnesses.

In 2007, more than 1.4 million new cancer cases were estimated to be diagnosed and more than half a million people were projected to succumb to the disease (ACS 2007). The diagnosis of cancer is often experienced as a life-altering, traumatic event. Treatments are harsh and disruptive, and uncertainty about the outcome and prognosis for survival provokes varying levels of anxiety. Many patients with cancer experience significant symptoms of distress at one or more points during their illness.

Resources and Coping

Consistent with our conceptual model, there are a variety of R/S resources and coping techniques utilized by individuals following a diagnosis of cancer. A review of the literature suggests that prayer is the most prevalent R/S means of coping with the cancer experience. Such prayer includes self-prayer as well as prayer offered by others within the patient's faith community. It is also common for cancer patients to pursue some form of spiritual healing. In a large survey of patients with cancers of the breast, lung, head, and neck; the genitourinary tract; or gynecological, hematological, or gastrointestinal cancers, 77 percent of participants reported using prayer to assist them in coping with diagnosis/treatment (Yates et al. 2005). Of these patients, 19 percent also reported spiritual healing. Similarly, interviews of outpatients concerning particular "complementary" therapies (i.e., music, breathing exercises, meditation, prayer, muscle relaxation, visualization/ imagery, hypnosis/self-hypnosis) revealed that of all the strategies presented, prayer was used by the highest percentage of participants (64 percent) (Zaza, Sellick, & Hillier 2005). Additional studies report that the prevalence of prayer in coping with cancer ranges from 49 percent to 76 percent, and spiritual healing is sought or experienced by 29 percent to 54 percent (Balneaves, Kristjanson, & Tataryn 1999; Lengacher et al. 2003; Vande-Creek, Rogers, & Lester 1999). Furthermore, patients have reported using personal faith, self-prayer, relationship/dialog with God, prayers from fellow church members and others, counseling from a religious leader, reading the Bible, attending religious services, meditation, and finding and spending time at locations of spiritual energy (i.e., churches, specific geographical locations, or certain natural settings) as means of coping with cancer and its treatment (Tatsumura et al. 2003).

Several studies have identified R/S as a key strategy in the adaptive coping repertoire of many patients with cancer. In several investigations with breast cancer patients, religious and spiritual faith were found to be important sources of emotional support in dealing with the disease (Heim et al. 1993; Sodestrom & Martinson 1987) and provided patients with the ability to find meaning in everyday life (Feher & Maly 1999). Other investigations revealed that R/S was not just "another" means of coping, but, rather, was the single most important strategy in dealing with cancer-related distress (Carver et al. 1993, Fredette 1995, Halstead & Fernsler 1994).

Outcomes of Religious or Spiritual Coping for Cancer

In following our conceptual model, what are some of the outcomes experienced by cancer patients who rely on R/S resources and coping activities? Based on the literature, cancer patients use R/S because it provides a sense of hope. Several studies have demonstrated a relationship between greater

R/S coping or higher levels of spiritual well-being and lower levels of hopelessness (Brandt 1987, Mickley et al. 1992). For example, in one study the majority of hospitalized cancer patients reported that their religious beliefs had given them support after they became ill with cancer (Ringdal 1996). Specifically, religiosity was associated with improved satisfaction with life and fewer feelings of hopelessness. In another study of women diagnosed with gynecological cancers, 93 percent of respondents reported that faith had increased their ability to be hopeful (Roberts et al. 1997). This relationship between R/S and hope is even stronger in the cancer palliative care setting, where R/S has been shown to offer some protection against end-of-life despair (McClain, Rosenfeld, & Breitbart 2003).

Studies suggest that R/S, as a means of coping, not only provides hopefulness for the cancer patient, but is significantly associated with measures of adjustment and management of disease-related symptoms (NCI 2006). As examples, R/S factors have been related to various aspects of adaptation to cancer, including self-reported physical well-being (Highfield 1992), general quality of life (Canada et al. 2006, Cotton et al. 1999), self-esteem and optimism (Gall, Miguez de Renart, & Boonstra 2000), positive appraisals and nonreligious coping (Gall 2000), and life satisfaction (Yates et al. 1981). R/S coping in patients with cancer has also been associated with lower levels of patient discomfort, reduced hostility, and less social isolation (McCullough et al. 2000; Acklin, Brown, & Mauger 1983), as well as decreased anxiety (Kaczorowski, 1989).

Furthermore, it has been suggested that R/S resources may serve multiple functions in long-term adjustment to cancer, including maintaining confidence, providing a sense of meaning or purpose in life, giving comfort, reducing emotional distress, increasing inner peace, and engendering a positive attitude toward life (Jenkins & Pargament 1995, Johnson & Spilka 1991, Levin 1994, Maton 1989). In one study, spiritual well-being, particularly a sense of meaning and peace, was significantly associated with an ability of cancer patients to continue to enjoy life despite high levels of pain or fatigue (Brady et al. 1999). Some survivors who had drawn on spiritual resources to cope with cancer even reported substantial personal growth as a consequence of their illness experience (Carpenter, Brockopp, & Andrykowski 1999). Although little of the research on the positive physiological effects of R/S has been specific to cancer patients, one study

(Sephton et al. 2001) found that helper and cytotoxic T-cell counts were higher (suggesting better immune function) among women with metastatic breast cancer who reported placing a greater emphasis on spirituality than their less spiritual counterparts.

Much of the literature in the field supports an association between positive R/S coping and better health status. Conversely, there is emerging evidence to suggest that negative R/S coping or religious struggle is linked to poorer mental and physical outcomes, including such outcomes in the oncology population. In an earlier cross-sectional examination of the prevalence and correlates of religious struggle in medical patients, including those with cancer, negative religious coping or religious struggle was associated with higher levels of emotional distress and depressive symptoms (Fitchett et al. 1999). More recently, religious struggle in multiple myeloma patients undergoing transplant workup was associated with greater levels of general distress and depression and, to a lesser extent, higher indices of pain and fatigue, and more difficulties with daily physical functioning (Sherman et al. 2005). Similarly, in women who had undergone surgery for breast cancer, religious struggle was associated with poorer overall quality of life and lower life satisfaction (Manning-Walsh 2005). In addition, among women diagnosed with gynecological cancer within the past year, those who used more negative spiritual coping, like thinking they were being punished by God, were more depressed and experienced greater levels of anxiety (Boscaglia et al. 2005).

Interventions

Such findings suggest that it may be important for health care providers to assess patients' level of spirituality and to intervene, when appropriate, in order to help patients deal with the adverse effects of chronic illness. This may be particularly true where religious struggle is involved. For example, a woman in her fifties with advanced cancer told a chaplain, "Why? Why me? I just can't figure it out. And I get so depressed that I just want to give up on life altogether, you know? And I'm so very angry at God. So angry. I refuse to speak to Him. You know what I mean?" (Fitchett & Roberts 2003). As people attempt to integrate the reality of grave illness or other adverse life events into their preexisting religious beliefs, they may ask, "God, why did you let this happen to me?" (Bradshaw & Fitchett 2003). For some, this period of religious struggle may be brief; for others it can be quite protracted. It may lead to growth and transformation for some people and to distress and despair for others (Carpenter, Brockopp, & Andrykowski 1999; Ingersoll-Dayton, Krause, & Morgan 2002). How then can we identify patients grappling with religious struggle and provide them with an opportunity to address it? One option is for health care professionals to listen for signs of religious struggle and to make a referral. Another option, currently being tested at our large urban medical center, is to include screening for religious struggle as a part of the admitting assessment process. The screening protocol we are using appears in Figure 8–2. When patients' responses to the screening questions indicate possible religious struggle, a referral should be made for a more in-depth spiritual assessment. We suggest that, if the screening protocol indicates possible religious struggle, the person doing the screening does not ask the patient if she wishes to undergo any further assessment for possible religious struggle. This may be a very sensitive question. We believe it is best left to a trained, certified chaplain to discuss it with the patient as part of the assessment visit. Often, the initial experience with a nonjudgmental chaplain may transform a patient's skepticism about religious authorities and allow a helpful relationship to develop.

Some patients may simply need support in mobilizing resources for positive R/S coping. To date, very little empirical evidence has addressed the value of explicitly religious or spiritual intervention in patients with cancer. Among the scant evidence, there are two published studies that, although in need of replication, suggest that R/S intervention in patients with cancer would likely be well-received and efficacious (Cole & Pargament 1999, Kristeller et al. 2005). As a way of presenting possible strategies for use in working with cancer patients, these two studies will be described in some detail below.

Cole and Pargament (1999) designed an intervention for patients with cancer that integrates psychotherapy and spirituality. It incorporates some of the coping components of cognitive-behavioral group interventions, documented as efficacious for patients with cancer (Fawzy et al. 1990, Greer 1992), and is supported by the literature that strongly suggests that spirituality is an important means of coping for religious people being

Figure 8–2   Protocol for Screening for Religious Struggle.

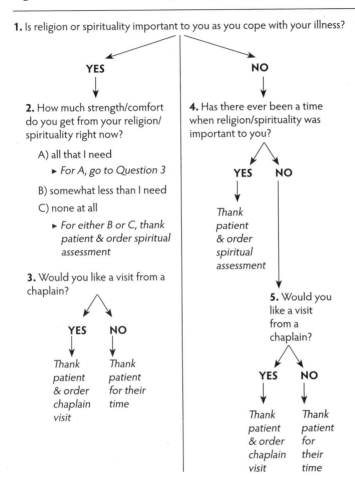

1. Is religion or spirituality important to you as you cope with your illness?

YES

2. How much strength/comfort do you get from your religion/spirituality right now?

A) all that I need
   ▸ *For A, go to Question 3*

B) somewhat less than I need

C) none at all
   ▸ *For either B or C, thank patient & order spiritual assessment*

3. Would you like a visit from a chaplain?

YES   **NO**

Thank patient & order chaplain visit   *Thank patient for their time*

NO

4. Has there ever been a time when religion/spirituality was important to you?

YES   **NO**

Thank patient & order spiritual assessment

5. Would you like a visit from a chaplain?

YES   **NO**

Thank patient & order chaplain visit   *Thank patient for their time*

treated for cancer. The goals of this intervention are to facilitate general adjustment to cancer, enhance spiritual coping, and resolve spiritual strain and struggle. Based on the authors' research, the specific components of this intervention were formulated around four existential issues: control, identity, relationships, and meaning.

In the control component of the R/S intervention, patients are assigned an exercise in which they place illness-related issues either "under my control" (e.g., choosing a doctor, eating well) or "under God's control" (e.g., final outcome of treatment). To address the issues "under God's control," patients are introduced to activities designed to help them "let go." Examples of such activities include visualizing religious imagery and contemplative prayer. Such techniques may be considered under the rubric of "emotion-focused coping" (Lazarus & Folkman 1984), which research suggests is more beneficial than problem-focused coping in low-control situations (e.g., chronic illness). Next, to address items that are "under my control," patients are taught to increase control by monitoring physiological arousal (through relaxation techniques), engaging in nurturing self-care, practicing assertive conflict management, and adapting a collaborative coping approach (i.e., viewing God as a partner).

The identity component of the intervention involves grief work. First, patients are asked to create a "loss list" in relation to their identity (e.g., changes in physical strength and appearance, work and familial roles, interpersonal relationships). Sharing the loss list with others helps desensitize the patient to his losses and facilitates the integration of changes into a new self-schema that reestablishes his sense of self-worth. The second exercise in grieving involves participant completion of an "I am" list, a list of things that continue to be valuable about him in spite of the cancer diagnosis. Introducing spirituality into such grief work involves the patient imagining the presence of God as a compassionate witness to his losses. Patients are then led through a sacred or "transformation" guided imagery exercise and encouraged to reaffirm their spiritual identity and worth, which transcend cancer.

The relationship component of the intervention addresses cancer-related disruptions in relationships with oneself, with others, and with God. Relationships with others are dealt with under the control component above. Relationship with the self is nourished in the intervention through: (1) listening to one's feelings (using self-monitoring forms throughout week); (2) positive self-talk and understanding of the cognitive-behavioral model; and (3) self-care (e.g., taking time out for play, rest, relaxation, reflection, exercise, and being spiritually present in the moment). Relationship with God is addressed through a "Circle of Light" guided imagery activity. God sits in the "empty chair" and the patient has an imagined conversation with the Divine. Through such enactment the patient is able to "reconstruct a relationship with the Sacred that integrates the negative affective response to the diagnosis and re-establish a sense of trust, mutual affection, and connectedness" (Cole & Pargament 1999, 403).

The meaning component of the intervention is designed to facilitate the resolution of inner conflict and to foster the development of positive meanings associated with the cancer experience. Included is a discussion of feelings that cancer is a punishment from God. If a participant holds such a view, intervention involves an exploration of paths for purification and forgiveness within the participant's religious tradition. Following the discussion, patients reflect on the spiritual meaning of their cancer experience through a guided imagery exercise. This task is followed by further discussion designed to help the patient find meaning through giving and receiving from others. A journaling assignment builds on the theme of making meaning through notation of meaningful moments experienced each day.

A pilot trial of this protocol (Cole 2005) with sixteen cancer patients revealed that participation in the intervention (as opposed to a no-treatment control condition) had a positive impact on pain severity and depression. Namely, those participants in the intervention group had relatively stable levels of pain and depression; however, those in the control group experienced greater pain and increased depression from pre- to post-treatment and two-month follow-up.

In the second published study, Kristeller and colleagues (2005) describe a five- to seven-minute physician-led spiritual intervention for patients with cancer. Oncologists introduce the intervention to patients in a neutral, inquiring manner, using language such as, "When dealing with a serious illness, many people draw on religious or spiritual beliefs to help cope. It would be helpful to me to know how you feel about this." Based on each participant's initial response to the topic, the oncologist inquires further, using one of four approaches. If the participant's response is judged to be indicative of "positive-active faith," the physician asks, "What have you found most helpful about your beliefs since your illness?" If the response is determined to be "neutral-receptive," the oncologist continues, "How might you draw on your faith or spiritual beliefs to help you?" A "spiritually distressed" response (e.g., anger or guilt) is met with a statement like this: "Many people feel that way. What might help you come to terms with this?" Finally, if the patient responds in a "defensive/rejecting" manner, the oncologist replies, "It sounds like you're uncomfortable that I brought this up. What I'm really interested in is how you are coping. Can you tell me about that?"

Based on the initial inquiry and response, the oncologist continues to briefly explore the patient's R/S coping methods, as indicated. Following this discussion, the physician queries about ways in which the patient finds meaning and a sense of peace in the midst of the cancer experience. Finally, after exploring resources, the oncologist offers assistance as appropriate and available (e.g., referral to a chaplain or a support group). The discussion concludes with the physician's expressing appreciation for the patient's willingness to discuss R/S issues.

A pilot of this study with 118 cancer patients revealed that oncologists were able to effectively address spiritual issues with patients using the brief, patient-centered intervention. The intervention was well-received, and those patients who participated (as compared to a control group) reported less depression, better quality of life, and a greater sense of interpersonal caring from their oncologist.

Conclusions

Based on the two studies described, as well as additional evidence from research with other health populations (Harris et al. 1999), it appears that there are many potential modes of R/S intervention (e.g., direct R/S inquiry and exploration, R/S-based cognitive-behavioral exercises). These may be offered by a variety of health care personnel (e.g., nurses, physicians, psychologists, chaplains), and they may facilitate adaptive coping and lead to better outcomes in the patient with cancer. Clearly, however, more rigorous research on such interventions is needed and, hopefully, will be forthcoming.

Regardless of intervention specifics, the following general modes of addressing R/S-related issues with cancer patients have been suggested (NCI 2006): (1) explore R/S concerns within the context of the patient's medical care; (2) encourage the patient to pursue assistance from his or her own clergy; (3) make formal referrals to a hospital chaplain; (4) refer patients to a religious or faith-based therapist; and (5) refer patients to support groups known to address religious/spiritual issues. Another mode of addressing R/S concerns in the outpatient environment is to make available R/S resources in the waiting room (NCI 2006). Many such resources exist, and those materials that address all potential faith backgrounds of patients are desirable.

Summary

The onset or persistent symptoms of a chronic illness—whether a mental illness or a physical illness—continually call on resources for coping. Religion and spirituality play an important role for many people in appraising the threats that may be associated with their illness. R/S also provide resources for coping with illness, such as social support, offering comfort, and ways of making meaning. We have seen that from 41 percent to 77 percent of patients turn to R/S to help them absorb the reality of having an illness, as well as cope with their symptoms. These people who turn to R/S tend to have better quality of life and better physical well-being than those who do not. For some people, illness can challenge established religious beliefs and lead to R/S struggle or spiritual distress. When this struggle goes unresolved, they may have poorer emotional and physical responses.

A spiritual assessment can inform the caregiver about the needs of the patient for support in processing concerns, or in celebrating gifts and new insights from the experience of illness. It will also raise awareness about patients who might be engaged in R/S struggle and are in need of intervention, perhaps through a referral to a professional chaplain. Research in the relationship of R/S and health continues to expand. We have offered both information about that research as well as implications for patient care. We hope the reader will continue to explore research-based interventions when providing for the spiritual needs of patients.

Reflective Activities

1. How does religion/spirituality influence your coping abilities when you are ill?
2. How would you want a health care professional to support you as you draw on religious supports?
3. Which of the spiritual interventions identified as useful with the patient with a mental illness would you be comfortable using? Why? What about with a patient diagnosed with cancer? What would impede you from intervening to support the religious or spiritual needs of patients?

References

Abramson, L. Y., Metalsky, G. I., & Alloy, L. B. (1989). Hopelessness depression: A theory-based subtype of depression. *Psychological Review* 96: 358–72.

Acklin, M. W., Brown, E. C., & Mauger, P. A. (1983). The role of religious values in coping with cancer. *Journal of Religion and Health* 22: 322–33.

Aleman, A., Hijman, R., de Haan, E. H. F., & Kahn, R. S. (1999). Memory impairment in schizophrenia: A metanalysis. *American Journal of Psychiatry* 156: 1358–66.

American Cancer Society (ACS). (2007). Cancer facts and figures 2007, Atlanta: American Cancer Society. http://www.cancer.org/downloads/STT/CAFF2007PWSecured .pdf. Accessed March 21, 2008.

American Psychiatric Association (APA). (1994). *Diagnostic and statistical manual of mental disorders*, 4th ed. Washington, D.C.: American Psychiatric Association.

Anandarajah, G., & Hight, E. (2001). Spirituality and medical practice: Using the HOPE questions as a practical tool for spiritual assessment. *American Family Physician* 63: 81–89.

Avants, S. K., Beitel, M., & Margolin, A. (2005). Making the shift from 'addict self' to 'spiritual self': Results from a stage I study of spiritual self-schema (3-S) therapy for the treatment of addiction and HIV risk behavior. *Mental Health, Religion & Culture* 8: 167–77.

Baetz, M., Larson, D. B., Marcoux, G., Bowen, R., & Griffin, R. (2002). Canadian psychiatric inpatient religious commitment: An association with mental health. *The Canadian Journal of Psychiatry* 47: 59–166.

Balneaves, L. G., Kristjanson, L. J., & Tataryn, D. (1999). Beyond convention: Describing complementary therapy use by women living with breast cancer. *Patient Education and Counseling* 38: 143–53.

Bauemeister, R. F. (1990). Suicide as escape from self. *Psychological Review* 97: 90–114.

Bennett, M. J. (2001). *The empathic healer: An endangered species?* San Diego: Academic Press.

Boscaglia, N., Clarke, D. M., Jobling, T. W., & Quinn, M. A. (2005). The contribution of spirituality and spiritual coping to anxiety and depression in women with a recent diagnosis of gynecological cancer. *International Journal of Gynecological Cancer* 15: 755–61.

Bosworth, H. B., Park, K., McQuoid, D. R., Hays, J. C., & Steffens, D. C. (2003). The impact of religious practice and religious coping on geriatric depression. *International Journal of Geriatric Psychiatry* 18: 905–14.

Braam, A. W., Hein, E., Deeg, D. J., Twisk, J. W. R., Beekman, A. T. F., & Tilburg, W. V. (2004). Religious involvement and 6-year course of depressive symptoms in older Dutch citizens: Results from the longitudinal aging study in Amsterdam. *Journal of Aging and Health* 16: 467–89.

Bradshaw, A., & Fitchett, G. (2003). "God, why did this happen to me?": Three perspectives on theodicy. *Journal of Pastoral Care and Counseling* 57, no. 2: 179–89.

Brady, M. J., Peterman, A. H., Fitchett, G., Mo, M., & Cella, D. (1999). A case for including spirituality in quality of life measurement in oncology. *Psycho-oncology* 8: 417–28.

Brandt, B. T. (1987). The relationship between hopelessness and selected variables in women receiving chemotherapy for breast cancer. *Oncology Nursing Forum* 14: 35–39.

Canada, A. L., Parker, P. A., de Moor, J. S., Basen-Engquist, K., Ramondetta, L. M., & Cohen, L. (2006). Active coping mediates the association between religion/spirituality and quality of life in ovarian cancer. *Gynecological Oncology* 101: 102–7.

Carpenter, J. S., Brockopp, D. Y., & Andrykowski, M. A. (1999). Self-transformation as a factor in the self-esteem and well-being of breast cancer survivors. *Journal of Advanced Nursing* 29: 1402–11.

Carson, V., Soeken, K. L., & Grimm, P. M. (1988). Hope and its relation to spiritual well-being. *Journal of Psychology and Theology* 16: 159–67.

Carson, V., Soeken, K. L., Shanty, J., Terry, L. (1990). Hope and spiritual well-being: Essentials for living with AIDS. *Perspectives in Psychiatric Care* 26, no. 2: 28–34.

Carver, C. S., et al. (1993). How coping mediates the effects of optimism on distress: A study of women with early stage breast cancer. *Journal of Personality and Social Psychology* 65: 375–90.

Chang, B., Skinner, K. M., Zhou, C., & Kazis, L. E. (2003). The relationship between sexual assault, religiosity and mental health among male veterans. *The International Journal of Psychiatry in Medicine* 33: 223–39.

Cole, B. S. (2005). Spiritually-focused psychotherapy for people diagnosed with cancer: A pilot outcome study. *Mental Health, Religion & Culture* 8: 217–26.

Cole, B., & Pargament, K. (1999). Re-creating your life: A spiritual/psychotherapeutic intervention for people diagnosed with cancer. *Psycho-oncology* 8: 395–407.

Cook, C. H. (2004). Addiction and spirituality. *Addiction* 99: 539–51.

Cotton, S. P., Levine, E. G., Fitzpatrick, C. M., Dold, K. H., & Targ, E. (1999). Exploring the relationships among spiritual well-being, quality of life, and psychological adjustment in women with breast cancer. *Psycho-oncology* 8: 429–38.

Dalmida, S. G. (2006). Spirituality, mental health, physical health, and health-related quality of life among women with HIV/AIDS: Integrating spirituality into mental health care. *Issues in Mental Health Nursing* 27: 185–98.

Eeles, J., Lowe, T., & Wellman, N. (2003). Spirituality or psychosis? An exploration of the criteria that nurses use to evaluate spiritual-type experiences reported by patients. *International Journal of Nursing Studies*, 40: 197–206.

Ellison, C. G., Boardman, J. D., Williams, D. R., & Jackson, J. S. (2001). Religious involvement, stress, and mental health: Findings from the 1995 Detroit area study. *Social Forces* 80: 215–49.

Fallott, R. D. (1998a). Assessment of spirituality and implications for service planning. In R. D. Fallott (ed.), *Spirituality and religion in recovery from mental illness*, 13–23. San Francisco: Jossey-Bass.

———. (1998b). Spiritual and religious dimensions of mental illness recovery narratives. In R. D. Fallott (ed.), *Spirituality and religion in recovery from mental illness*, 35–44. San Francisco: Jossey-Bass.

Fallott, R. D., & Heckman, J. P. (2005). Religious/spiritual coping among women trauma survivors with mental health and substance use disorders. *Journal of Behavioral Health Services & Research* 32: 215–26.

Fawzy, F. I., et al. (1990). A structured psychiatric intervention for cancer patients: I. Changes over time in methods of coping and affective disturbance. *Archives of General Psychiatry* 47: 720–25.

Feher, S. & Maly, R. C. (1999). Coping with breast cancer in later life: The role of religious faith. *Psycho-oncology* 8: 408–16.

Fitchett, G. (1999a). Screening for spiritual risk. *Chaplaincy Today* 15, no. 1: 2–12.

———. (1999b). Selected resources for screening for spiritual risk. *Chaplaincy Today* 15, no. 1: 13–26.

Fitchett, George. (1993/2002). *Assessing Spiritual Needs: A Guide for Caregivers*. Original edition, Minneapolis: Augsburg, 1993; reprint edition, Lima, Ohio: Academic Renewal Press, 2002.

Fitchett, G., Burton, L. A., & Sivan, A. B. (1997). The religious needs and resources of psychiatric inpatients. *Journal of Nervous and Mental Disorders* 185: 320–26.

Fitchett, G., Murphy, P. E., Kim, J., Gibbons, J. L., Cameron, J. R., & Davis, J. A. (2004). Religious struggle: Prevalence, correlates and mental health risks in diabetic, congestive heart failure, and oncology patients. *The International Journal of Psychiatry in Medicine* 34: 179–96.

Fitchett, G., & Risk, J. L. (In Press). Screening for spiritual struggle. *Journal of Pastoral Care and Counseling*.

Fitchett, G., & Roberts, P. A. (2003). In the garden with Andrea: Spiritual assessment in end of life care. In C. M. Puchalski (ed.), *Walking together: Physicians, chaplains and clergy caring for the sick*. Washington, D.C.: The George Washington Institute for Spirituality and Health.

Fitchett, G., Rybarczyk, B. D., DeMarco, G. A., & Nicholas, J. J. (1999). The role of religion in medical rehabilitation outcomes: A longitudinal study. *Rehabilitation Psychology* 44: 333–53.

Flynn, P. M., Joe, G. W., Broome, K. M., Simpson, D. D., & Brown, B. S. (2003). Recovery from opioid addiction in DATOS. *Journal of Substance Abuse Treatment*, 25: 177–86.

Fowler, J. W. (1981). *Stages of faith*. San Francisco: Harper & Row.

Fredette, S. L. (1995). Breast cancer survivors: Concerns and coping. *Cancer Nursing*, http://www.norc.org/GSS+Website/Download/SPSS+Format/, 18: 35–46.

Gall, T. L. (2000). Integrating religious resources within a general model of stress and coping: Long-term adjustment to breast cancer. *Journal of Religion and Health* 39: 167–82.

Gall, T. L., Miguez de Renart, R. M., & Boonstra, B. (2000). Religious resources in long-term adjustment to breast cancer. *Journal of Psychosocial Oncology*, 18: 21–38.

Goeders, N. E. (2003). The impact of stress on addiction. *European Neuropsychopharmacology* 13: 435–41.

Greer, S. (1992). Adjuvant psychological therapy for women with breast cancer. *Boletin de Psicologia* 36: 71–83.

General Social Survey (GSS). (2007). (1972-2006) GSS Cumulative Data Set. http://www.norc.org/GSS+Website/Download/SPSS+Format/. Accessed March 21, 2008.

Halstead, M. T., & Fernsler, J. I. (1994). Coping strategies of long-term cancer survivors. *Cancer Nursing* 17: 94–100.

Harris, A. H. S., Thoresen, C. E., McCullough, M. E., & Larson, D. B. (1999). Spiritually and religiously oriented health interventions. *Journal of Health Psychology*, 4: 413–33.

Heim, E., Augustiny, K. F., Shaffner, L., & Valach, L. (1993). Coping with breast cancer over time and situation. *Journal of Psychosomatic Research* 37: 523–42.

Highfield, M. F. (1992). Spiritual health of oncology patients: Nurse and patient perspectives. *Cancer Nursing*, 15: 1–8.

Hout, M., & Fisher, C. S. (2002). Why more Americans have no religious preference: Politics and generations. *American Sociological Review* 67: 165–90.

Idler, E. L., & Kasl, S. (1992). Religion, disability, and the timing of death. *American Journal of Sociology* 97: 1052–79.

Ingersoll-Dayton, B., Krause, N., & Morgan, D. (2002). Religious trajectories and transitions over the life course. *International Journal of Aging* 55: 51–70.

Jacobson, C. J., Jr., Luckhaupt, S. E., Delaney, S., & Tsevat, J. (2006). Religio-biography, coping, and meaning-making among persons with HIV/AIDS. *Journal for the Scientific Study of Religion* 45: 39–56.

Jamison, K. (1995). *An unquiet mind: A memoir of moods and madness*. New York: Vintage Books.

Jenkins, R. A., & Pargament, K. I. (1995). Religion and spirituality as resources for coping with cancer. *Journal of Psychosocial Oncology*, 13: 51–73.

Johnson, S. C., & Spilka, B. (1991). Coping with breast cancer: The role of clergy and faith. *Journal of Religion and Health* 30: 21–33.

Josephson, A. M., & Peteet, J. R. (eds.). (2004). *Handbook of spirituality and worldview in clinical practice*. Washington, D.C.: American Psychiatric Publishing, Inc.

Kabat-Zinn, J., et al. (1992). Effectiveness of a meditation-based stress reduction program in the treatment of anxiety disorders. *The American Journal of Psychiatry* 149: 936–43.

Kaczorowski, J. M. (1989). Spiritual well-being and anxiety in adults diagnosed with cancer. *Hospice Journal* 5: 105–16.

Kendler, K. S., Gardner, C. O., & Prescott, C. A. (1997). Religion, psychopathology, and substance use and abuse: A multimeasure, genetic-epidemiologic study. *The American Journal of Psychiatry* 154: 322–29.

Kessler, R. C., Berglund, P., Demler, O., Jin, R., Merijangas, K. R., & Walters, E. E. (2005). Lifetime prevalence and age-of-onset distributions of DSM-IV disorders in the national comorbidity survey replication. *Archives of General Psychiatry* 62: 593–602.

Kessler, R. C., Nelson, C. B., McGonagle, K. A., Edlund, M. J., Frank, R. G., & Leaf, P. J. (1996). The epidemiology of co-occuring addictive and mental disorders: Implications for prevention and service utilization. *American Journal of Orthopsychiatry* 66: 17–31.

Kirkbride, J. B., et al. (2006). Heterogenity in incidence rates of schizophrenia and other psychotic syndromes: Findings from the 3-center AeSOP study. *Archives of General Psychiatry* 63: 250–58.

Kirkpatrick, L. A., & Shaver, P. R. (1990). Attachment theory and religions: Childhood attachments, religious beliefs and conversion. *Journal for the Scientific Study of Religion* 29: 315–34.

Kirov, G., Kemp, R., Kirov, K., & David, A. S. (1998). Religious faith after psychotic illness. *Psychopathology* 31: 234–45.

Koenig, H. (2001). Religion and medicine II: Religion, mental health, and related behaviors. *The International Journal of Psychiatry in Medicine* 31: 97–109.

Koenig, H. G., George, L. K., & Peterson, B. L. (1998). Religiosity and remission of depression in medically ill older patients. *The American Journal of Psychiatry* 155: 536–42.

Koenig, H. G., McCullough, M. E., & Larson, D. B. (2001). *Handbook of religion and health*. New York: Oxford University Press.

Kohut, H. (1987). *The Kohut Seminars, on self psychology and psychotherapy with adolescents and young adults*, M. Elson (ed.). New York: Norton.

Krause, N., & Van Tran, T. (1989). Stress and religious involvement among older Blacks. *Journals of Gerontology* 44: S4–13.

Kristeller, J. L., Rhodes, M., Cripe, L. D., & Sheets, V. (2005). Oncologist Assisted Spiritual Intervention (OASIS): Patient acceptability and initial evidence of effects. *The International Journal of Psychiatry in Medicine* 34: 329–47.

Kroll, J., & Sheehan, W. (1989). Religious beliefs and practices among 52 psychiatric inpatients in Minnesota. *The American Journal of Psychiatry*, 146: 67–72.

Laudet, A. B. (2003). Attitudes and beliefs about 12-step groups among addiction treatment clients and clinicians: Toward identifying obstacles in participation. *Substance Use and Misuse* 38: 2017–47.

Lawson, R., Drebing, C., Berg, G., Vincellette, A., & Penk, W. (1998). The long term impact of child abuse on religious behavior and spirituality in men. *Child Abuse & Neglect* 22: 369–80.

Lazarus, R. S., & Folkman, S. (1984). *Stress, apprisal, and coping*. New York: Springer.

Lengacher, C. A., et al. (2003). Design and testing of the use of a complementary and alternative therapies survey in women with breast cancer. *Oncology Nursing Forum*, 30: 811–21.

Levin, J. S. (1994). Religion and health: Is there an association, is it valid and is it causal? *Social Science & Medicine* 38: 1475–82.

Levin, J. S., & Chatters, L. M. (1998). Religion, health, and psychological well-being in older adults: Findings from three national surveys. *Journal of Aging and Health* 10: 504–31.

Lindgren, K. N., & Coursey, R. D. (1995). Spirituality and serious mental illness: A two-part study. *Psychosocial Rehabilitaton Journal* 18, no. 3: 93–111.

Lucas, A. M. (2001). The discipline for pastoral care giving. In L. VandeCreek and A. M. Lucas (eds.), *Introduction to the discipline for pastoral care giving*, 1–33. Binghamton, N.Y.: Haworth Press, Inc.

Manheimer, E., Anderson, B. J., & Stein, M.D. (2003). Use and assessment of complementary and alternative therapies by intravenous drug users. *The American Journal of Drug and Alcohol Abuse* 29: 401–13.

Matri, S. (2001). *Spiritual dimensions of the Enneagram: Nine faces of the soul*. New York: Barnes and Noble.

Manning-Walsh, J. (2005). Spiritual struggle: Effect on quality of life and life satisfaction in women with breast cancer. *Journal of Holistic Nursing* 23: 120–40.

Maton, K. I. (1989). The stress-buffering role of spiritual support: Cross-sectional and prospective investigations. *Journal for the Scientific Study of Religion* 28: 310–33.

McClain, C. S., Rosenfeld, B., & Breitbart, W. (2003). Effect of spiritual well-being on end-of-life despair in terminally-ill cancer patients. *Lancet* 361: 1603–7.

McCullough, M. E., Hoyt, W. T., Larson, D. B., Koenig, H. G., & Thoresen, C. (2000). Religious involvement and mortality: A meta-analytic review. *Health Psychology* 19: 211–22.

McCullough, M. E., & Larson, D. B. (1999). Religion and depression: A review of the literature. *Twin Research* 2: 126–36.

Mickley, J. R., Carson, V., & Soeken, K. I. (1995). Religion and adult mental health: State of the science in nursing. *Issues in Mental Health Nursing* 16: 345–60.

Mickley, J. R., Soeken, K., & Belcher, A. (1992). Spiritual well-being, religiousness and hope among women with breast cancer. *IMAGE: Journal of Nursing Scholarship* 24: 267–72.

Miller, W. R. (1998). Researching the spiritual dimensions of alcohol and other drug problems. *Addiction* 93: 979–90.

Mitchell, L., & Romans, S. (2003). Spiritual beliefs in bipolar affective disorder: Their relevance for illness management. *Journal of Affective Disorders* 75: 247–57.

Mohr, S., & Huguelet, P. (2004). The relationship between schizophrenia and religion and its implications for care. *Swiss Medical Weekly* 134: 369–76.

Murphy, P. E., Ciarrocchi, J. W., Piedmont, R. L., Cheston, S., Peyrot, M., & Fitchett, G. (2000). The relation of religious belief and practices, depression, and hopelessness in persons with clinical depression. *Journal of Clinical and Consulting Psychology* 68: 1102–6.

Murphy, P. E., & Fitchett, G. (2006). The impact of religious belief on response to treatment for clinical depression: A longitudinal analysis. *Psychosomatic Medicine* 68, no. 1: A-86.

Murray-Swank N., & Pargament, K. I. (2005). God, where are you? Evaluating a spiritually integrated intervention for sexual abuse. *Mental Health, Religion, & Culture* 8: 191–203.

National Cancer Institute (NCI). (2006). *Physician Data Query: Spirituality in cancer care.* http://www.nci.nih.gov/cancerinfo/pdq/supprtivecare/spirituality/healthprofessional. Accessed June 1, 2006.

Neelman, J., & Lewis, G. (1994). Religious identity and comfort beliefs in three groups of psychiatric patients and a group of medical controls. *International Journal of Social Psychiatry* 40: 124–34.

Nielsen, S. L., Ridley, C. R., & Johnson, W. B. (2000). Religiously sensitive rational emotive behavior therapy: Theory, techniques, and brief excerpts from a case. *Professional Psychology: Research and Practice* 31: 21–28.

Pardini, D. A., Plante, T. G., Sherman, A., & Stump, J. E. (2000). Religioius faith and spirituality in substance abuse recovery: Determining the mental health benefits. *Journal of Substance Abuse Treatment* 9: 347–54.

Pargament, K. I. (1997). *The psychology of religion and coping: Theory, research, practice.* New York: The Guilford Press.

Pargament, K. I., Koenig, H. G., Tarakeshwar, N., & Hahn, J. (2004). Religious coping methods as predictors of psychological, physical and spiritual outcomes among medically ill elderly patients: A two-year longitudinal study. *Journal of Health Psychology* 9: 713–30.

Pargament. K. I., et al. (2004). Religion and HIV: A review of the literature and clinical implications. *Swiss Medical Journal* 97: 1201–9.

Park, C. (2005). Religion and meaning. In R. F. Paloutzian and C. L. Park (eds.), *Handbook of the psychology of religion and spirituality*, 295–314. New York: The Guilford Press.

Pollner, M. (1995). Divine relations, social relations, and well-being. *Journal of Health and Social Behavior* 30: 92–104.

Poloma, M. M., & Pendleton, B. F. (1991). The effects of prayer and prayer experiences on measures of general well-being. *Journal of Psychology and Theology* 19: 71–83.

Propst, R., Ostrom, R., Watkins, P., Dean, T., & Mashburn, D. (1992). Comparative efficacy of religious and nonreligious cognitive-behavioral therapy for treatment of clinical depression in religious individuals. *Journal of Consulting and Clinical Psychology* 60: 94–103.

Pruyser, P. W. (1976). *The Minister as Diagnostician.* Philadelphia: The Westminster Press.

Puchalski, C., & Romer, A. L. (2000). Taking a spiritual history allows clinicians to understand patients more fully. *Journal of Palliative Medicine* 3: 129–37.

Rector, N. A., & Beck, A. T. (2001). Cognitive behavioral therapy for schizophrenia: An empirical review. *The Journal of Nervous and Mental Disease* 189: 278–87.

Reger, G. M., & Rogers, S. A. (2002). Diagnostic differences in religious coping among individuals with persistent mental illness. *Journal of Psychology and Christianity* 21: 314–48.

Ringdal, G. I. (1996). Religiosity, quality of life, and survival in cancer patients. *Social Indicators Research* 38: 193–211.

Rizutto, A. M. (1979). *The birth of the living God: A psychoanalytic study*. Chicago: University of Chicago Press.

Roberts, J. A., et al. (1997). Factors influencing views of patients with gynecological cancer about end-of-life decisions. *American Journal of Obstetrics and Gynecology* 176: 166–72.

Russinova, Z., Wiorski, N. J., & Cash, D. (2002). Use of alternative health care practices by persons with serious mental illness: Perceived benefits. *American Journal of Public Health* 92: 1600–1603.

Scott, J., Paykel, E., Morriss, R., Bentall, R., Kinderman, P., Johnson, T., Abbott, R., & Hayhurst, H. (2006). Cognitive-behavioural therapy for bipolar disorder. *The British Journal of Psychiatry* 188: 488–89.

Sephton, S., Koopman, C., Schaal, M., Thoresen, C., & Spiegel, D. (2001). Spiritual expression and immune status in women with metastatic breast cancer: An exploratory study. *The Breast Journal* 7: 345–53.

Sherman, A. C., Simonton, S., Latif, U., Spohn, R., & Tricot, G. (2005). Religious struggle and religious comfort in response to illness: Health outcomes among stem cell transplant patients. *Journal of Behavioral Medicine* 28: 359–67.

Smith, T. B., McCullough, M. E., & Poll, J. (2003). Religiousness and depression: Evidence for a main effect and the moderating influence of stressful life events. *Psychological Bulletin* 129: 614–36.

Sodestrom, K. E., & Martinson, I. M. (1987). Patients' spiritual coping strategies: A study of nurse and patient perspectives. *Oncology Nursing Forum* 14: 41–46.

Stern, D. N. (1985). *The interpersonal world of the infant: A view from psychoanalysis and developmental psychology*. New York: Basic Books, Inc.

Strawbridge, W. J., Shema, S. J., Cohen, R. D., & Kaplan, G.A. (2001). Religious attendance increases survival by improving and maintaining good health behaviors, mental health, and social support. *Annals of Behavioral Medicine* 23: 58–74.

Strawbridge, W. J., Shema, S. J., Cohen, R. D., Roberts, R. E., & Kaplan, G. A. (1998). Religion buffers effects of some stressors on depression but exacerbates others. *Journals of Gerontology: Series B: Psychological Sciences and Social Sciences* 53B: S118–26.

Strozier, C. B. (2001). *Heinz Kohut: The making of a psychoanalyst*. New York: Farrar, Straus & Giroux.

Sullivan, W. P. (1998). Recoiling, regrouping, and recovering: First-person accounts of the role of spirituality in the course of serious mental illness. In R. D. Fallot (ed.), *Spirituality and religion in recovery from mental illness*, 25–33. San Francisco: Jossey-Bass.

Tatsumura, Y., Maskarinec, G., Shumay, D. M., & Kakai, H. (2003). Religious and spiritual resources, CAM, and conventional treatment in the lives of cancer patients. *Alternative Therapies in Health and Medicine* 9: 64–71.

Tepper, L., Rogers, S. A., Coleman, E. M., & Malony, H. N. (2001). The prevalence of religious coping among persons with persistent mental illness. *Psychiatric Services* 52: 660–65.

Turner, R. P., Lukoff, D., Barnhouse, R. T., & Lu, F. G. (1995). Religious or spiritual problem: A culturally sensitive diagnostic category in the DSM-IV. *Journal of Nervous and Mental Disease* 183: 435–44.

VandeCreek, L., Rogers, E., & Lester, J. (1999). Use of alternative therapies among breast cancer outpatients compared with the general population. *Alternative Therapies in Health and Medicine* 5: 71–76.

Ventis, W. L. (1995). The relationship between religion and mental health. *Journal of Social Issues* 51, no. 2: 33–48.

Vidal, C. N., et al. (2006). Dynamically spreading frontal and cingulated deficits mapped in adolescents with schizophrenia. *Archives of General Psychiatry* 63: 25–34.

Westerhoff, J. H., III. (1976). *Will our children have faith?* New York: The Seabury Press.

Yates, J. S., Mustian, K. M., Morrow, G. R., Gillies, L. J., Padmanaban, D., Atkins, J. N., Issell, B., Kirshner, J. J., & Colman, L. K. (2005). Prevalence of complementary and alternative medicine use in cancer patients during treatment. *Supportive Care in Cancer* 13: 806–11.

Yates, J. W., Chalmer, B. J., St. James, P. , Follansbee, M., & McKegney, F. P. (1981). Religion in patients with advanced cancer. *Medical and Pediatric Oncology* 9: 121–28.

Zaza, C., Sellick, S. M., & Hillier, L. M. (2005). Coping with cancer: What do patients do? *Journal of Psychosocial Oncology* 23: 55–73.

9

SPIRITUALITY AND ELDER CARE

THOMAS E. DELOUGHRY

> *Love never fails.*
> —1 Corinthians 13:8

Introduction

Growing old is harder than growing up. Loss looms. Cherished roles and loved ones disappear. Vitality fades—gradually or suddenly. The purpose for living may be challenged or shattered.

Yet we are never too old to be well (DeLoughry & Levy 2006), despite diminished roles, declining abilities, and serious illness. The elder who sits alone in a kitchen that once bustled with life, the ninety-year-old who has reluctantly moved to a nursing home, and the newly diagnosed cancer patient can all find greater happiness—and so can those who care for them.

Lasting peace of mind can be found by prioritizing the pursuit of love. The goal is not to rekindle the physical passions of youth. Instead, deep satisfaction can be found by growing in selfless love, or agape.

Agape is articulated in the golden rule, expressed by Jesus Christ as "loving your neighbor as yourself." It also is common to all the great religions, including Buddhism, Islam, Christianity, Hinduism, and Confucianism (Armstrong 2006). Hillel the Elder, a Jewish religious leader who lived during the time of King Herod, expressed it by saying: "Whatever is hateful to you, do not do to your neighbor. That is the whole Torah. The rest is commentary" (Weinstein 2006).

"Every religion emphasizes human improvement, love, respect for others and sharing other people's suffering," according to the Dalai Lama (Robinson 2006). Thus, these common values are a good starting point for a consideration of spirituality in elder care, since they are held by people of every faith or no faith.

Studies indicate that spirituality is a consistent predictor of well-being, regardless of physical functioning (Daaleman et al. 2004) or degree of frailty (Kirby et al. 2004). Spirituality is an important aspect of elder care, yet approaching it in elder care is complicated by the variety of religions.

Spirituality is good medicine for the challenges and disappointments of aging. "I've had to accept that I'm not important anymore," said Isabelle Reilly, a ninety-six-year-old sister of St. Francis. Her responsibilities had included the direction of more than five hundred nuns who operated two large hospitals and ran twenty-five schools in five East Coast states. "But now I have more time to experience love," she added with a quiet smile.

Spirituality is simple—it's about love, caring, and being connected. But it's also complex, because everyone has a different view of it, which needs to be respected. Religion can guide us to spirituality and love. But since we're all different, it's important to respect individual beliefs and different ways of finding love, with or without religion.

Most of the same steps that can help the elderly can help each of us. Thus, this chapter is aimed at helping the elderly and family caregivers as well as the professionals and aides who serve them.

In this chapter, love—held up as the greatest of virtues by St. Paul—will be a particular focus. Love is both a spiritual goal (e.g., experiencing the love of God) and a path to reach that goal (e.g., "Love one another").

Although love will be used as a theme to explore spirituality in elder care, we must realize that no words—let alone one single concept—can ever capture the majesty, wonder, and mystery of the Spirit. God is often described as love. For example, Thomas Merton has written: "He is none of our idols, none of our figments, nothing that we can imagine anyway. He is Love itself. And if we realize this . . . life itself is transformed" (Merton 1994).

Love will be discussed as a "sense of oneness"—an experience that includes the intimacies of friendship, the ties within a family, a connection to nature, and the union with the Spirit. It is also the caring that draws professionals and aides to the patients they serve.

There is, of course, both a quantative and a qualitative difference between the love or "oneness" someone might feel for a friend, a family member, or nature. And there may be an infinite difference between the love of God and other expressions of "oneness" we may experience. However, "oneness" remains a useful concept as we explore the varying dimensions of love.

This chapter will also describe love as a behavior. Thus, love is also the service of the aging volunteer who delivers meals on wheels, serves as a foster grandparent, or makes phone calls to lonely shut-ins.

Viewing love as a behavior will allow us to explore cognitive-behavioral strategies, health behavioral concepts, and community intervention principles (Green & Kreuter 1991) in the quest to promote greater peace of mind.

Some, who would otherwise be reluctant to interject spirituality into elder care, should find it easy to discuss love as a relationship issue. This perspective also allows the rich literature and related strategies for enhancing social support to be considered.

What if the goal of "experiencing more love" were incorporated into the care plans of the elderly as well as wellness plans of their caregivers? And what if these plans addressed physical, emotional, and spiritual needs through a community program that reached out—through newspapers, newsletters, television, community workshops, staff training, and the Internet—to touch everyone who touched the elderly?

In western New York, a Niagara County program (DeLoughry & DeLoughry 2002) has been answering these questions for the past six years. Goals for the mind, body, and spirit are being supported by the County Office for the Aging, the County Department of Health, the Coalition of Agencies in Service to the Elderly (CASE), the Council on Aging (COA), and other elder care organizations. This approach to continuous-improvement care planning meets federal training and mandated accreditation requirements, while teaching relevant cognitive-behavioral skills. Organizational policies and procedures are also considered in an effort to improve both quality and outcomes.

Bridging the Separate Silos of Care

"Optimal physical, emotional and spiritual well-being are our goals for elder care," says John Kinner, executive director of the Health Association of Niagara County, Inc. (HANCI). For the past seventy-five years, HANCI has promoted quality of life for well seniors, frail elders, and their caregivers through its social, home health, and adult day care programs. It touches more than fifty thousand seniors each year through its support of the Council on Aging, Golden Age Clubs, Foster Grandparents programs, Senior Companion program, and Retired Senior Volunteer Program (RSVP).

"We are taking steps to bridge the separate silos of care," Kinner says, "by developing care plans that address the needs of the mind, body, and spirit. And we're doing that within the context of a community program that coordinates staff training and presentations at senior centers with newspaper, television, and Internet campaigns. We want everyone—professionals, aides, seniors, elders, family caregivers—to speak the same language."

The Niagara Caregivers Network, which HANCI sponsors and Kinner helped launch, coordinates much of Niagara's mind-body-spirit program. The same simple poem (DeLoughry & Levy 2006) is used for care planning, organizational planning, and community planning to achieve medical, emotional, and spiritual goals:

> Remember goals and
> Check the signs.
> Take some steps and
> Learn each time.

The progression described in this poem will be used in this chapter to discuss the medical, emotional, and spiritual issues of elder care. It outlines a universal process that can help well seniors, frail elders, caregivers, organizations, and communities to achieve their goals.

Are We Ever Too Sick to Be Well?

During her early seventies, Loretta was an active senior, despite the beginnings of emphysema and occasional episodes of angina and depression.

At seventy-four, she suddenly became ill and was admitted to the hospital. She declined quickly, as all treatments failed. Her daughter packed her black dress and flew home.

"How much love can we experience?" Since medicine wasn't helping, that question guided the family. Her husband, son, and daughter held her hand and talked

about the good times. Music softened the sterility of her hospital room. They prayed together, thanking God for a life where the good outweighed the bad.

The next day she was better, and three days later she was discharged. The doctors never diagnosed the cause of her illness.

She recommitted herself to the Catholicism that had been an important part of her life, becoming a Eucharistic minister and volunteering at a nursing home. Her physical health declined as emphysema took its toll, but her spiritual wellness grew.

"I know why I got so sick," Loretta said. It was three years later and she was picnicking with her son by a creek behind her assisted living home.

"I flunked my high school equivalency exam," she began. Her son was shocked into silence.

"It always bothered me that I had to drop out of high school during the Depression and I wanted that diploma," Loretta explained. "So I swore your Dad to secrecy and enrolled in a high school equivalency program. I thought I did pretty well, but when they mailed me the test results I saw that I had failed—by just two points! The next day I started to get sick, and three days later the ambulance took me to the hospital."

A disappointment caused her illness. Perhaps her family's love was the cure.

"During her final months, there was a glow about my mother I had never seen before," her son recalled. "She had terrible falls and was always short of breath. Yet mostly she was happy and peaceful."

"My mother was well in the months before she died," he continued. "It's odd to say that because physically she was such a mess."

What makes us well? (See Figure 9–1.) Loretta's emotional and spiritual well-being outshone her physical limitations. Her story shows what research demonstrates: Spirituality is an important factor in well-being.

You're never too old to be well—regardless of the physical illnesses or limitations you have. You do not have to stop being well, just because your body is sick. In fact, peace of mind can always grow.

Because there is such a strong connection between physical, emotional, and spiritual health, this chapter will address each type of wellness as it affects the goals of elder care, the assessment of needs, and the development of care plans.

Spiritual and emotional outcomes can continue to improve up until the moment of death.

In elder care we expect that sooner or later a patient's physical well-

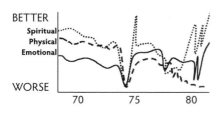

What Makes Us Well?

Figure 9–1   Loretta's spiritual and emotional health improved, despite a decline in physical health.

being will wane, and a major goal of medicine and related therapies is to delay this decline. Equal, or greater, attention should be paid to enhancing the wellness of the mind and the spirit.

The spiritual values of love and compassion may be the best hope for addressing the individual, organizational, and community challenges of aging. As baby boomers age, it is widely anticipated that resources will shrink as demand increases, forcing communities to make difficult choices.

A crisis is looming for many families and most communities. Thus, this chapter will also discuss how spirituality can guide our choices as professionals, administrators, and policy makers.

The Goals of the Elderly

Aging is a tough battle, fought with fewer and fewer resources. Earlier allies, like self-esteem and usefulness, may be weak or absent. Former strategies to conquer depression, such as visiting friends, attending a church supper, or even walking, are difficult or impossible when you're in a wheelchair, worried about incontinence, or tethered to an oxygen concentrator.

The words of Jesus on the cross, "My God, my God, why have you forsaken me?" are echoed every day by millions of elders. Some lie bed-bound in nursing homes or hospitals. Others stare out windows of empty homes. Too few grow in love and wisdom. Too many never grasp the godly graces that surround them, or the blessings that await them.

Physical impairments and emotional problems make activities of daily living more and more challenging. A sense of meaning, or a purpose for living, is hard to find. Freedom from family responsibilities creates feelings of futility. The ending of a career may seem like the end of usefulness.

Yet, as expressed earlier by Sister Isabelle, the quieter times and slower rhythms of the elder years can be a time to hear the harmonies of nature and see the light of love.

Goals for elders might include:

PHYSICAL

Taking care of all, or most, of your own needs at home

Feeling well enough to garden, dance, or enjoy some other hobbies

Having the mobility to visit friends and family

SOCIAL/SPIRITUAL

Experiencing as much love as possible—perhaps the most important goal?

Maintaining contact with friends, family, and relatives

Maintaining or restoring a sense of being needed and recognized

Having a sense of purpose (e.g., passing on wisdom; sharing more love)

Finding meaning and comfort in life

EMOTIONAL

Feeling content, despite declining abilities

Maintaining control and choice

Overcoming depression and stress

Experiencing love and joy

How Much Love Can We Experience?

"'How much love can we experience?' That was the question that turned the tide," recalled Loretta's son. *"We still pushed the doctors to do more tests and to try new therapies. But a lot of our focus shifted to treasuring what we thought would be Mom's final days. We wanted to celebrate our love. Apparently that was the medicine she needed."*

Love is a useful starting point in exploring spiritual goals in elder care because of:

The universality of love in the world's major religions.

The value of love as both a goal (e.g., being loved by God) as well as a means to that goal (e.g., loving God and others).

The perception of love as both a social experience and a spiritual experience. Thus, a health professional can comfortably discuss love even with a confirmed atheist.

The importance of love in:
Goal setting.
Assessments.
Individual care plans and organizational initiatives.
The measure of our own personal ministries.

This chapter will explore four strategies to help elders, caregivers, and professionals to enhance their spirituality by experiencing more love. These are:

To employ the ministries of word, action, and presence, as presented by Dr. Verna Benner Carson in chapter 6.

To use the "satisfaction skills"—four cognitive behavioral skills (i.e., awareness, affirmations, assertiveness, and acceptance) that will be detailed later in this chapter.

To implement organizational policies, training programs, and other initiatives.

To practice the golden rule.

The Goals of Caregivers

It is as difficult to help the elderly without considering their caregivers as it is to help children without involving their parents.

Most babies smile and giggle when their diapers are changed. However, an elderly person, faced with this indignity, is more likely to be curt than cute. Thus, caregivers have the responsibilities of parenting with few of the rewards.

Viewing caregiving as a spiritual ministry can help a significant proportion of our population, as approximately one out of every five adults is engaged in elder care. Family caregivers are the most important part of our long-term care system. They provide about 80 percent of the care for people who need help with daily activities, such as bathing and dressing, taking medications, and paying bills.

What issues are faced by caregivers? Burnout, frustration, disappointment, and the questioning of God's will. Regardless of education and role, these issues must be addressed whether the caregiver is paid or unpaid.

Goals for family caregivers might include:

Finding spiritual meaning in their caregiving

Becoming actively involved in care planning

Avoiding burnout through the use of available resources as well as communication and coping skills

Organizational Goals

"For a long time the spiritual piece was left out of care planning because we were uncomfortable with it," says HANCI's Kinner. "But we conducted a community survey and learned that 87 percent of seniors felt that their spiritual needs were as or more important than their medical needs; and that 94 percent found their emotional needs to be as or more important than their medical needs.

"The needs of the whole person were rarely integrated into one treatment plan when we started to look at spirituality from the organizational perspective."

Organizations are likely to see controlling costs or increasing market share as more important goals than caring. Yet, caring—a goal with spiritual dimensions—can make a crucial contribution to these "more important" goals. This is true because the spiritual values of love and compassion are associated with better communication. This leads to more satisfied patients who are less likely to sue for malpractice or "jump" to services provided by another organization.

Love, compassion, and communication are also crucial factors in reducing costly turnover of elder care aides and professionals. The top three reasons associated with turnover are poor communication (Davidson & Folcarelli 1997, Buelow et al. 1999); high stress (Gaddy & Bechtel 1995);

and lack of involvement in care planning (Caudill & Patrick 1991). These issues can be effectively addressed in an organization where staff truly cares for one other.

The integration of spirituality into the workplace is not just restricted to health care organizations, nor should it be restricted just to those who "touch" patients. As reported in the *New York Times* (Shorto 2004), work-sites ranging from the federal Centers for Disease Control and Prevention to Intel, the technology giant, allow employees to discuss religious issues on their premises.

Organizational goals may include the integration of spiritual values into mission statements, policies and procedures, supervisory sessions, training programs, and strategic plans (Artis 2005, Smessaert 1989, Woods 2001) in order to achieve:

Improved medical, emotional, and spiritual outcomes

Greater patient and family satisfaction

Reduction of staff turnover

Compliance with Medicare/Medicaid standards and the Joint Commission on Accreditation of Healthcare Organizations (JCAHO) accreditation standards

Improved quality of care

Community Goals

"Niagara County is resource rich. The problem is that people don't know where to go for services," says Christopher Richbart, director of Niagara County's Office for the Aging. "We want them to be able to access all the resources that might help them, whether they be medical, emotional, social, or spiritual services."

Communication about the services and the development of care plans that utilize all appropriate services are important goals for most communities. Because health is cocreated—it is important to engage the whole community in developing pathways to care.

In planning sessions sponsored by the Niagara Caregivers Network, two important coalitions have worked together to examine how spirituality can be integrated into elder care. They are:

1. The Coalition of Agencies in Service to the Elderly (CASE), consisting of more than thirty traditional elder care organizations, which has been invaluable in providing professional leadership.
2. The Council on Aging (COA), which has lent grassroots support and practical advice in program planning, while representing over fifty senior clubs and centers throughout the county.

The initial collaboration of COA and CASE on a mind-body-spirit initiative was the launching of Sharing Your Wishes—an end-of-life care planning program that was developed and funded through the Community Health Foundation of Western and Central New York. Four steps are suggested:

1. Think about what's important to you and how you want to receive your care.
2. Select a person to speak for you if you are unable to speak for yourself.
3. Talk about your health care wishes.
4. Put your choices in writing, using a state-approved health care proxy form.

Although much of Sharing Your Wishes is focused on planning for your medical needs if you are unable to speak for yourself, the Niagara County initiative also encourages participants to plan for their emotional and spiritual goals.

It has been integrated with the Never Too Old initiative because:

Both programs support the same patient-centered goals espoused by the Community Health Foundation, and

The health care agent (appointed by the proxy form to represent the patient's wishes if the patient is unable to speak for herself) is also likely to be the primary family caregiver, whom Never Too Old enlists as a health care partner.

"It's all about the conversation," says Laurie Marshanke, CASE chairperson and a Sharing Your Wishes trainer, who also assisted in the development of Never Too Old. "We're encouraging discussions that focus on medical needs, but also on what people want emotionally and spiritually in their final days.

"Conversations about mind-body-spirit goals in Never Too Old are equally or even more important because our goal there is quality of life, rather than respecting wishes at end of life," she added.

Never Too Old is funded by the Niagara County Office for the Aging. It uses an interactive CD, which includes forty-five minutes of video, introducing families to elder care services while stressing the importance of considering goals for the whole person. An accompanying booklet, "Never Too Old to Be Well: Improving the Physical, Emotional and Spiritual Health of Elders and their Families" (DeLoughry & Levy 2006), communicates:

The range of elder care services and how to access them.

Two concepts:
Wellness depends on physical, emotional, and spiritual health.
The choices we make determine how we age.

Two processes:
A care planning system, which can be used to enhance physical, emotional, and spiritual health, as expressed through a simple poem (introduced earlier) that encourages continuous quality improvement:
Remember goals and
Check your signs.
Choose your steps and
Learn each time.

A communication cycle, called "satisfaction skills," that teaches four cognitive-behavioral skills (i.e., awareness, affirmations, assertiveness, acceptance), which can be used to improve communication, manage stress, and/or enhance spirituality.

Never Too Old pilot participants (i.e., elders, family caregivers, professionals, aides) report that the satisfaction skills help them with the goals of improving communication, reducing stress, and enhancing spirituality:

One hundred percent of professionals (n = 65) and caregivers (n = 211) agreed that the satisfaction skills could help to improve communication and manage stress.

Ninety-seven percent of professionals (n = 63) and 95 percent of caregivers (n = 201) agreed that the satisfaction skills could enhance their spirituality.

Figure 9–2   A coordinated community approach to improving quality of life.

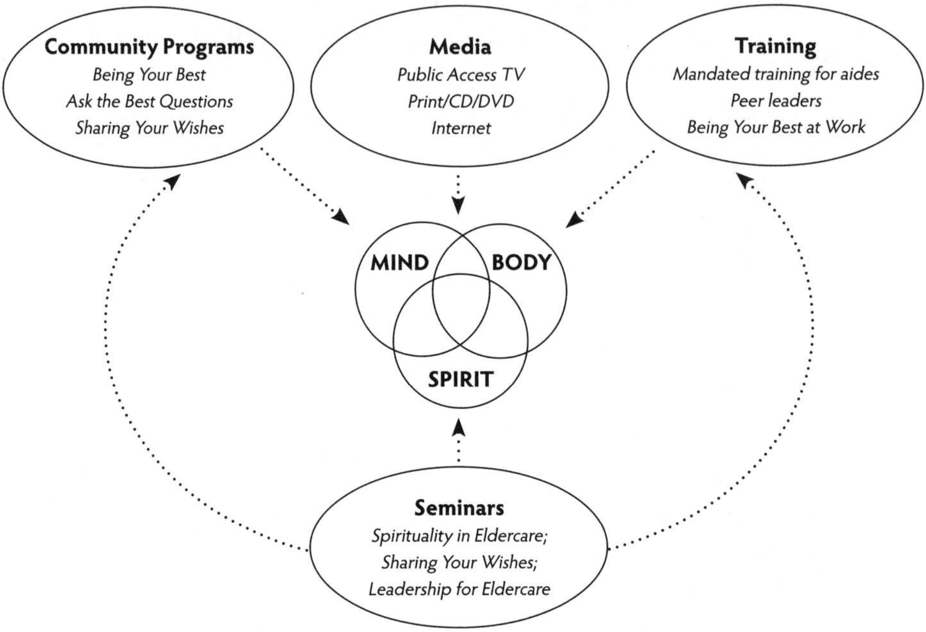

One hundred percent of aides in home health (n = 64) and long-term care (n = 59) agreed that the satisfaction skills could improve communication, while 94 percent of aides agreed that it could help in managing stress; and 88 percent agreed that it could enhance their spirituality.

Never Too Old has been developed as a communitywide intervention (Green & Kreuter 1991) that integrates patient and caregiver education with staff training and organizational policies and procedures, while coordinating a community newspaper, Internet, and television campaigns that link people to existing programs and services. As shown in Figure 9–2, a series of professional seminars have also been used to reinforce program activities.

Never Too Old is based, in part, on federally mandated training requirements for aides,[1] as well as quality-improvement protocols mandated by the Centers for Medicare and Medicaid Services and the Joint Commission on Accreditation of Healthcare Organizations (JCAHO). It also addresses goals of Project 2015: State Agencies Prepare for an Aging New York.

"The best way to serve our home health patients is to address the full range of their needs," says Paulette Kline, director of Niagara County's Health Department. "Our Long-Term Home Health Care program is sometimes called a 'nursing home without walls.' Our staff is incorporating Never Too Old materials into their care plans because we see it as a way to address the needs of the whole patient, while encouraging a closer collaboration between the Health Department and the Office for Aging."

The establishment of a Leadership for Elder Care forum, a final community goal, has yet to be accomplished. The intent is to bring the business community, insurance carriers, legislators, and professionals who provide emotional, medical, and spiritual care to the same table to discuss how to improve the quality of life for seniors, elders, and their caregivers. The business community has a strong voice in determining legislation, regulations, and funding for elder care initiatives. Thus, it is important to engage them in a dialogue that considers the needs of the whole person.

Spirituality and the golden rule can also be good for business, as the "marketplace ministry" movement contends by viewing work as a spiritual path (Stevens & Banks 2005). Thus, we hope that engaging business and insurance leaders in a mind-body-spirit initiative may have multiple benefits as the spiritual values of love and compassion begin to influence decisions about elder care and a wide range of other issues.

Be Alert, But Don't Convert

The committee members had been spinning their wheels for the last half-hour. "When should assessments be done?" "Who should do them?" And, most difficult of all, "What should be done if spiritual issues do surface?"

The questions went back and forth between the members of HANCI's Policies and Procedures for Spirituality Committee, but no progress was being made. Then, a quiet voice spoke up: "Be alert, but don't convert."

Sister Marietta Miller, OSF, paused as her words were absorbed around the table. A small woman with deep insights, she is a Franciscan sister who is a certified spiritual director and has worked for HANCI's Retired Senior Volunteer Program (RSVP).

Her five words had captured the essence of the issue: Staff should be sensitive to spiritual needs without preaching or proselytizing.

Required Spiritual Assessments: CMS and JCAHO

The Centers for Medicare and Medicaid Services (CMS) and the Joint Commission on the Accreditation of Healthcare Organizations (JCAHO) both indicate that spirituality should be assessed in certain circumstances. However, few specifics are provided as to how the assessment should be conducted, or what should be done if spiritual needs are identified.

CMS states that hospice patients, including those in nursing homes, need to have their spiritual needs assessed (CMS: 42 CFR Parts §418.70[f] and §418.88[c]), but no further guidance is presented.

CMS also states, in its Resident Assessment Protocols (RAPs) for Long-Term Care, that "religious needs . . . should be assessed" if any of these psychosocial well-being "triggers" occur:

Conflict with staff, family, or friends

Withdrawal from activities of interest

Grief over lost status or roles

Changes in the current daily routine

JCAHO broadens the settings in which spiritual assessments must be performed, and provides examples as to the type of questions that should be asked. JCAHO sets standards for a broad array of health- and mental health–related settings. These include hospitals, home health, long-term care, and the like. In each of these settings, JCAHO standards state that

Spiritual assessment should determine the patient's denomination, beliefs, and important spiritual practices.

Organizations must define the content and scope of spiritual assessments and the qualifications of the individual(s) performing the assessment.

Examples provided by JCAHO include:

Who or what provides the patient with strength and hope?

Does the patient use prayer in his life?

How does the patient express her spirituality?

What type of spiritual/religious support does the patient desire?

What do suffering and dying mean to the patient?

Does a particular house of worship or faith community play a role in the patient's life?

Individual Assessments

From HOPE to COPE

An individual's spiritual needs can be assessed through the systematic process described by Dr. Carson in chapter 6, whether that person is a well senior, a frail elder, or a family caregiver. In addition, other tools are available to assist the practitioner in conducting a spiritual assessment (Koenig 2002a).

One of the simplest is the "HOPE questions" (Anandarajah & Hight 2001), which introduce the following concepts for discussion:

H—sources of Hope, strength, comfort, meaning, peace, love, and connection.
O—the role of Organized religion for the patient.
P— Personal spirituality and practices.
E— Effects on medical care and end-of-life decisions.

In Niagara's mind-body-spirit project, HOPE has been adapted so that it is presented as COPE in the Never Too Old booklet (DeLoughry & Levy 2006) and the wallet card that accompanies the program (see Figure 9–3).

COPE, as an acronym, is more compatible with a cognitive-behavioral approach to aging, since COPE focuses on current behaviors and "connections," whereas HOPE focuses on more of a future orientation.

An expanded focus on "social/spiritual practices" in COPE, rather than the more narrow "personal spirituality and practices" in HOPE, prompts a discussion of both social support and/or spiritual support.

Figure 9–3 A wallet card summarizes the COPE assessment and the other strategies used in the program.

Use the Satisfaction Skills For Communication and Stress Management *(and—if you want—Steps Toward Spirituality)*	**It's BEST to ASK . . .** Don't assume a problem is "just" physical. Consider how each of these factors may help or hurt:
• Awareness •Focus inside and outside of yourself • Affirmations •Compliment, praise, and be thankful • Assertiveness •Say what you think, need and feel • Acceptance •Listen, relax, forgive yourself and others	• **B**ehaviors (communication, depression, motivation) • **E**nvironment (e.g., hazards, lighting, noise, home setting) • **S**ocial/**S**piritual (e.g., isolation, support, peace of mind) • **T**reatment (e.g., medications, surgeries, therapies)

BEING YOUR BEST	**Questions to COPE Better** Ask these questions to consider needs, then plan for social or spiritual support
Decide your **goals** (physical, emotional, spiritual) and Check your **signs** (blood pressure, stress, peace of mind) Take some **steps** (resources, meds, lifestyle, communicate) **Learn** each time (What steps work for you?)	• **C** Sources of comfort, connections, peace, love • **O** Role of organized religion and other activities • **P** Personal spirituality and social/spiritual practices • **E** Effects on medical care and end-of-life decisions

Niagara Caregivers Network	
Health Association of Niagara County	716-285-8224
Niagara County Office of the Aging	716-438-4020
Erie County Dept. of Senior Services	716-868-8526
The Dale Association	716-754-7376

Adapted from: Anandarajah et al. (2001) HOPE Assessment Questions

www.NiagaraCaregivers.org

This may be particularly helpful for patients who are agnostics or atheists. It also provides a more familiar starting point for health professionals experienced in assessing social support, but unfamiliar with spiritual assessments.

The wallet card is provided to elders and caregivers, as well as professionals and paraprofessionals. The goals of the Niagara County program are to encourage:

A discussion of spiritual issues (i.e., COPE) and a plan for support.

The use of the "goals, signs, steps, and learn" care planning system.

The use of the "satisfaction skills."

A discussion of the BESST Questions, as described later in this chapter.

An understanding of the above factors can help us to be sensitive to the type of spiritual issues that someone is struggling with. The factors (i.e., beliefs) discussed in the next section can guide us in the development of care plans.

Assessing Beliefs

Beliefs are more than just a spiritual creed—they are a determinant of all of our behaviors, such as prayer and worship as well as exercise, eating habits, and compliance with medication regimens. Thus, beliefs have great importance for understanding not only spiritual health, but also emotional and physical health.

Practitioners wishing to help patients to move toward greater spiritual health may be wise to take a lesson from what has been learned about promoting physical health. Compliance (e.g., the actions that a patient and/or the family caregiver take to achieve a goal) is directly correlated with a number of well-researched beliefs, including:

Seriousness, susceptibility, benefits, barriers (Rosenstock 1985).

Self-efficacy (Grembowski et al. 1993).

For example, we are more likely to act if we believe that:

A problem is serious.

We are susceptible to even worse problems if we do nothing.

There are helpful benefits in taking a particular action.

The value of these benefits outweighs any barriers (e.g., fears, cost, inconvenience) we may encounter.

We have the personal capability (i.e., self-efficacy) to do what is required.

Table 9–1 provides examples of beliefs that might affect medical outcomes (e.g., taking medications to control diabetes) or spiritual outcomes (e.g., using prayer to enhance spirituality).

Individual movement toward a spiritual goal, then, could be affected by:

the belief in a heavenly or earthly reward.

the barriers (e.g., fear of "confessing"; "it's 'too late' to seek forgiveness").

Table 9–1   Beliefs Affect Progress toward Medical and Spiritual Goals.

Type of Belief	Medical	Spiritual
	I believe. . . .	
Seriousness	. . . untreated diabetes can cause blindness, amputations, or an early death.	. . . spiritual problems can cause deep pain for me and anguish for others.
Susceptibility	. . . if I don't follow prescribed treatments, my illness will get much worse.	. . . if I don't pray, go to church, or seek spiritual counseling, my pain will get much (or eternally) worse.
Benefit	. . . this medication can really help me.	. . . prayer can result in peace of mind.
Barriers	. . . the side effects are worse than the illness; . . . medications are too expensive.	. . . I'll be embarrassed if I talk to a chaplain or pray; . . . A spiritual path is too hard to follow . . . I don't have time.
Support	. . . my friends and family want me to follow doctor's orders.	. . . my friends and family want me to pray and/or go to church.
Self-Efficacy	. . . I could never stick to a diet and/ or remember everything I need to do to manage my diabetes.	. . . I could never be a "good" person; that is because God and/or my family could never forgive me.

self-efficacy or confidence (e.g., "I'm condemned as a sinner" vs. "God loves me").

support (e.g., personal encouragement, spiritual direction, faith community).

resources (e.g., availability of sacred texts, worship services).

It is best for health professionals not to impose their own beliefs on a patient. However, sensitivity to the importance of the above beliefs could allow a professional to say something like:

It sounds like you believe that spirituality is important to you and that prayer might have some benefits. Would you like to discuss this in more detail with a chaplain? Or

It sounds like you don't believe that spirituality is important or that prayer is particularly helpful. Are there any steps that might bring you more peace of mind? If so, could I suggest some people or organizations that could help you with these steps?

Beliefs can be modified through education, role modeling, and other strategies.

Organizational Assessments

"We've got to change the way we're doing business," says John Kinner, HANCI's executive director. "An aide came up to me after we did an in-service on Spirituality and Elder Care. She pointed out that our Employee Handbook states that 'no political or spiritual discussions should take place in the home.' Our logo says 'HANCI . . . where caring counts.' But what does 'caring' mean when you look at it from a spiritual perspective?

"Our community survey, plus JCAHO guidelines, tell us that spirituality is important," Kinner continued, "so we formed a committee to reassess our written policies and procedures. We're also taking a closer look at our mission statement."

As Kinner suggests, organizations should reassess their mission statement, policies, procedures, and training programs to consider how spirituality can be integrated with elder care. The beliefs that an organization has about its mission are a good starting point.

Organizational Beliefs

Beliefs (sometimes called the "corporate culture") influence organizational behaviors as well as individual behaviors. Thus, an organization's movement toward a spiritual goal (such as the inclusion of *love, caring,* or *spirituality*) in a mission statement or care plan could be affected by:

The belief that a mission statement and/or training program could really make a difference.

The barriers (e.g., fear of being judged as "unprofessional" or a "zealot").

Self-efficacy or confidence (e.g., I [or we] don't have the ability/ influence to change my organization).

Support (e.g., the attitudes and behaviors of other staff and upper management).

Resources (e.g., the examples cited in this chapter or found in other books).

Community Assessments

What If We Collaborated to Improve the Quality of Life?

In February 2003, eighteen professionals engaged in medical, emotional, or spiritual care met at the Center of Renewal at Stella Niagara, a Franciscan Retreat Center about ten minutes north of Niagara Falls. Their goal was to discuss how a collaboration of medical, emotional, and spiritual organizations might improve the quality of life for elders in Niagara County.

"One community organization had done a study a few years earlier that showed that elders tended to stay with the first agency they were referred to, regardless of the nature of the problem. We hope that somehow these meetings would help to avoid someone getting stuck in a particular 'silo of care,'" said Kinner.

The group, which was to become the Niagara Caregivers Network (NCN), shared the belief that physical, emotional, and social factors are interrelated, as expressed by leading medical organizations (American Academy of Family Physicians 1995) and stated by the World Health Organization (WHO), which views health as: "a state of complete physical, mental and social well-being, and not merely the absence of disease or infirmity."

Figure 9–4 Quality of life goals, as viewed by the Niagara Caregivers Network.

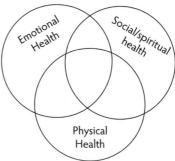

The group decided that "spiritual well-being" was an essential dimension to include after reviewing JCAHO accreditation requirements, as well as evidence that spirituality is important to patients (Mueller 2001) and may contribute to better health (Koenig 1999, Harris 1999). It was linked with "social well-being" because love can be viewed as both a spiritual and a social concept.

Just as the mind, body, and spirit are connected on a personal level, it was concluded that connecting the "silos," or systems, of emotional, medical, social, and spiritual care would benefit the community. This "social assessment" was to serve as Phase 1 in the community planning model illustrated in Figure 9–4.

Using a Systems Approach to Achieve Goals

The group used a community-assessment model (Green & Kreuter 1991), which asks which factors (e.g., administrative, educational, behavioral) need to be adjusted to achieve program goals, as illustrated in Figure 9–5.

For example, quality of life (which the NCN defined as emotional, physical, social, and spiritual well-being in its Phase 1 assessment) is affected by patient behaviors (e.g., physical exercise, prayer) as well as cognitive-behavioral strategies (e.g., assertiveness, acceptance). These behaviors are influenced by educational factors (such as knowledge about exercise and prayer) and by the predisposing beliefs discussed above (e.g., seriousness, benefits). Support from family and friends is another important factor, as is the availability of community education, staff training, media, and Internet programs. Administrative policies are also influential, such as accreditation guidelines and organizational policies and procedures.

In their initial epidemiological assessment in Phase 2, the Niagara group reviewed evidence regarding the relationship of spirituality and well-being. There was considerable discussion about targeting adolescents. However, the group decided to focus their attention on well seniors and frail elders because they believed that people sixty years of age and older would be more receptive to the spiritual component of the anticipated programs.

The systems approach (Capra 1996) views quality of life as a cocreation of both the professionals' and the patient's behavior, as well as administrative, organizational, and community influences. This systems approach,

Figure 9–5   Community assessment to improve spiritual health, conducted by the Niagara Caregivers Network.

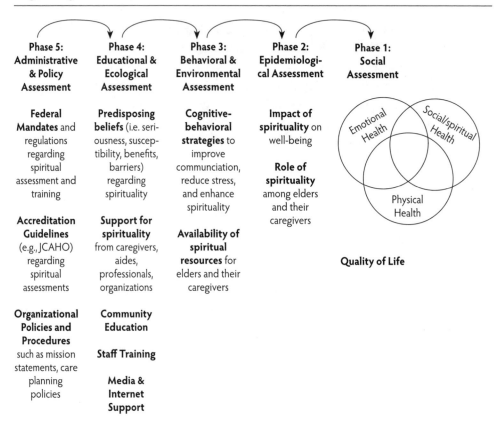

when integrated with the community planning model described above, became the framework for Niagara County's Never Too Old program, which was launched to improve the well-being of elders, family caregivers, and their aides.

Financial Support

The initial community program was approved for coverage as a wellness benefit by three local managed care organizations and was supported by a mailing from the American Association of Retired Persons (AARP). The strong backing was due, in part, to the research and assessment that had shaped the program, as well as its broad focus on physical, emotional, social, and (nondenominational) spiritual well-being.

However, few caregivers came to the initial workshops because they were too busy providing care, and few frail elders attended because they were too frail to travel. Thus, the group began preparing videos to bring the workshops into living rooms, waiting rooms, and hospital rooms.

The Niagara County Office for the Aging agreed to fund this revised program, which included a video DVD and an interactive computer CD (DeLoughry 2006). Both contain forty-five minutes of video designed for staff training and family discussions. The "Peace of Mind" segment focuses on "love" as a suggested goal for care planning, featuring an interview with Dr. Verna Carson (Carson and Koenig, 2004). The "Fun, Friendship and More" segment focuses on the importance of voluntarism and a "sense of purpose" (Koenig, 2002) through an interview with Dr. Koenig. The "Planning and Cooperation" segment suggests that family conflicts can be resolved through communication, stress management, and prayer, using the satisfaction skills described below.

TAKE SOME STEPS . . .

> Preach the Gospel always, use words when necessary.
> —St. Francis of Assisi

Preliminary Considerations

This section will explore three strategies to help elders, caregivers, and professionals to enhance their spirituality by experiencing more love:

Utilize the ministries of word, action, and presence, as presented by Dr. Carson in chapter 6.

Practice the "satisfaction skills"—four cognitive-behavioral skills (i.e., awareness, affirmations, assertiveness, and acceptance) that will be detailed below.

Implement organizational policies, training programs, and other initiatives.

Before that, however, we will briefly review:

How four people play a role in creating wellness.

The value of the golden rule.

The importance of a care plan to improve physical, emotional, and spiritual well-being.

How to address the needs of the whole person by asking the BESST (behavioral, environmental, social, spiritual, and treatment) questions

Wellness Is Cocreated

Three other people play an essential role in cocreating spiritual wellness, in addition to the professionals who provide medical, emotional, and spiritual care. They are:

The elder—who must remain the primary focus—especially in any organization that offers patient-centered care.

The family caregiver—whose own well-being is the best predictor as to whether an elder can stay in the community.

The aide—who has more day-to-day contact with the elder than the professionals.

In elder care, the aide and the family caregiver are crucial in ensuring that the care plan is followed. These "allies" can provide detailed feedback to the care team leader and/or the physician regarding what medical, emotional, and/or spiritual strategies are most effective, as will be discussed when the BESST questions are addressed below.

Aides, family caregivers, and health professionals should be encouraged to follow that same continuous-improvement process (i.e., remember goals, check your signs, choose your steps, and learn each time) that is being prescribed for the elder. The benefits include reduced stress and burnout, as well as improved relationships and better quality of care.

The Golden Years Need the Golden Rule

> *"Whoever called these the golden years ought to be shot."*
> —Overheard at a senior center

For many, the elder years are far from a rich experience that gleams with grace. To them, the promised "golden years" are little more than a well-meaning Santa tale told to brighten a child's Christmas.

Yet, the retirement years can be golden, enriched with blessings and deepened by love. Although the next two sections will detail strategies to enhance this love, the best suggestion may be the simplest—just follow the golden rule.

This simple spiritual instruction—Do unto others as you would have them do unto you—is a good compass to navigate the complexities of various theologies and/or administrative polices and procedures. As detailed in Table 9–2, the notion of "doing unto others . . ." is central to all major religions (Armstrong 2006).

The heart of spirituality in elder care, therefore, may be found in the aides, professionals, friends, and family who are simply treating the elder the way they would like to be cared for.

Table 9–2 The Golden Rule as Expressed in Major Faiths

Buddhism	Hurt not others in ways that you yourself would find hurtful. —Udana-Varga 5, 1
Christianity	Do to others as you would have them do to you. —Jesus (5 BCE–33 CE) in Luke 6:31, 10:27; Matthew 7:12
Confucianism	What you do not want others to do to you, do not do to others. —Confucius (ca. 551–479 BCE)
Hinduism	This is the sum of duty; do naught onto others what you would not have them do unto you. —Mahabharata 5, 1517
Islam	Hurt no one so that no one may hurt you. —Muhammad, The Last Sermon (570–632 CE)
Judaism	Whatever is hateful to you, do not do to your neighbor. That is the whole Torah. The rest is commentary. —Hillel the Elder (50 BCE–10 CE)

Figure 9–6   *Plan with a Partner* encourages support for a continuous-improvement care plan.

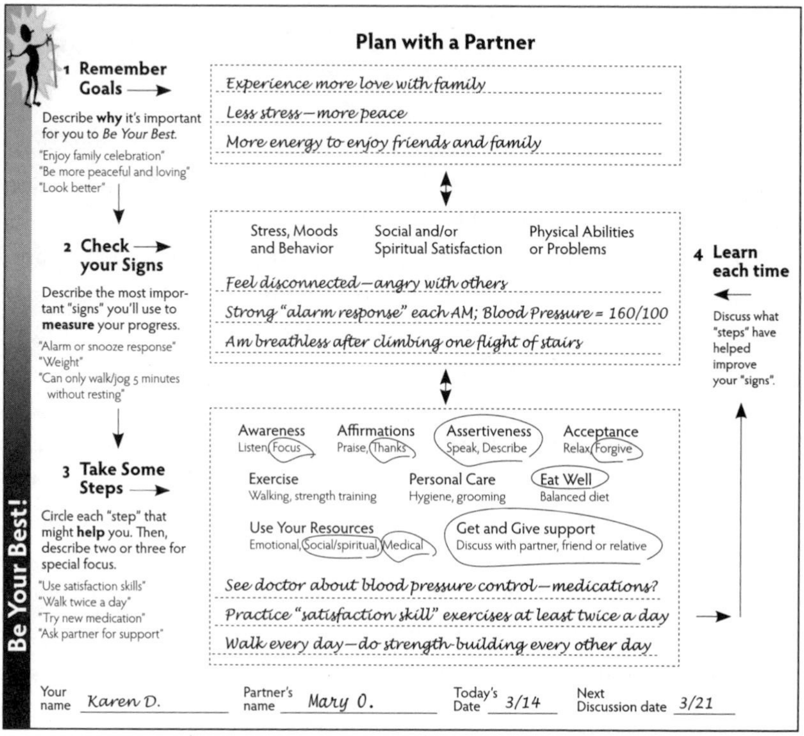

Using a Care Plan

Never Too Old engages elders, family caregivers, aides, and professionals in following a care plan that addresses the needs of the whole person.

Most health care professionals have been trained in the use of care plans. This may be the SOAP (symptoms, observations, analysis, plan) used by many physicians or some other model. Fewer paraprofessionals, who have the closest contact with elders, have received such training. And few family caregivers ever get to see a written care plan, or make a contribution to it.

Never Too Old changes that process by teaching a care plan based on a poem that stresses the importance of continuous improvement (DeLoughry & Levy 2006). As can be seen in Figure 9–6, a sample care plan, this kind of plan:

Can be used to reach medical, emotional, and spiritual goals.

Encourages motivational discussions about goals.

Establishes "signs," or benchmarks, by which to measure programs.

Prompts a consideration of "steps" that include:
Communication, stress management, and prayer skills.
Positive lifestyle behaviors (i.e., exercise, nutrition, personal care).
Use of medical, emotional, social, and spiritual resources.
Getting and giving support.

Encourages the continuous-quality improvement of care by "learning each time" (i.e., rechecking signs) which strategies are most effective.

Active support from a "wellness partner" is encouraged by her signature on the form.

The "Plan with a Partner" care planning form (see Figure 9–6) is useful for motivation, communication, and the tracking of a few key factors. A more in-depth "Signs and Steps Learning Log" is also provided for the more detailed tracking of many factors.

Asking the BESST Questions

All Never Too Old participants are also trained to ask the BESST questions, an acronym that stands for each of the aspects that may either contribute to a problem, or may help to cure it.

B—Behaviors
E—Environmental
S—Social
S—Spiritual
T—Treatment

The twenty most common problems of the elderly (e.g., dementia, incontinence, falls) are the focus of a detailed guide (DeLoughry & Levy 2006) that outlines "Warning Signs" and "BESST Questions" to address the needs of the whole person. They are adapted from the Resident Assessment Protocols (RAPs) that are mandated by the Centers for Medicare and Medicaid for long-term-care facilities.

Improving the Quality of Care

It is anticipated that this approach can make a significant contribution to improving the quality of care because:

> It encourages the application of the golden rule. By encouraging the spiritual values of love and compassion, it is anticipated that incidents of elder abuse will decrease.

> It teaches the basic principle of continuous-quality improvement through the "learn each time" component of the Being Your Best care plan.

> It enables elders, family caregivers, and aides in home settings (where the great majority of older citizens reside) to use a quality-improvement tool (i.e., the BESST Questions) derived from the Resident Assessment Protocols that are mandated in the long-term-care settings by the Centers for Medicare and Medicaid.

Individual Steps

After the elder's goals are understood and "signs" have been identified for benchmarks, it is important to consider what "steps" may help him to achieve his chosen medical, emotional, and spiritual goals. This can be determined through the ministries of word, presence, and action and the satisfaction skills, in addition to other strategies (e.g., exercise, nutrition, medications, and therapies) that are part of the care plan.

The Ministries of Word, Presence, and Action

The ministries of word, presence, and action, described by Dr. Carson in chapter 6, should not be restricted to professionals. This is especially true in elder care, when the elderly are looking for meaning and family care-givers, as well as aides, might benefit from a spiritual perspective on their work.

The ministry of presence is more than just physical presence. Rather, it is a connection that is established through a commitment to, and practice of, active listening and empathy.

"Our 'presence' may be the most important part of our ministry," says Anne Marie MacIsaac, who is president of the Western New York Parish Nurse Institute. "And it's not just being fully present when the patient and I are in the same room. It's also being available for the patient. For example, I have a patient who calls me every Thursday at 9:30 a.m., just to say hello. It gives her comfort, I think, for her to know that I really am there for her."

The ministry of word includes the discussion of spiritual issues, the support and encouragement of spiritual beliefs, referrals to a chaplain or spiritual leader, as well as the sharing of prayer and sacred texts.

"Sometimes the 'ministry of word' is a very casual thing," says MacIsaac. "I might reference a scripture passage in passing as a comment on a personal experience I'm having. Sometimes, though, it's the sharing of a sacred text that may bring some comfort to a troubled patient."

The ministry of action is simply what you do on behalf of the patient and your attitude while doing it.

"Sometimes—or maybe most of the time—the action isn't 'overtly' spiritual. It may be helping someone find some food when they are hungry or arranging for a ride. It's not so much what you do, it's your reason for doing it," MacIsaac adds.

These ministries are also important considerations for "well seniors" who could benefit from the spiritual sense of purpose that is expressed through these ministries as they volunteer to help the community, a friend, or a family member. Also, these ministries are not just the province of professionals who provide medical, emotional, or spiritual care. They are also a path for aides—the paraprofessionals who, in many ways, work harder for fewer rewards.

The Satisfaction Skills: A Cognitive-Behavioral Approach to Communication, Stress Management, and Prayer

Cognitive-behavioral techniques have demonstrated their effectiveness in helping caregivers of elders suffering from Alzheimer's disease (Livingston et al. 2005) and Parkinson's (Secker & Brown 2005). This approach, which recognizes the importance of our thoughts in how we feel and what we do, has also been effective in reducing anxiety in family caregivers (Akkerman & Ostwald 2004).

In Niagara's Never Too Old program, four cognitive-behavioral skills are being used to improve communication, reduce stress, and enhance spirituality, while also playing an important role in fostering forgiveness. They are: awareness, affirmations, assertiveness, and acceptance (DeLoughry & Levy 2006).

The role of each of these skills in improving communication will be addressed below, as well as the role of each in reducing stress. First, however, we will address their use as prayer skills.

If prayer is "any thought or action that connects us to God and God's creations," as suggested earlier in this chapter, then each of these skills addresses a different form of prayer:

> *Awareness:* Awareness of the Spirit in each of us and all of creation is a form of contemplative prayer. Awareness, as taught in Never Too Old, uses focusing as a meditation technique to focus attention in the present moment, a strategy employed in many mystical traditions.

> *Affirmations:* "Praise worship," in which the wonders of the Spirit are appreciated and God is thanked for blessings, is a common form of worship. Hallelujah!

> *Assertiveness:* Assertiveness is useful as a "petitioner's prayer," as exemplified by "Give us this day our daily bread" in the Lord's Prayer. Although physical healing may be possible, Never Too Old especially encourages people to pray for an awareness of God's love and peace of mind, two goals that are rarely denied.

> *Acceptance:* "Thy will be done" from the Lord's Prayer captures the essence of acceptance. It is a crucial step in forgiving oneself, others, or God.

"Anger at God blocks many people from experiencing the Spirit or His love," says Sister Isabelle Reilly, OSF, whose comments about love introduced this chapter.

"The essence of peace, joy, and contentment is accepting God's will, which sometimes means we need to 'forgive' him. The Spirit is loving, but his plan and wisdom are beyond our understanding," she added.

Prayer, whether it is the recitation of a familiar passage learned in childhood, or a more personal communication with the Spirit as suggested by the satisfaction skills, can move us toward forgiveness and joy. It may also reduce caregiver burnout, especially if these spiritual expressions are practiced on a daily basis (Holland & Neimeyer 2005).

We can reduce stress by focusing our awareness on the present, affirming the good things about ourselves, and communicating our needs and feeling, while accepting what cannot be changed. Thus, the following steps concurrently reduce stress while enhancing communication.

Acceptance and Forgiveness

Forgiveness of self, others, and God is a crucial task at any age, but especially in our final years. Forgiveness can be defined:

Behaviorally: as attention to the present rather the past.
Emotionally: as a reduction of anger, fear, or guilt.
Spiritually: as an acceptance of God's love.

Forgiveness can be enhanced by the following cognitive-behavioral skills:

Becoming *aware* of resentments, anger, guilt, and strengths.

Affirming oneself and others for strengths, successes, and positive qualities.

Asserting our needs, feelings, and goals.

Accepting what can't be changed by focusing on the present.

Acceptance can be the "saving grace" when, despite everyone's best efforts, a situation gets worse instead of better. It also helps when people are frustrated with others or disappointed in themselves.

Acceptance doesn't mean giving up, just as forgiving doesn't mean forgetting. Instead, acceptance, as taught through Never Too Old, means letting go of your anger, fear, or guilt. When you accept or forgive, the goal isn't to "forget" what happened. Instead, the goal is not to dwell on past actions or future fears, so goodness or beauty might be seen in the present moment.

It is easier to see goodness and love when we are not feeling stressed, fearful, angry, or guilty. Focusing and relaxation are skills that make it easier to let go of negative feelings and accept what is. Focusing helps you keep your mind in the present, and relaxation calms both your body and your mind.

To get better at acceptance and forgiveness, practice all the satisfaction skills, plus relaxation and focusing on a daily basis.

The behavioral skill of relaxation (i.e., the physical easing of muscle tension) and the cognitive skill of focusing (i.e., returning one's attention to the present moment) can be easily taught through a relaxation tape, CD, or DVD. These skills have been successfully incorporated into the American Lung Association's national program for emphysema and chronic bronchitis (DeLoughry 1983) as well as a stress management program (DeLoughry & DeLoughry 1991) created by a large managed care organization. Video instruction in both of these skills is included in Niagara's Never Too Old program (DeLoughry 2006).

Communicating with the Elderly

Examples as to how each skill can be used in communicating with the elderly include:

Awareness: Make sure you note the abilities and potential of the senior you care for, as well as the handicaps and barriers that make change difficult. Ask questions.

Affirmations: Offer encouragement by reminding the senior of her past accomplishments and successes, as well as more current qualities she displays or can draw on.

Assertiveness: Encourage the elder to follow the steps that are part of the comprehensive care plan. Use short, direct phrases to minimize confusion. Share your thoughts and feelings. Encourage her to be assertive.

Acceptance: Tolerate mistakes, setbacks, and missed goals. Accept that progress and/or benefits may not be as great, or may be different, from what you had hoped.

The Satisfaction Cycle: When? . . . How?

Any one of the satisfaction steps may be helpful at any time. However, for the most success, it may be most helpful to use them in this order (as shown in Figure 9–7):

1. *Awareness:* Take a few deep breaths and focus on the present moment. Let go of past problems or future fears and pay attention to right now.

2. *Affirmations:* Start your discussion with some compliments or "thanks" to help reduce the fear and anger the other person may have. Then they can listen better to the rest of what you have to say. Remember also to affirm yourself!

3. *Assertiveness:* Say what's on your mind, using "I" statements, described below.

4. *Acceptance:* Relax and listen. What is true about the other's point of view?

In summary, the following steps can help elders, family caregivers, aides, and professionals integrate spirituality into elder care:

Consider the ministries of word, action, and presence as a guide to your interactions.

Use a continuous-improvement care plan, such as: "Remember goals, check your signs, choose your steps, and learn each time."

Figure 9–7   The Satisfaction Cycle consists of four cognitive-behavioral skills that can improve communication, reduce stress, and enhance spirituality.

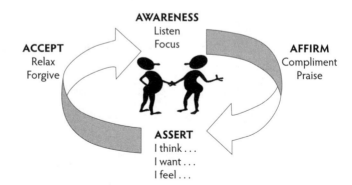

Use the satisfaction skills of awareness, affirmations, assertiveness, and acceptance to improve communication, reduce stress, and enhance your spirituality.

Utilize the spiritual resources within your organization and community, such as chaplains; ministers, priests, rabbis, or imams; churches, synagogues, or mosques; and the parish nurse.

Steps for Organizations

"Sometimes I wish that we had something, like a Hippocratic Oath that physicians follow, to guide our staff," says John Kinner, reflecting on the steps that HANCI is taking to integrate spirituality into its care plans. But, then, I suppose that we do. It's the golden rule, and it's respected by everyone.

"But caring needs to be something more than being nice to each other and our clients at work and on home visits. We are a family here, and we need to have a presence at the milestones in each other's lives. For example, if volunteers have lost a loved one, we should have a presence at the wake or the funeral. They've helped us deal with our crises; we should be there for theirs."

The steps that an organization can take to integrate spirituality into elder care include:

Discuss the issue of spirituality and elder care with staff, clients, and the board of directors.
> Consider how the values of love and compassion might promote the achievement of other important goals (e.g., patient satisfaction, decreased staff turnover, increased market share, better communication, better outcomes).

Survey staff and clients to learn more from their perspectives.

Establish a committee or task force to review or examine your organization's
> Mission statement.
> Policies and procedure.
> Employee handbook.
> Relevant accreditation and training mandates.

Reach outside your organization to others (e.g., hospice, spiritual directors, hospital chaplains) who are integrating spirituality with elder care.

Integrate staff training with patient education and caregiver support, so that a common vocabulary and set of skills can enhance communication as well as improve the quality and outcomes of care.

Steps for Communities

The following steps may be helpful in developing a community approach toward integrating spirituality into elder care:

Contact the officers of relevant professional organizations (e.g., parish nurses, discharge planners, human resource managers) to determine their interest in these issues.

Contact the officers of relevant grassroots and professional coalitions (e.g., Council on Aging, Golden Age Clubs, Network in Aging) to determine their interest in these issues.

Contact the directors of local government organizations (e.g., Office for Aging, Department of Health, Department of Social Services, Department of Mental Health) to determine their interest in these issues.

Contact the directors of relevant elder care organizations (e.g., home health care, adult day care, long-term care, managed care) to determine their interest in these issues.

Organize a conference on Spirituality and Elder Care to start a community discussion and identify interested individuals from other organizations who are interested in these issues.

Convene a community planning session of interested parties to examine the behavioral, educational, predisposing, administrative, and other factors that can influence your success (Green & Kreuter 1991).

Establish pilot programs and evaluate results.

Seek grants and governmental support.

. . . and LEARN EACH TIME

Individual Lessons

> There is, after all, something eternal that lies beyond the hand of fate and of all human delusions. And such eternals lie closer to an older person than to a younger one oscillating between fear and hope. For us there remains the privilege of experiencing beauty and truth in their purest forms.
>
> —Letter from Albert Einstein to Queen Elizabeth of Belgium, sent March 20, 1936

Beauty was once described by Samuel Taylor Coleridge (Perry 1999) as "the many seen as one." In doing so, he distinguished the beautiful from the agreeable (which is merely "pleasant"). His definition of beauty embraces a mystical understanding of spirituality, and also encompasses the definition of love (i.e., "a sense of oneness") that has been used in this chapter.

A sense of beauty, a sense of meaning, or a sense of love can all be seen as measures of spiritual understanding. The degree to which they are present, or absent, are "signs" that can help each individual to "learn each time" which "steps" or strategies are most successful.

How much beauty do elders see around them? The trillions of cells that work as one to produce a flower—or a smile—hint at an eternal wisdom within the cycle of life. This can be appreciated even by those, like Einstein, who do not believe in a personal God who intervenes in human affairs (Dukas 1989).

The spiritual path is different for everyone, and some may see it only as a social or a moral experience. But the rewards of love, beauty, and peace of mind await everyone who seeks them, regardless of their theology or philosophy.

"You can never take anyone higher than you are," said Ram Dass, a spiritual teacher who devoted his life to the teaching of Hinduism as an alternative to the excesses of LSD and other drugs. His comment illustrates how easily professionals can overlook a spiritual issue faced by the elder.

The blinding effect of our own limitations can restrict our grasp of the spiritual lessons the elder is learning. It is quite possible that a patient may be "stuck" in a "higher" stage of spiritual development than the professional has achieved. This reinforces the importance of listening and encouraging, rather than judging, as the elder "learns each time" what spiritual strategies work the best for him.

In some Eastern cultures, old age is a time for these spiritual reflections. In caring for our elderly patients, we can encourage these reflections by helping elders to use the process and the skills presented in this chapter, and by modeling these behaviors ourselves.

The process of "remembering goals, checking signs, taking steps, and learning each time" is an unending cycle. It can take us ever closer to our goals, although the experience of God is beyond words, and an understanding of the Spirit is beyond the human mind.

The satisfaction cycle of awareness, affirmations, assertiveness, and acceptance is another process of steps that never ends. But we are never too old to appreciate more of the beauty, love, and peace that the Spirit brings.

Each time individuals remeasure the signs (e.g., blood pressure, alarm response, peace of mind) that mark progress toward their goals, they learn an important lesson about what strategies are most helpful.

Organizational Lessons

"We're not there yet, but we're on the path toward achieving a goal we're comfortable with," Kinner said as he reflected on HANCI's future. "Right now, we're a little jittery because it's new and it's important. But whenever we've been challenged in the past, our staff has shown great facility in reaching beyond the walls of our organization for answers.

"Regarding the integration of spirituality and elder care, there are some organizations that have already accomplished this, such as hospice. And we're asking for advice from spiritual directors, ministers, and others who have more experience than we do.

"We think we're facing a future with shrinking resources, but the spiritual values of love and compassion have helped us in the past, and they'll help HANCI in the future."

No one professional (no matter whether she provides medical, emotional, or spiritual care) has the power to confer spiritual health. Instead, the enhancement of spiritual wellness occurs within the context of the patient's personal, medical, social, and spiritual environment. The greater the organizational support, the greater the likelihood that spiritual values can be integrated into elder care.

Striving toward an enhanced sense of spirituality is an unending process for organizations, as well as for individuals. The organizational steps suggested above may be helpful for organizations that want to "learn each time" which strategies are most successful.

Community Lessons

Professionals work within the context of the community where the patient lives. Thus, the role of the entire "system" must be considered if we wish to enhance spiritual well-being. The steps suggested above might be considered by those who wish to help communities "learn each time" what strategies may be most effective.

In working with community projects, as well as large organizational initiatives, it is easy to become distracted by politics and turf wars. Thus, it may be helpful to recall the words of St. Francis of Assisi: "Preach the gospel always. Use words when necessary."

In that regard, greater personal satisfaction will likely come from placing a higher priority on "how much love you can experience" rather than "how many objectives you can achieve." And, in the paradox common to many spiritual endeavors, focusing more on love and less on the task may actually lead to a greater integration of spirituality and elder care in your organization, your community, and your life.

Reflective Questions

For professionals providing medical, emotional, and spiritual care:

In your personal life: What are the five most important goals in your life? Is spirituality or "experiencing more love" included? Should they be ranked higher or lower?

In serving patients: How important is spirituality or "experiencing" more love to the patients you serve? Have you discussed it? Is it part of a written care plan? What are the barriers to including it in the plan? What are the benefits of including it in the care plan?

In dealing with coworkers: What role would you like love or spirituality to play in your relationships with your peers? With your supervisor? With those you supervise?

What professional forums (or conferences) exist to discuss these issues with your professional peers from other organizations?

For organizations:

What do you think are the top five values within the culture of your organization?

Is love, spirituality, and/or caring among them?

Should they be ranked higher or lower?

How would greater expressions of love and caring affect the following within your organization:

satisfaction with care?
market share?
malpractice complaints?
the quality of care?
health outcomes?
costs?

Review your organization's mission statement. Are spiritual values, such as love and compassion, included?

How is love or spirituality reflected in the culture of your organization?

What professional forums (or conferences) exist to discuss these issues with other elder care organizations?

How are the values of love and caring integrated into:

care plans?
staff training?
supervisory sessions?

For communities:

How does your community help elders and their caregivers to bridge the separate silos of emotional, medical, and spiritual care?

What steps (e.g., seminars, consortiums, directories) might help the community to bridge them?

What professional and community forums currently exist to discuss these issues as a community?

What conferences or ongoing forums could be organized to stimulate discussion about these goals?

Acknowledgment

This chapter is adapted from T. DeLoughry, *Never Too Old to Be Well: Improving the Medical, Emotional and Spiritual Health of Elders, Their Families and Their Aides* and the *Eldercare Professional Guide* (Grand Island, NY: Center for Health Management, 2007). Reprinted by permission.

Note

1. Centers for Medicare and Medicaid Regulations: CHF §483.152 Requirements for approval of nurse aide training and competency evaluation for long-term care; and §484.36 Home Health Aides Services.

References

Akkerman, R. L., & S. K. Ostwald (2004). Reducing anxiety in Alzheimer's disease family caregivers: The effectiveness of a nine-week cognitive-behavioral intervention. *American Journal of Alzheimer's Disease and Other Dementias* 19(2): 117–23.

American Academy of Family Physicians (1995). Human behavior and mental health: Recommended core educational guidelines for family practice residents. *American Family Physician* 51(6): 1599–1602.

Anandarajah, G., & E. Hight (2001). Spirituality and medical practice: Using the HOPE questions as a practical tool for spiritual assessment. *American Family Physician* 63(1): 81–89.

Armstrong, K. (2006). *The Great Transformation: The Beginning of Our Religious Traditions.* New York: Knopf Publishing Group.

Artis, B. (2005). Promoting health, building community. *Health Progress* 86(2): 27–31.

Buelow, J. R., et al. (1999). Job satisfaction of home care assistants related to managerial practices. *Home Health Care Services Quarterly* 17(4): 59–71.

Capra, F. (1996). *The Web of Life*. New York: Simon & Schuster.

Carson, V. B., and H. G. Koenig (2004). *Spiritual Caregiving: Healthcare as Ministry*. Philadelphia: Templeton Foundation Press.

Caudill, M. E., & M. Patrick (1991). Turnover among nursing assistants: Why they leave and why they stay. *Journal of Long Term Care Administration* 19(4): 29–32.

Daaleman, T. P., et al. (2004). Religion, spirituality, and health status in geriatric outpatients. *Annals of Family Medicine* 2(1): 49–53.

Davidson, H., & P. Folcarelli (1997). The effects of health care reforms on job satisfaction and voluntary turnover among hospital-based nurses. *Medical Care* 35(6): 634–45.

DeLoughry, T. E. (1983). *Help Patients to Better Breathing*. New York: American Lung Association.

———. (2006). *Never Too Old: Help for You and Your Aging Parents* (Interactive CD). Grand Island, NY: Center for Health Managment.

———. (2006). *Never Too Old: Help for You and Your Aging Parents* (Video DVD). Grand Island, NY: Center for Health Management.

DeLoughry, T. E., & K. B. DeLoughry (1991). *Feeling Fit at Work and School*. Buffalo, NY: Independent Health Association.

———. (2002). *Improving Satisfaction and the Quality of Care: A Program Manual for Home Health and Long-Term Care Organizations*. Grand Island, NY: Center for Health Management.

DeLoughry, T. E., & S. Levy (2006). *Never Too Old to Be Well: Improving the Medical, Emotional and Spiritual Health of Elders, Their Families and Their Aides*. Grand Island, NY: Center for Health Management.

Dukas, H. (1989). *Albert Einstein: The Human Side*. Princeton, NJ: Princeton University Press.

Gaddy, T., & G. A. Bechtel (1995). Nonlicensed employee turnover in a long-term-care facility. *The Health Care Supervisor* 13(4): 54–60.

Green, L. W., & M. W. Kreuter (1991). *Health Promotion Planning: An Educational and Environmental Approach*. Toronto: Mayfield Publishing Company.

Grembowski, D., et al. (1993). Self-efficacy and health behavior among older adults. *The Journal of Health and Social Behavior* 34(2): 89–104.

Harris, W. S. (1999). A randomized, controlled trial of the effects of remote, intercessory prayer on outcomes in patients admitted to the coronary care unit. *Archives of Internal Medicine* 159(19): 2273–78.

Holland, J. M., & R. A. Neimeyer (2005). Reducing the risk of burnout in end-of-life care settings: The role of daily spiritual experiences and training. *Palliative & Supportive Care* 3(3): 173–81.

Kirby, S. E., et al. (2004). Spirituality and well-being in frail and nonfrail older adults. *The Journals of Gerontology. Series B, Psychological Sciences and Social Sciences* 59(3): P123–29.

Koenig, H. G. (1999). How does religious faith contribute to recovery from depression? *The Harvard Mental Health Letter* 15(8): 8.

———. (2002a). *Spirituality in Patient Care: Why, How, When, and What*. Philadelphia: Templeton Foundation Press.

———. (2002b). *Purpose and Power in Retirement*. Philadelphia: Templeton Foundation Press

Livingston, G., et al. (2005). Systematic review of psychological approaches to the management of neuropsychiatric symptoms of dementia. *The American Journal of Psychiatry* 162(11): 1996–2021.

Merton, T. (1994). *Freedom to Witness: Letters in Time of Crisis*. Selected and edited by William H. Shannon. New York: Farrar, Straus & Giroux.

Mueller, P. S. (2001). Religious involvement, spirituality, and medicine: Implications for clinical practice. *Mayo Clinic Proceedings* 76(12): 1225–35.

Perry, S. (1999). *Coleridge and the Uses of Division.* Oxford: Oxford University Press.

Robinson, B. A. (2006). Shared Belief in the Golden Rule: Ethics of Reciprocity. http://www.religioustolerance.org/reciproc.htm; accessed June 10, 2006.

Rosenstock, I. (1985). Understanding and enhancing patient compliance with diabetic regimens. *Diabetes Care* 8(6): 610–16.

Secker, D. L., & R. G. Brown (2005). Cognitive behavioural therapy (CBT) for carers of patients with Parkinson's disease: A preliminary randomised controlled trial. *Journal of Neurology, Neurosurgery, and Psychiatry* 76(4): 491–97.

Shorto, R. (2004). Faith at Work. *New York Times.* October 31. http://www.nytimes.com/2004/10/31/magazine/31FAITH.html (accessed November 1, 2004).

Smessaert, A. H. (1989). Focusing efforts toward the poor. A system raises its consciousness. *Health Progress* 70(7): 28–31.

Stevens, R.P. & R. Banks (eds.) (2005). *The Marketplace Ministry Handbook: A Manual for Work, Money and Business.* Vancouver: Regent College Publishing.

Weinstein, A. (2006). Jewish Learning: Being Loving to Your Neighbor. http://www.jewishvirtuallibrary.org/jsource/Judaism/loving1.html; accessed June 10, 2006.

Woods, S. L. (2001). Using evidence-based approaches to strategically respond to the nursing shortage. *Critical Care Nursing Clinics of North America* 13(4): 511–19.

10

SPIRITUALITY IN DEATH AND BEREAVEMENT

MIRIAM JACIK

> For everything its season, and for everything under heaven its time:
> a time to be born and a time to die,
> a time to plant and a time to uproot,
> a time to kill and a time to heal,
> a time to pull down and a time to build up,
> a time for mourning and a time for dancing,
> a time for silence and a time for speech.
>
> —Ecclesiastes 3:1–7

Facing the Inevitability of Death

Death has a way of making us keenly aware of our mortality and vulnerability. It also points up the fragility of human existence. Loss of any kind leads us to take an honest look at the ultimate loss, which is death. Of all the methods employed by humankind to deal with death, the one most subject to failure is the effort to ignore death or deny its existence. To many, especially adolescents and young adults in our society, death is still an event "out there" and "far away." Likewise, it always affects "somebody else."

Americans take pride in claiming that nothing is unattainable in our advanced, truly progressive society. Technological advances and scientific discoveries have permitted us to explore the moon and the planets, transplant vital organs, unlock the mysteries of the human heart and mind, bring forth life through implanted embryos, and so on. As a society in

279

> **Box 10–1   Lessons Many People Learn about Loss, Death, and Grieving**
>
> ---
>
> Don't feel bad—don't cry or be sad.
>
> Replace the loss quickly—you'll soon get something in place of what you lost.
>
> Grieve alone—don't upset others with your grieving.
>
> Just give it time—in time your wounds will be healed.
>
> Be strong for others—if you are male, this is definitely your message.
>
> Keep busy—busyness is a distraction and a deterrent to grieving.
>
> ---
>
> Source: Adapted from James & Friedman (1998, 26–35).

general, and within the field of medical technology in particular, Americans feel confident that we can control life and death. We try to do this, perhaps, because we fear death so and that fear is largely a spiritual issue. Death raises questions about the meaning of life; the hereafter; and forgiveness, hope, and the nature of God.

Being very much a part of the life process, death comes to each one of us whether we accept it or not. Its arrival is inevitable at some point in our lives. People suffer many small deaths through loss during a single lifetime. These losses are but a prelude to the final event of physical death. Abandoning familiar ways of doing things, launching out on new adventures, and taking risks that may lead to success or failure often involve loss, and are ways of facing some form of dying. Losing friends, family members, pets, an important position, status, or money puts us personally in touch with tangible expressions of the dying process. Everyone can identify with one or more of the events of life just listed.

Dr. Elisabeth Kübler-Ross (1975) offers the invitation to befriend death when she writes: "Dying is something we human beings do continuously, and not just at the end of our physical lives on earth. If you can begin to see death as an invisible but friendly companion on life's journey, then you can learn to truly live your life rather than simply pass through it" (145).

Attitudes toward death are also affected by our exposure to death, as presented by our families during our formative years. If the issue of death is not discussed, and children are kept from encountering it, death becomes secretive, foreboding, and fear-filled. Children permitted to face the death of a loved one, to have their questions or concerns candidly addressed by the adults in their lives, and encouraged to say their good-byes, regard death in a very different light. They grow up knowing that death is a sad event, but nonetheless, a part of life. James and Friedman (1998), in a chapter of their book titled *We Are Ill-Prepared to Deal with Loss*, reflect on the lessons about loss, death, and grieving that people often learn as they grow up. A summary of these lessons are outlined in Box 10–1.

The Role of Nursing in the Dying Process

Although many nurses face loss and death in their work setting on a daily basis, most feel woefully unprepared to undertake the awesome responsibility of assisting those confronted with loss and death. In general, only chaplains have the expertise needed in this area. Most nurses are influenced by the prevailing attitude of society that death should be denied as long as possible. For the nurse, this attitude may translate into behaviors that offer false hope to patients and families, heroic measures that forestall the inevitable, and avoidance of the dying patient when there are no more physical interventions to be offered. These are hardly the behaviors of someone who is not only expected to recognize the inevitability of death but to provide physical as well as spiritual ministrations.

Nurses, by nature of their professional responsibilities, are called upon to:

explore their personal attitudes toward death and dying so as to be more comfortable in addressing similar issues with the people for whom they care.

come to know the losses that dying people and their families face.

assess and meet the needs confronting dying people and grieving families.

provide whole person care to others, giving adequate attention to spiritual needs.

This does seem like a monumental task. Many of these responsibilities are addressed in this chapter.

Dr. Elisabeth Kübler-Ross (1969) spent many years working with and assisting dying people. She encouraged clinicians to become more in touch with their personal attitudes and feelings about death, and more particularly about their own deaths. She believed that if health care providers were uncomfortable thinking about their personal death issues, they would be ineffective in helping others to do so. To help nurses get in touch with some of their own fears and concerns related to dying, a questionnaire titled "A Personal Look at Death and Dying" is provided in Box 10–2.

Where Do People Die?

In a study by Teno et al. (2004), published in the *Journal of the American Medical Association*, the issue of end-of-life care was explored. The study indicated that 67 percent of deaths occurred in health care institutions, with the remainder occurring in the home. There was a focus in the study on the presence of hospice care within the home. Of the group studied, 15 percent had the services of some hospice organization assisting with care before death. The families who received assistance from hospice were very satisfied with the whole experience.

The hospice concept endorses palliative care, effective pain management, comfort measures, respect for the wishes of dying people, an honest exchange of information with dying people and their families, as well as death with respect and dignity. The hospice team places a high value on meeting the spiritual needs of the dying person and his family. Hospice teams are composed of nurses, doctors, chaplains, therapists, social workers, nutritionists, health aides, homemakers, and hospice volunteers. The dying person and the family caregivers are also considered vital members of the team. The hospice team succeeds in providing care that is more

Box 10–2   A Personal Look at Death and Dying

When you were a child, how was the issue of death dealt with?

What does death mean to you? (Use phrases or words to express how you feel about your own death.)

Do you believe that psychological factors like stress can predispose you to a premature death? How?

In your thinking, what role does God or a Higher Power play in the areas of illness, suffering, and death?

Have there been times in your life when you wanted to die? When?

What do you believe might be the cause of your own death?

What aspect of your own death is most uncomfortable or frightening to you?

Do frequent natural disasters and wars influence you personally to reflect upon death? Why? Why not?

If you could choose, when would you want to die? Do you think you would be ready for this event?

Do you believe in a life after death? How does this influence your attitude toward death?

cohesive, more holistic, and less fragmented than the care being offered in health care institutions, other than inpatient hospices. Many who are dying wish to die within the comfort and security of their own homes. This desire may not be honored because of varying circumstances: the inability of families to participate in care, fears that emergencies or crises may arise and not be able to be handled properly, exacerbating symptoms related to the terminal condition, and the like.

As indicated earlier, a greater percentage of people die in some form of a health care institution than at home, including acute care hospitals, skilled nursing facilities, and long-term care and assisted living facilities. Generally, these settings are not oriented to providing holistic care. The focus of acute care is on treating the seriously ill, trauma victims, those requiring surgery, or those with worsening medical conditions. Health care delivery within acute care settings is fast-paced, less personal, and controlled by insurers so as to be cost-effective. Those who are dying often spend their last days in intensive care units, where care is the most sophisticated and technologically proficient, but frequently the most impersonal. Is this environment, which is so focused on advanced treatment modalities and curing health care problems, the ideal place to meet the needs of the dying?

The care of dying people in other health care institutions is also limited. Poor staffing, less qualified health care personnel, an institutionalized environment, and deficits in personalized care are all factors that contribute to the less-than-optimal care dying people receive in these settings. It is not unusual to see terminally ill persons who have had a medical emergency or who are closer to dying being sent to the hospital, where they will either be stabilized or die. It seems that we could do a better job of ministering to the dying.

Holistic Care of Dying Persons

In describing the type of care offered by hospice organizations, we get a glimpse of holistic care. Holistic care focuses on all the dimensions of the person—biological, psychological, social/relational, and spiritual. As nurses we are called on to give holistic care.

The reader is encouraged to review chapter 1 for the conceptual model of human beings that illustrates the centrality of the spirit. This model makes it clear that the spirit is expressed through the body, the mind, and the emotions. Likewise, the spirit is touched through ministrations to the body, the emotions, and the mind. The care of the dying provides the perfect opportunity to implement the spiritual interventions of ministry of presence, ministry of action, and ministry of word (see chapter 6). When we provide loving physical care and try to alleviate pain, we not only minister to the body but we minister to the spirit. Likewise, when we listen to the patient's deepest concerns and offer our presence instead of false reassurances, we are not only ministering to the emotional needs of the patient, we are ministering to his spirit. When we offer to pray with a patient, we touch his spirit, which, in turn, leads to a more relaxed body and calmer emotions.

The call to wholeness reaches each individual personally in the depths of her being. To heed that call is to respond to the Creator's invitation to live life fully, with purpose, in wellness, and with a totality of our personhood. So many hear the call to wholeness but cannot or do not respond. Instead of experiencing growth, integration, and actualization they experience neutral living, lack of wellness, and lack of fulfillment. In holistic living a person is motivated especially by the power of love—love of life, love of oneself, love of others, love of the Creator, and love of all of the gifts of this earth. A challenge for nurses is to embrace holism and a holistic view of life, first for themselves and then to integrate that holistic way of being into the care given to others. The call to wholeness leads the health care provider to guide others out of disease and a lack of wellness into a state of well-being. This focus changes somewhat when death is the presumed outcome. It is important for health care providers to believe that we can help others to die well, much as we help others to live well.

As we now explore the needs of dying people, we are encouraged to remember the reality that human life is temporary, that human beings are mortal, and that the journey through life is transient. "For here we have no lasting city, we are seeking one which is to come" (Hebrews 13:14).

Assessing the Needs of the Dying and Their Families

To accompany another through his dying process, it is important for nurses to know what is happening to and within the dying person's world. It is equally as important for them to understand what the family is experiencing at this time, for they stand by their loved one sorrowing and in need of care and concern.

Meeting people who are dying at their own level of need is accom-

Table 10–1   Needs of Dying People from a Holistic Perspective

Physical	Emotional	Social	Spiritual
Adequate treatment & care	Hope	Presence of loved ones	Forgiveness/ reconciliation
Caring health clinicians	Respect	Time with family/ friends	Prayer/religious services
Prudent medical management	Control	Permission to die	Spiritual assistance at death
Comfort	Honesty/Open communication	Complete unfinished business	Peace

Source: Carson (1989, 266).

plished by respecting their individuality, their personal preferences, and their unique means of coping with the dying process. Table 10–1 outlines some of the important needs of dying people—needs that are physical, emotional, social or relational, and spiritual. These needs are holistic in nature.

Physical Needs

ADEQUATE TREATMENT AND CARE

Often people fear being abandoned to die alone and without treatment and care once it is determined that their condition is terminal. They hope that the nurses who have so diligently cared for them will not forsake them once there is no longer hope for a cure or for recovery.

CARING CLINICIAN

Dying is one of our most difficult experiences. It can be so much easier when dying people know that they are receiving the best and the most loving assistance possible from those caring for them. This can make the difference between a frightening, lonely exit from this earthly life and a warm, loving departure among friends.

PRUDENT MEDICAL MANAGEMENT

With the advent of advance directives, stated in a living will, and a better recognition of their importance, the call for prudent medical management of dying people has become clearer and louder. For so long the orientation in health care has been to cure, heal, and expend any effort to save lives. Medical management has often taken a turn toward the use of heroic, life-saving measures to prolong life and delay death. Undue expense, unnecessary grief for those who are dying and their families, as well as a prolongation of the dying process, are often the outcomes of such decisions. Bringing physicians and distraught families into dialogue, through which prudent decisions can be made, is an invaluable service that nurses can render to the dying.

COMFORT

Death is often linked with pain, suffering, and physical disintegration. Dying people fear being overcome by unbearable pain at the time of their death. They welcome any measures that will keep them comfortable during the last days and weeks of their lives. Human presence is a priceless source of comfort to the dying as well. Most people do not want to die alone. If there is a universal, yet often unspoken, request that dying people make, it is that significant others, health care providers, and friends be there during their final hours. A presence that comforts and supports is what is needed.

A clinical example that captures how the physical needs of a dying person were met might be helpful at this point.

Case Example #1

Sally Jacket was a nurse working in a large skilled nursing facility. She was happy to be able to follow the progress and care of her father. She hoped that he would be a good rehabilitation candidate when he was transferred to her facility. However, he never did recover his strength and mobility. His condition continued to decline further with each passing day. The physician who provided care to Mr. Jacket began limiting his daily visits, in light of his patient's weakening condition. Sally knew that her father looked forward to those daily visits from his doctor. Sally arranged a meeting with her father's physician and requested that the daily contacts continue because they had been so important to her father. The physician agreed and began seeing Mr. Jacket daily until the day of his death.

Emotional Needs

HOPE

People face an illness with the hope of a recovery and the best possible care while it is happening. As a disease progresses, bringing them to the end of their lives, hope changes its focus to some extent. For some, there is hope for a hereafter that is free of pain and suffering; for others, hope may mean holding on for a special family event; still others, who don't believe in an afterlife, may hope to receive support and assistance while making the transition from life to death. Nurses are called upon to foster hope in whatever form is beneficial to the dying person.

RESPECT

People who are ill expect to be treated with dignity. They hope for competent care, loving concern, as well as the freedom to make their own choices. Dying people also cherish the right to express their final wishes. Nurses give dying people the respect they desire by honoring their requests and wishes.

CONTROL

Illness and treatment within our present health care system have a way of fostering dependence in the recipients of care. Control is easily relinquished when illness makes the patient feel weak, vulnerable, and helpless. Yet those being cared for are, for the most part, thinking, judging, and choosing human beings, as are the nurses who serve them. Nurses, aware of the need people have to control the final phase of life, can advocate for the person's freedom to question, disagree, contradict, or decide against any form of care being offered.

OPEN COMMUNICATION/HONESTY

Initiating a conversation with a dying person will often open the way for subjects that are difficult to discuss, such as a definitive prognosis, the circumstances of her dying, health care measures still available to her, and the like. Dying people expect nurses to tell them the truth. They expect to hear information that they can readily understand. When nurses refuse to listen or respond honestly to questions voiced by the person who is dying, they cast the dying person into a state of isolation, silence, and aloneness.

Another clinical example demonstrates the manner in which the emotional needs of a dying person can be met.

Case Example #2

John Smith has been feeling weaker and more tired since he became sick. Visiting the doctor with his wife was very unsettling. The questions that Mr. Smith asked were vaguely answered by his doctor. His wife made efforts during their visit to make light of what the doctor was telling her husband. Mr. Smith knew by the way he felt that his ALS was worsening. What he didn't know was that his wife had begged the doctor to keep "the truth" from her husband regarding his condition. She felt the truth would take away his hope. In a conversation with his physician, outside the presence of his frightened wife, Mr. Smith was able to acquire the candid information he needed to help him begin his slow preparation for death.

Social Needs

PRESENCE OF LOVED ONES

Human beings are social beings placed, since birth, within a primary social unit, the family. We learn to trust the support and concern of family members during all of life's events—whether happy or tragic. Dying people and their families suffer a grave injustice if denied each other's supportive, caring presence as death approaches. Loved ones should never be considered a bother or "in the way" by nursing staff. How fortunate is the person who can die with family and loved ones present at his side during the final hours of life.

TIME TO SHARE WITH FAMILY/FRIENDS

Too many people die never having said the things that they most wanted to say to their loved ones. Many family members carry in their hearts, for years, the regret of never having said good-bye, never having forgiven, never having said thank-you, or never having expressed appreciation to a loved one. Dying people need to spend time with those closest to them to share last concerns as well as hopes and wishes for those they are leaving behind. Within the busy hospital routine, so heavily scheduled with activity, nurses are challenged to provide for this social need of dying persons.

PERMISSION TO DIE

Each of us has the innate instinct to preserve life at all costs, once it is endangered. People grappling with serious illnesses often make the difficult decision to accept long and painful periods of treatment just to have more time. There comes a point, however, when fighting to stay alive becomes burdensome and futile. The terminally ill know this, even when their loved ones do not. They may be afraid, however, to stop fighting and to let death ensue, for fear of disappointing their caregivers and those who want them to live. Nurses can advocate for the dying with their families as well as with the members of the health care team so that permission to die is granted by all.

UNFINISHED BUSINESS

Dr. Elisabeth Kübler Ross often made mention in her writings of the need of the dying to take care of unfinished business. *Unfinished business* can mean a lot of things, including strained relationships that need to be mended, business deals that must be closed, familial silences that must be broken, projects that must be completed, wills that must be drawn up, and promises that must be kept. In death we must let go of so much. Encouraging the dying person to complete unfinished business guarantees her a more peaceful leave-taking, a smoother disengagement from loved ones, and a greater sense of accomplishment for her lifetime.

A third clinical example demonstrates how the social needs of dying persons might be met.

Case Example #3

Sue Margolis, a registered nurse, was called out of state to the bedside of her terminally ill father. She sat with him all night, planning in her mind the things she wanted to tell him before he died. By morning her courage was waxing and waning. She found herself leaving the hospital with her words unspoken. Not comfortable with this situation, Sue gathered the other family members and returned to the hospital a few hours later. Sitting at her father's bedside, she courageously made the first statement. "Dad, we know that you are very ill. What words of wisdom and advice would you leave with each of us?" A whole stream of heart-rending, soul-lifting communication followed. Many tears were shed, memories were recaptured, joys and sorrows were remembered, and the requested advice and counsel was forthcoming. At the end of two and a half hours of sharing, each family member felt that he or she had said, "Good-bye, Dad. We love you. Thank you for being you. We'll miss you."

Spiritual Needs

Spiritual needs will be explored more fully toward the end of this chapter. At this point a cursory look at these needs and how they may be met by nurses is provided.

FORGIVENESS/RECONCILIATION

People can deeply wound or greatly offend others by the selfish or insensitive things they do or say. The outcome of this is often broken ties, separation, silence, bitterness, or deep-seated pain. Dying people can often approach death overwhelmed or deeply troubled by the fact that in certain relationships they have never granted forgiveness or been forgiven. Mending of broken ties and reconciliation has never occurred. Facilitating this process of reconciliation is an important form of care that nurses can offer to dying persons.

PRAYER/RELIGIOUS SERVICES

A more complete discussion of the importance of prayer as a form of spiritual care will be provided later. Prayer is recognized, however, as a source of comfort and strength to the dying. In the face of impending death we can often be at a loss for the proper, most helpful words to say. Religious services, such as the reception of sacraments, anointing with oil, or receiving a blessing of departure, are very meaningful to dying people and their families. Sometimes the patient and his family may be unaware that such services are available. Nurses, familiar with chaplaincy services or the

Pastoral Care Department of a health care institution, can arrange for religious services to be provided for those desiring them.

The following example illustrates the use of prayer with a dying patient.

Case Example #4

Praying with Larry was a real challenge. He had hoped for a cure, but
instead he was anxiously awaiting death. As the pastoral visitor prayed
with him, the words came haltingly. He prayed, "Lord God, it is so hard
to understand why things have happened as they did. Larry had so much
hoped for a cure, or at least a period of respite from his disease. He wanted
more time with his family. Please accept the confusion, the disappointment, the unsettled feelings that we both feel because this hasn't happened. Be with Larry; help him as he prepares to leave his family and to
come home to you."

The pastoral visitor knew that trying to express in prayer the feelings
that Larry was experiencing was the appropriate thing to do.

SPIRITUAL ASSISTANCE AT DEATH

Spiritual assistance at the time of death sometimes requires nothing more
from the nurse than caring words and respect for what is about to ensue.
Feeling helpless, saddened, and unable to do more for the dying person are
difficult and sobering experiences for nurses. Their physical presence and
loving concern, however, are invaluable, not only to the dying but also to
their grieving families. Spiritual assistance at death can also mean having
our spiritual leader, friends from our house of worship, and family members joined in prayer at our deathbed. What better way to be sent forth from
this earth into the loving care of our God than surrounded by those who
have shared common beliefs and faith!

PEACE

We may question whether peace is a blessing as well as a need. Actually it
can be and is both. Dying persons do need to know peace and tranquility
of spirit so that they can courageously depart from this world to the next.
When the needs of the dying, as discussed thus far, have been met, peace
can be expected to follow. Peace comes with the assurance that life has

been lived well. As St. Paul has said, one has truly run the race, the battle against evil and illness was courageously fought, and now one has reached the finish line (adapted from Philippians 3:12–14).

Needs of Grieving Families

To conclude this discussion of needs, let us consider the needs of grieving families. As has been suggested, the family plays a vital role in each person's life. A period of illness or the experience of death can, in no way, diminish or negate that role. People learned to trust and depend on their loved ones long before they came to know their health care providers. Why should the family not continue to furnish loving assistance during illness and at the time of death?

Many of the needs of grieving family members were already mentioned when the needs of dying people were outlined. For clarity, these needs are now reiterated.

Hope—for betterment, for the best care possible, for a hereafter where suffering and pain cease.

To be informed—to have periodic encounters with health care providers, to make decisions together with the dying person, to have the right to question.

Participation—to be a part, in some way, of what is happening, to be able to render some form of care, to be free to come to or leave the bedside.

Emotional support—to have fears and concerns accepted and understood; to be helped to cope with changes; to feel free to be angry, tearful, confused, or enraged; and to be close to the loved one who is dying.

Spiritual assistance—to be comforted by those who share a common faith, to be supported with prayer, to experience God's presence and strength through others, including the nurses who are providing care.

Time to grieve—to have private time and space with the deceased loved one, to have time to let go, to have sufficient opportunity to say good-bye and to express regrets, to linger with the deceased, as need dictates.

Grieving families are often forgotten once the body of the deceased person leaves the area where care has been given. Families are then abandoned to their process of bereavement, through which they often struggle unassisted. This, fortunately, is not the case when hospice services are being provided. Hospices offer supportive care to grieving families on an ongoing basis, at least for the first year after a loved one's death. It is helpful to briefly consider what families experience as they gather the personal belongings and some prized possessions of their deceased loved one who has been in a hospital or another health care facility. They start the journey home, enveloped in sorrow, as they carry a filled suitcase, whose owner, however, does not accompany them. They leave with vivid memories of all that has transpired within the last few hours, days, or weeks.

Unfortunately, the nurses who have come to know the family quickly lose contact and break ties with that family once death has occurred. Support groups for grieving families are very helpful to them, and nurses can encourage families to avail themselves of such services. Grief support groups are available within local communities, are provided by church or synagogue groups, or are sponsored by hospice groups.

Grieving: A Response to Loss

Grieving is a process that follows a loss of any significance. It involves painful feelings of separation from that which one has lost. Although grieving is most often linked with death experiences, it is a necessary process for all the losses we confront. The greater the importance or investment we have in a person, object, project, or pursuit, the greater the sense of loss.

One of the major concerns regarding the grieving process is how long it will last. Table 10–2 outlines the stages of grieving, the predominant characteristics of each stage, and an estimated time frame for each stage, as described by Veninga (1985).

Diets (1988) indicated that because grieving and our recovery from it are demanding, people often look for any way to escape this process. To move through grieving requires patience and stamina. The process is longer than we would desire, and it is difficult. Fitzgerald (1994) writes about the importance of expressing our grief. Efforts to ignore grieving can result in physiological disturbances such as flare-ups of chronic health prob-

Table 10–2   The Stages of Grieving

Stages	Characteristics	Duration
Stage 1: Shock and Disbelief	Shock, numbness, disbelief, can't make decisions, short attention span, difficulty carrying on conversations, anxious, physical symptoms such as nausea, vomiting, shortness of breath.	Several hours, days, or weeks
Stage 2: Attempts at Denial, Illusion of Normalcy	Seems anesthetized; begins to reestablish order; stabilizing his or her life; appears as if all is as before; makes decisions; greets friends, tries to fill void.	A few weeks
Stage 3: Feeling Lonely and Empty	Begins painful journey into darkest areas of life; expresses strong emotions, such as intense anger, loneliness, guilt; expresses negative themes—"My life will never be the same"; "It's impossible to ever be happy again." Some are stoic and logical; others feel the hurt deeply and show it; still others dwell on the loss; while some counterattack to dispel the anger (e.g., join Mothers Against Drunk Driving) and some become physically and/or psychologically ill.	Many months
Stage 4: New Awareness	A search for meaning begins; can find hopeful events once again. There is the belief that life can be happy, a view of self and the world is refashioned; a sense that he or she will make it.	Many months
Stage 5: Acceptance	Accepting but not forgetting the loss, reinvestment in life's undertakings and social events, letting go and moving on.	A year or two (maybe longer)

Source: Adapted from Veninga (1985, 112).

lems; weight loss; sleep abnormalities, gastrointestinal disturbances, and the like; or psychological disturbances, such as depression, bouts of anger, relational problems, anxiety, and so on (37). Grief is experienced holistically, with disruptions in physical, emotional, relational, and spiritual dimensions of life. It is not uncommon for the grieving person to wonder where God is as she moves through the pain of grief (Guntzelman 2001).

Major Tasks of Grieving

Worden (2002) outlined the major tasks or challenges that grieving people face. These include:

accepting the reality of the loss—believing the loss has really occurred.

knowing the situation will not reverse itself.

experiencing the emotional pain—knowing the disappointment, the loneliness, the emptiness, the absence of what was, and experiencing the emotions that accompany these realizations.

adjusting to life without the "lost object"—recognizing that one's life is not over or totally destroyed, knowing that one can go on.

letting go and moving on—reinvesting one's energies into new relationships.

beginning new undertakings; discovering a new purpose and meaning for one's life.

Each of these tasks is accomplished as the grief process unfolds. The reality of the loss is felt as acute emotional pain. Energies are poured into coping with the loss. The person wonders whether he will ever feel better. As the months of grieving pass, the person slowly begins to believe that he is adjusting. However, the arrival and passing of a holiday or special occasion can rekindle the emotional pain and deep longing once again. In time, however, more emotional energy becomes available for the person to face challenges, meet responsibilities, and accept new undertakings. Normal grieving, if it is allowed to progress through this series of tasks, will prepare the grieving person to accept the many possibilities that the future holds (Wolfelt 2003).

Grieving that becomes incapacitating and unusually prolonged is regarded as complicated grieving, which requires professional help for the griever (Rando 1993).

It might be mentioned that depression is often seen as a component of both normal and complicated grief reactions. The helplessness and hopelessness of depression often rob the grieving person of the emotional energy needed to do grief work. Thus, the need to address the depression.

Life is forever changed for those who have lost loved ones and much more. The grieving families are left to pick up the pieces and move forward with their lives. The slow, progressive loss of life, caused by many illnesses, leaves families with time to prepare for the inevitability of death. During the "waiting period," families experience "anticipatory grieving." There is time to slowly let go and release their loved ones to death. Families see the progressive decline and increased dependence as the illness advances; involvement in family life waxes and wanes until it is seen as being nonexistent (Noel & Blair 2000).

Through all these experiences, family members are forced to recognize the many losses that are befalling them. Their responses are varied and range from anger at the unfairness of the situation, disbelief that they are losing a vital member of their family, rage that health care professionals aren't doing enough, sadness that someone so loved is being snatched by death from their midst, and a sense of helplessness that they cannot reverse what is happening. "Letting go" of a dying loved one is not always an easy process.

Whether the grieving is characterized as a normal grief reaction or complicated grieving, there are strategies that nurses can use as they reach out to the dying or their grieving family members. Again the reader is referred to chapter 6 for a discussion of the interventions of ministry of presence, ministry of word, and ministry of action—each is appropriate to assist those who are grieving (Carson 1989, Carson & Koenig 2004, Soder-Alderfer 1994). These are outlined in Box 10–3.

Working through grief provides an opportunity for tremendous spiritual growth (Sittser 1995).

Box 10–3   Strategies for Helping Grieving People and Their Families

Reach out with genuine concern.

Speak words of understanding.

Encourage the grieving person or family members to talk about their pain.

Offer physical and emotional presence.

Try to view losses from the grieving person's perspective.

Encourage talking, a retelling of the loss event, even periods of silence, without demonstrating personal discomfort.

(box continues)

(Box 10–3 continued)

Provide necessary information about the grief process.

Allow tears and volatile feelings to surface while providing a safe environment for this to happen.

Encourage the person/family to grieve for as long as necessary.

Help those who are grieving to identify unfinished business that needs their attention.

Hold out to grievers the expectation and the hope that they will heal and recover.

Recognize your inability to eliminate, abbreviate, or lighten the pain of grieving.

Discuss the importance of having a strong support system while grieving.

Invite all who are grieving to maintain good self-care practices.

Encourage grieving people and families to draw on their personal faith and religious beliefs as a source of strength.

Avoid efforts to console, using false reassurances, such as "Feel better, your loved one is with God," "You can have a bright future before you," or "At your age there are plenty of opportunities to have more children, to find a new husband [and the like]."

Grief affects the body, mind, spirit, and relationships; thus the need for gentle care of self while grieving.

Relaxation strategies, physical exercise, and good health practices can help promote physical and emotional well-being.

Ongoing grief therapy, provided by a psychiatrist, a psychologist, a psychiatric nurse, a social worker, or a grief counselor, is indicated when the grief process has become long and incapacitating.

A grief support group can facilitate grief work by providing grief education and the caring support of other grieving persons.

Unfinished business often includes resolving differences with others, granting forgiveness, reconciling with estranged friends or family members, taking care of financial affairs, or fulfilling a lifelong dream. It is important to put closure to unfinished business.

Be aware of daily needs: Supply meals, offer to baby-sit, provide transportation, offer to clean house, polish shoes, and run errands.

Providing Spiritual Assistance to Those Facing the Reality of Death

Exploring the Realm of Spirituality

As the topic of spiritual care for the dying and bereaved is explored, we may question whether the seriously ill and dying are concerned about religious matters and issues of a spiritual nature. Illness has a way of putting people in touch with the spiritual. It may lead them to think not only about their dying, but also about their lives and a life hereafter.

As people use the long quiet hours that illness imposes on them, they may enter into a life review in which they ponder the deeper issues of their lives. They examine who they are or have become, where life has taken them, what their purpose or mission in life was and whether they fulfilled this purpose, how illness has affected their life goals, what death has come to mean for them, why they have to face a serious illness and the possibility of death at this time, where God is in this process, and what comes after death. Life reviews also incorporate some of the values that people desire for their lives. These may include honesty, caring, a sense of justice, concern for the earth and its beauty, kindness, compassion for the poor and struggling, and the like. The dying person may question what expression these values have had for her.

When people face the possibility of death and grieve the losses being imposed upon them, they often wrestle with their beliefs and with their God or Higher Being. They may be angry or disappointed with the God who seems to have abandoned them. They question where the miracles or the cures are for them. Some believe that their illness and impending death are a punishment from God for past wrongdoing.

By nature we are all spiritual beings. At the core of our being is a yearning for association with and reliance upon a presence greater than ourselves. We may come to know that presence as God, a Higher Power, or some spiritual force. Many will find comfort and solace in their relationship with their God, even in the midst of crises, tragedies, a serious illness, and the prospect of death.

We might conclude, then, that terminally ill and dying people are concerned about issues of a spiritual nature. They may choose to ponder their weighty concerns during the long hours of a sleepless night or during the

---

Box 10–4   Personal Spiritual Survey

Explain in a few brief sentences who God is for you and what God means to you

Of what does your belief system consist?

If prayer is a part of your life, what form does it take?

When you question the meaning of life for yourself, what convictions strike you most clearly or deeply?

When you try to fathom the "why" of illness and suffering, what ideas or feelings are aroused within you?

If you have spent some time considering your own death, what strong thoughts or sentiments about it do you have? If you haven't, where would a consideration of your own dying take you?

What do you do to live out your spiritual beliefs?

---

quiet moments of their lives. Often, at these times, family members, the clergy, close friends, or the professional staff are not available to listen. The hope is for someone to be there and to comfort them.

In exploring the area of spirituality, it is important for nurses to take an honest look at their own spirituality. The Personal Spiritual Survey provided in Box 10–4 will help the health care professional to examine his personal beliefs and to discover the truths and religious principles by which his life is guided. Taking an honest look at our own spirituality will not only be personally beneficial, but will also make the us more attuned to and respectful of another's spirituality.

Restricting the spiritual care of dying people to those who are theologically prepared is a questionable practice. Experience proves that, in a time of need, most of us are eager and willing to share our spiritual concerns and discuss our personal issues with anyone who will provide genuine caring, acceptance, understanding, and trust. As indicated, dying people question their beliefs, reveal their religious concerns, and discuss their relationship with a Higher Being. They do not expect theological answers from their listeners. It is not even necessary for the listener to share the same religious affiliation to be able to reach out and comfort at this time. What is needed most is a listener who is attentive, empathetic, and fully present.

Spiritual Care of Dying People and Their Families

As nurses undertake the task of providing spiritual care for their patients, they are cognizant of the fact that such care is not reserved for the hours prior to death. Spiritual care should encompass the whole period of illness, much as physical care does. Dying people are often too incapacitated for conversation or for many personal exchanges at the time of their death. As health care providers offer assistance, sensing that death may only be a few days away, the family is encouraged to say and do those things that may be necessary to prepare for the separation that death will impose.

A practice used in hospice is to invite families to engage in a meaningful conversation with the person who is preparing to die. During that conversation, truly a sacred time shared among family members, each person is invited to share what he or she feels is important and should be said. During the many workshops given by Dr. Elisabeth Kübler-Ross, she observed family members laying aside anger, resentments, and strained relationships to become more loving, warm, and close to each other (Varcarolis, Carson, & Shoemaker 2006). What Dr. Kübler-Ross hoped to accomplish can be summarized in the process of giving four gifts to each other. In this process, outlined in Box 10–5, the blessings are reciprocal. The giver receives healing, as does the receiver.

Assessing Spiritual Needs

Before we can reach out to provide spiritual assistance and care to dying people and their grieving families, it is important to know the areas of spiritual need or spiritual distress. As a point of reference, people who have a sense of spiritual well-being know the experience of feeling alive, purposeful, and fulfilled. They have a sense of a peace and serenity. There is a certain reverence for life, feelings of compassion for others, and a deep gratitude toward the God who sustains us with good gifts. Needless to say, not everyone enjoys this kind of well-being.

Spiritual needs abound in the lives of many. These needs are manifested through an inability to establish a meaningful relationship with a Higher Power, the members of our family, and the friends we meet along the

---

Box 10-5   The Four Gifts of Healing Dying People Await

Forgiveness (I'm sorry, I forgive you.)

These statements lead to truly pardoning and then releasing the pent-up hurt. Letting go of pain and anger can then follow.

Love (I love you.)

The message is that we are loved just for being who we are, not just for what we have done or achieved.

Gratitude (Thank you.)

A statement of appreciation for what another has been in our life—a gift, a mentor, a lover, a listener, a "soft place to fall."

Farewell (Good-bye! I'll be okay, although I'll miss you.)

These words acknowledge and honor the importance and depth of the relationship.

Source: Adapted from the writings of Elisabeth Kübler-Ross by B. Ryan, LCSW, of the Hospice of Twin Cities in Minnesota.

---

path of life. We encounter difficulty in sharing love, trust, and forgiveness.

Spiritual distress is manifested as disharmony within the human spirit. It involves a person's belief system, religious practices, value system, and meaningful relationships. Spiritual distress is evidenced through concerns about life, death, and suffering. There is discomfort surrounding issues of a religious nature, such as the existence of God or some form of Higher Power, the fairness (or, more likely, the unfairness) of life, religious practices, faith, and a personal spirituality.

People who exhibit spiritual need and demonstrate clear signs of spiritual distress are often in need of healing, forgiveness, personal catharsis, a life review, an empathic listener, or someone who reaches out in love and caring to them. A terminal condition or the approach of death leaves people fearful about the brokenness and incompleteness of their lives and vulnerable to bouts of depression. To come to know the spiritual concerns of the grief-stricken and dying, a spiritual assessment is necessary. It entails learning about a person's belief in God, her religious beliefs and practices, a sense of purpose and meaning in her life, her ability to cope with illness and the adversities of life, her capacity to give and receive love, her personal and spiritual values, and sources of her hope and strength (Shelly 2000, 109–11).

Providing Spiritual Interventions

As Carson & Koenig (2004) indicate, the primary task of the nurse who sets out to provide spiritual assistance is to offer compassion and caring. These are coupled with professional knowledge and skill. Nurses look at interventions that will bring comfort and peace, hope and support, an easing of pain and fear, and a loving presence for the journey beyond this life. Nurses who hold spiritual values, and who act on their own religious beliefs by attending worship services or other forms of spiritual activity, will provide spiritual care more readily and more consistently. Spiritual activities that are readily accepted by people who are ill and nearing death are outlined in Box 10–6.

There are barriers to healing and well-being about which nurses should be aware. These are outlined in Box 10–7.

Box 10–6   Spiritual Activities That Minister to the Grieving and Dying

---

Reading from the Bible or other sacred literature.

Praying for the persons involved.

Receiving communion or being anointed.

Listening to religious television programs, music, or tapes.

Reading inspirational books or pamphlets.

Receiving spiritual resource persons, such as the pastoral care minister, a pastor or another spiritual leader, or members of one's faith community.

Being ministered to through the presence, loving words, and actions of nurses.

Box 10-7   Spiritual Barriers to Wellness

Unresolved or trapped emotions with the pain they bring.

Repressed anger and resentments.

Lack of forgiveness of self and others.

Guilt and depression.

Hopelessness and despair.

Lack of peace and harmony within oneself.

Far too many people die estranged from those they once knew well and loved. They die with lack of forgiveness and much regret. Many carry personal burdens and hurts that they have accumulated over a lifetime. They have never dealt with the pain and hurt. They die with many unresolved issues in an embittered and resentful state.

A clinical example might be helpful in demonstrating how the spiritual needs of a dying person can be assessed by a health care provider.

Case Example #5

Nurse Michaels had attended some classes provided by the Pastoral Care Department of her hospital. They taught the participants how they could be ministering persons. Nurse Michaels was always motivated by a strong desire to help dying people in the most effective way. She entered Mary's hospital room, fired with enthusiasm and ready to put into practice all that she had learned.

Mary readily engaged in conversation with her nurse. She had been in the hospital for weeks now, and her condition was continually declining. Her failing liver and generalized state of weakness were the result of a long history of substance abuse. Nurse Michaels looked at this once-beautiful woman and wondered how she had come to this point in her life.

Mary slept a lot, had few visitors, and spent a portion of her time consulting with her financial advisor. She was busy reinvesting her financial resources. The nurse knew that Mary had a grown son, and that recently she had her lawyer come in to draw up a will. She made her son the sole beneficiary of her assets. This was a reasonable thing for a dying woman to do, a part of the unfinished business that needs to be handled before death. But was Mary dealing with the more personal issues of her dying? Had she completed a life review during this long period of hospitalization? Did she have regrets about the direction her life had taken? Where was God for her? Why wasn't Mary spending her last days with her son? Was there a problem with their relationship? Troubled by these questions, the nurse tried to engage Mary in a conversation that would spark some concern about these issues. Her efforts were unsuccessful. Nurse Michaels found herself getting upset because Mary seemed to be skirting these important issues. She looked for opportunities to initiate a conversation about dying, Mary's life choices, God, the hereafter, and Mary's relationship with her son. The opportunities never came.

Nurse Michaels made an appointment to see the chaplain who had offered the workshop on ministering to dying persons, assessing their spiritual needs, and reaching out to meet those needs. In conversing with him, she learned that ministering to Mary meant respecting her feelings, her agenda. It meant being available to explore spiritual issues only if that is what Mary indicated she wanted. Reaching out to Mary meant being present to Mary each day, listening to her talk about her business, offering her supportive care, and loving her as the unique and special person that she was.

Summary

In summary, the issue of death and its inevitability has been explored. The prevailing attitudes toward death point to the trend within our society to fear, dread, and avoid death's reality. Nurses encounter many dying persons in the care they give to others. There is a challenge placed before them to be comfortable with their own dying. This will allow them to reach out with understanding to persons and family members confronting the experience of death.

Whole person care—care that is ultimately spiritual in nature—is the form of health care that professionals are called upon to provide. It permits them to be attentive to the physical, emotional, social, and spiritual needs of others. This is in lieu of a focus solely on physical needs and physical care. The needs of the dying and their families were outlined and discussed from a holistic perspective.

Terminal illness and death itself cause people to face many losses. The major loss, of course, is death itself. Loss calls forth the process of grieving. How the grieving process unfolds was discussed. Grief responds to the same holistic care that is used to assist the dying in their journey.

The often ignored areas of spiritual needs and spiritual care of those awaiting death were explored. Spiritual interventions were outlined so that needed spiritual assistance might be given to the dying and bereaved.

Reflective Activities

1. Review the sections of chapters 3 and 4 regarding the beliefs and practices of various religions, representing theistic and pantheistic worldviews. Ask yourself how a patient's worldview and/or religion would impact on the care offered to him through the dying process.
2. Reflect on your responses to the various questionnaires included in this chapter. What did you learn about yourself; your attitudes toward death; your attitudes toward spirituality? How can this self-knowledge be used to improve your health care practice?
3. Reflect on the ministries of presence, word, and action. Do these ministries move you out of your comfort zone as a health care professional? Are you challenged to work through your discomfort, or are you inclined to dismiss these interventions as "not part of your role"?

References

Bishops' Committee of the Confraternity of Christian Doctrine. (1983). *The New American Bible*. New York: Thomas Nelson Publishers.

Carson, V. B. (1989). *Spiritual Dimensions of Nursing Practice*. Philadelphia: W. B. Saunders Co.

Carson, V. B., & Koenig, H. (2004). *Spiritual Caregiving: Health Care as a Ministry*. Philadelphia: Templeton Foundation Press.

Diets, B. (1988). *Life after Loss*. Tucson, Ariz.: Fischer Books.

Fitzgerald, H. (1994). *The Mourning Handbook*. New York: Simon and Schuster Publishers.

Guntzelman, J. (2001). *God Knows You're Grieving*. South Bend, Ind.: Sorin Books.

James, J. W., & Friedman, R. (1998). *The Grief Recovery Handbook*. New York: HarperCollins Publications.

Kübler-Ross, E. (1969). *On Death and Dying*. New York: Macmillan Press.

———. (1975). *Death—The Final Stage of Growth*. Englewood Cliffs, N.J.: Prentice-Hall, Inc.

Noel, B., & Blair, P., (2000). *I Wasn't Ready to Say Good-bye*. Milwaukee: Champion Press.

Rando, T. (1993). *Treatment of Complicated Mourning*. Champaign, Ill.: Research Press.

Shelly, J. A. (2000). *Spiritual Care: A Guide for Caregivers*. Downers Grove, Ill.: InterVarsity Press.

Sittser, J. (1995). *A Grace Disguised—How the Soul Grows Through Loss*. Grand Rapids: Zondervan Press.

Soder-Alderfer, K. (1994). *With Those Who Grieve*. Elgin, Ill.: Lion Publishing.

Teno, J., et al. (2004). Family Perspectives on End-of-Life Care at the Last Place of Care. *Journal of the American Medical Association* 291, no. 1: 88–93.

Varcarolis, E., Carson, V., & Shoemaker, N. (2006). *Foundations of Psychiatric Mental Health Nursing*, 5th ed. St. Louis: Saunders/Elsevier Publishers.

Veninga, R. (1985). *The Gift of Hope: How We Survive Our Tragedies*. New York: Little Brown and Co.

Wolfelt, A. (2003). *Understanding Your Grief*. Fort Collins, Colo.: Companion Press.

Worden, W. (2002). *Grief Counseling and Grief Therapy*, 3rd ed. New York: Springer.

PART IV

THE THREAD OF SPIRITUALITY THROUGH COMMUNITY, ETHICS WORK, AND EDUCATION

The final section of the book defies easy categorization, yet the issues addressed here are critical ones. The chapters in this section move beyond the application of spiritual principles to the care of the individual patient and family, and invite the reader to consider broader applications of spirituality. Chapter 11 examines a variety of community endeavors, such as parish nursing and faith-based clinics, that integrate spirituality into the delivery of health care. In chapter 12 the reader is introduced to the concept of ethical decision making as a spiritual concern. Ethical decisions are weighty, and must be made not only with careful deliberation but with much soul searching. Chapter 13 posits that spirituality woven throughout the educational system as well as the workplace is essential to the development of caring and committed nurses and other health care professionals. These strands of spirituality allow nurses to find meaning, to experience joy, to overcome discouragement, and to stave off burnout as they continue to serve the neediest among us.

11

SPIRITUAL CARE IN COMMUNITIES

NANCY CHRISTINE SHOEMAKER

> We must delight in each other, make others' conditions our own, rejoice
> together, mourn together, labor and suffer together, always having before
> our eyes our community as members of the same body.
>> —John Winthrop, first governor of the
>> Massachusetts Bay Colony, speaking in 1630[1]

Recognizing the challenge of increasing and unmet health care needs, and realizing the potential of faith communities to promote health, churches and other religious groups are developing innovative partnerships to improve the health of their communities. There are multiple economic and demographic factors that create a problem with service delivery in our health care system. Faith organizations have inherent strengths, which can promote optimal health, as well as a long tradition of caring for the sick and needy. This chapter identifies the reasons for increasing the involvement of houses of worship in health care activities, provides examples of successful community partnerships, and examines potential barriers to desired outcomes.

Increasing and Unmet Health Care Needs

As spiritual leaders face their congregations in churches, synagogues, mosques, and temples, they see myriad unmet health care needs. In 2005, there were approximately 46 million uninsured Americans (Center on Budget and Policy Priorities, 2006, 1). Without insurance, individuals do not receive preventive care or early treatment for illness. Instead, they seek emergency care only when necessary, with greater risk to their health and increased costs in the health care system.

Health care costs continue to climb every year, and it is not clear how the government will keep up with the demand for mandated services. For example, Medicare costs have increased from less than $5 billion per year in the mid-1960s to a projected $444 billion by 2010 (Henry J. Kaiser Family Foundation 2005, 2). This figure does not include the cost for 75 million retiring baby boomers starting in 2011 (Hale & Koenig 2003, 2–3). With advances in medicine, Americans are living longer with higher risk for chronic illnesses, such as cardiac, respiratory, and endocrine disorders. By 2040, it is predicted that 80–100 million people over the age of sixty-five will require medical treatment covered by Medicare (Hale & Koenig 2003, 3). To cope with this huge demand, the health care system will have to focus more on preventing illness and improving disease management. Health care agencies will have to increase education programs for patients and their families to support improved screening and monitoring of medical conditions (Hale & Bennett 2000).

The Effect of the Faith Community on Health

Churches and other faith groups possess certain attributes that make them ideal for partnering with health care providers to promote optimal health. Americans are deeply committed to and influenced by their faith. In a 2005 national survey, 79 percent of respondents described themselves as "spiritual" and 64 percent called themselves "religious" (Adler et al. 2005, 48). Out of 1,004 adults aged 18–60+ years, 45 percent reported weekly attendance at worship services (Adler et al. 2005, 49). A place of worship provides contact with multiple age groups from youth to old age. It is especially useful to access people fifty years and older, who cannot usually be reached through public health campaigns in schools and work sites (Hale & Bennett, 2000, 4).

Hale & Koenig (2003) identify three specific factors that enable churches

> **Box 11–1   Seven Ways That Faith Communities Have a Positive Impact on Health**
>
> 1. Influence personality development.
>
> 2. Moderate unhealthy behaviors, such as smoking and use of alcohol.
>
> 3. Influence perceptions of pain and disability.
>
> 4. Convey hope and motivation.
>
> 5. Assist in coping with stress.
>
> 6. Encourage altruistic behaviors.
>
> 7. Provide a framework that gives meaning and purpose to life.
>
> *Source:* Adapted from Buijs & Olson (2001, 16).

to be prime sites for public health education. First, places of worship are located within the community and trusted local residents run their daily activities. Second, they have an existing structure for communication, such as announcements, bulletins, e-mail alerts, and the like. Third, these institutions have a strong history of altruism and volunteer service to others. In such an environment, a health screening or teaching event is easily advertised, and has a high probability of attendance with a ready supply of helpers to carry out necessary tasks.

Buijs & Olson (2001) also document unique characteristics of faith communities that support healthy lifestyles. Box 11–1 lists seven ways that churches may have a positive impact on health.

Federal Government Funding Initiative

The federal government clearly recognizes the benefit of an increased role for faith groups in community health. In 2001, President George W. Bush issued an executive order to establish Centers for Faith-Based and Community Initiatives in five cabinet departments, including Health and Human Services (White House 2001). The mission of these centers is to encourage faith-based and community-based organizations to collaborate with the government to provide services to vulnerable populations (U.S. Department of Health & Human Services 2006). Federal funding is available for religious groups that provide health-related services as long as they meet certain regulatory requirements.

Yet, an audit by the five centers in 2001 found that there were significant barriers to faith-based groups seeking federal support. Fifteen obstacles were found, revealing a bias against faith-based groups, especially small or first-time applicants (White House 2001). The major themes were excessive requirements beyond the budget of a small organization, and lack of access to grant information with preference for previous grantees; see Box 11–2 for more details on the obstacles. Faith groups are persevering through these difficulties, especially via formula grants to state and local governments.

Role of the Parish Nurse

There is a growing body of literature describing collaboration between faith groups and health care providers to offer health services. One of the most visible signs of this partnership is the increasing number of parish nurses: in 2002, there were an estimated six thousand parish nurses in the United States (Hugg 2002, 3). Parish nursing is a specialty in community nursing practice as defined by the American Nurses Association (ANA) and the Health Ministries Association. The parish nurse performs independent functions of professional nursing as a member of the health ministry of a faith community to promote health and healing within the context of faith practices (American Nurses Association & Health Ministries Association 1998). Belonging to the health ministry means that the parish nurse, either as a volunteer or as a paid employee, collaborates with other ministry staff in the mission to improve the health of the congregation and its surrounding community. In this context, the promotion of health and healing goes beyond the public health concepts of illness prevention to incorporate spiritual care. Health is defined as "the integration of the physical, psychological, social and spiritual aspects of the patient system and harmony with self, others, the environment and God." Illness also has a special defini-

Box 11–2 Barriers to Faith Groups Seeking Federal Funding

1. Government suspicion about faith-based organizations.

2. Exclusion of faith-based organizations from certain federal programs.

3. Excessive limits on religious activities.

4. Inappropriate application of obsolete religious restrictions to new programs.

5. Denial of faith groups' established right to consider religion in employment decisions.

6. Thwarting Charitable Choice (a congressional provision to support faith-based organizations by clarifying constitutional requirements for collaborating with the government).

7. Limited access to federal grant information.

8. Weight of multiple regulations and other requirements.

9. Preliminary requirements to meet even before applying for support.

10. Complex nature of grant applications and agreements.

11. Occasional favoritism for particular faith-based organizations.

12. Bias in favor of previous grantees.

13. Inappropriate requirement to apply in collaboration with a potential competitor.

14. Requiring formal Internal Revenue code status 501(c)(3) —without statutory authority.

15. Lack of attention to faith-based and community organizations in streamlining the federal grant process.

Source: White House (2001).

tion as "the experience of brokenness: disintegration of body, mind, spirit; and dis-harmony with others, the environment, and God" (ANA & Health Ministries Association 1998, 6).

Interventions of the Parish Nurse

There are seven specific interventions used by parish nurses, providing direct or indirect patient care to individuals or congregations (see Box 11–3). In one study, parish nurses described the unique rewards of their role in congregations. In health promotion activities, such as blood pressure screening, individuals with undiagnosed hypertension can be identified and referred for medical treatment. One nurse stated, "At work I'm taking care of people who are sick. At church, I keep people well via screening" (Chase-Ziolek & Iris 2002, 177). As an advocate, the nurse encourages patients to visit their health care providers and helps them to process the information they receive. If necessary, the nurse may contact the physician directly about a potentially dangerous symptom. One nurse remarked about advocacy, "The value in this was that I was able to educate and help people to be their own advocate. I also go to bat for people" (Chase-Ziolek & Iris 2002, 178). In health education, nurses teach about wellness topics through newsletters or health fairs. They describe feeling more relaxed and autonomous teaching in the congregation environment, and perceive patients to be more comfortable participating as a result of their relationship of trust. Finally, with health counseling, the nurse helps patients cope with feelings related to health problems and can freely include spirituality in the discussion. One nurse commented, "I make the most difference by counseling. . . . They trust me. If people have anxiety about surgery or a fall, they call me" (Chase-Ziolek & Iris 2002, 180).

NANDA Diagnoses and NIC Interventions for Congregations

Another study examined the most frequent nursing diagnoses and interventions used by parish nurses for congregations (Weis et al. 2002). The standard classification systems of the North American Nursing Diagnosis

---

Box 11–3   Primary Interventions of the Parish Nurse

1. Enhancing self-care and care-giving abilities.

2. Health teaching.

3. Primary, secondary, and tertiary health promotion.

4. Health counseling.

5. Collaborating with health care providers.

6. Providing information about and referral to community resources.

7. Advocacy for services and health policies.

Source: American Nurses Association & Health Ministries Association, Inc. (1998, 13).

Table 11–1   Most Frequent Parish Nurse NIC Interventions for Two NANDA Diagnoses

Health-Seeking Behavior	Potential for Enhanced Spiritual Well-Being
Active listening	Active listening
Health screening	Spiritual support
Support system enhancement	Emotional support
Presence	Learning facilitation
Self-esteem enhancement	Self-esteem enhancement
Learning facilitation	
Health education	

Source: Weis et al. (2002, 109).

Association (NANDA) and Nursing Interventions Classification (NIC) were used. There were three frequent NANDA diagnoses that varied according to age group: health-seeking behavior for members eighteen years old and younger; knowledge deficit for members nineteen to fifty-nine years old; and potential for enhanced spiritual well-being, for members sixty years old and older. In response to the diagnoses of health-seeking behavior and potential for enhanced spiritual well-being, certain interventions were utilized most often (see Table 11–1).

Multidisciplinary Collaboration

The parish nurse does not replace or duplicate the services of other health care providers. Rather, collaboration with other members of the multidisciplinary team is essential for the role. Collaboration is defined as "teamwork, partnership, group effort, alliance and relationship" (Habermeier 2004, 278). In the context of promoting optimal health, the parties may include the patient, family, parish nurse, community nurse, physician, and others. Originally called the "five gifts of collaboration," elements of successful collaboration for a team ministry include (Kelley 1994):

1. Respect.
2. Positive regard for others.
3. Setting clear goals.
4. Listening.
5. Dedication to caring for the whole person.

Other Examples of Successful Collaboration between Faith Groups and Health Providers

There are numerous examples of successful collaborative projects between multidisciplinary health care providers and faith groups. The leader or initiator of a project may be from a congregation—a pastor, a congregation member, or parish nurse. Alternatively, the leader may be drawn from the health care community—a doctor, a nurse, a pharmacist, a psychologist, a hospital, or an academic center. Regardless of how large or small the health activity becomes, it usually starts with the calling of one individual or a personal health event.

Hale and Koenig (2003) described ten different case studies of collaborative partnerships in Florida, offering practical guidelines so others could develop similar programs. Five selected examples of these ventures, as well as other notable projects, are summarized below.

Five Case Studies in Florida

#1 Free Clinic

In Orlando, a pastor felt a strong calling to establish a clinic for the uninsured people in his community. He turned to two church members for assistance—a practicing physician and a retired business executive. Through teamwork with other members and community leaders, they founded a free clinic in a nearby school. They were able to obtain donated equipment, supplies, and even medications. Health professionals agreed to volunteer their time.

#2 Medical Day Care Program

A parishioner with advancing Parkinson's disease and his wife were growing desperate about maintaining his safety at home during the day. They searched for an appropriate medical day care center but could only find a site for Alzheimer's patients. Then they learned that their church had a plan to open a medical day care program for the community. Two nurses in the congregation were hired to oversee the center, which was established near the church school and the children's day care program. This unique medical day care center provided for interactions with children and youth, as well as spiritual services for all participants.

#3 Lay Health Educators

The Halifax Medical Center contacted pastors to seek people who might be interested in training as lay health educators. Physicians and other hospital professionals volunteered to teach an eight-week course for interested participants; the course focused on disease and techniques to conduct health teaching. For at least one church, this resulted in ongoing screening programs for skin cancer, cholesterol, and diabetes; annual flu vaccinations; a walking club; CPR training; and classes on depression, medications, and living wills.

#4 Programs on End-of-Life Issues

One Sunday morning, an elderly congregant suffered cardiac arrest in church. He received prompt CPR from a nurse and two physicians in the church and survived. In the following months, he experienced many physical and spiritual challenges, along with his caregiver wife. As congregation members volunteered multiple services to them, the pastor realized the need for teaching about end-of-life issues. Fortunately, two of the congregants had received training as lay health educators. They chose the topic of advance directives for their first program, and got assistance from an attorney member in the congregation and a community social worker.

#5 Health Care Support Groups

A retired, eighty-year-old woman was suffering from increasing disabilities due to Parkinson's disease. She could no longer do her artwork and was in a wheelchair. One day at church, she and her husband learned of a Parkinson's support group held in a nearby church of another faith. This support group met monthly and had guest speakers talking about illness and treatment. After joining this group, the patient found out about another group at the same church focused on exercise. The weekly exercise group was led by a retired exercise science professor who encouraged patients to improve their strength and balance. The patient attended both of these support groups and credited them with her eventual ability to walk again and resume her painting.

Health Fairs

In a small midwestern city, a community health nurse identified cardiovascular disease as the community's main health concern, based on data from the health department and community leaders. She planned a series of three health fairs, to be held right after services at three different churches (Wilson 2000). She obtained free literature and a video from the American Heart Association and the Centers for Disease Control and Prevention. She evaluated each fair and offered four recommendations for improving participation at future health fairs.

1. Involve church members to greet people and assist with evaluation forms.
2. Seek donations from local businesses for refreshments.
3. Hand out literature individually rather than just leaving it on tables to be picked up.
4. Have enough staff to perform the screening so that people do not have a long wait.

Multidisciplinary Medication Education

A multidisciplinary medication education program was presented to twenty congregations in central Ohio (Schommer et al. 2002). Initiated through the Riverside Methodist Hospital–Church Partnership Department, the collaborative effort involved the hospital pharmacy department, the hospital-based parish nurse program, and two colleges of pharmacy. Parish nurses advertised the program to their congregations, and there were two hundred participants with an average age of sixty-nine.

The pastor and parish nurse started the program with introductions, and then the pharmacist and the nurse taught the members in groups and one on one. They found that a significant number of participants were not taking their medications appropriately: 57 percent had medicines that should have been discarded; 23 percent were storing their medicines improperly (Schommer et al. 2002, 4). In addition, there were adverse drug effects and drug interactions that had gone unreported. Although evaluations were positive, a follow-up study six months later showed no improvement in the number of people who always took their medication as ordered. The authors concluded that teaching only the patients was not enough to change behavior in this population. Instead, they recommended contact with caregivers or physicians or pharmacists to reinforce necessary corrections in medication management.

Wellness Services at Local Pharmacies

Two pharmacy professors noted that community pharmacists share responsibility with other health care professionals to educate patients about health. They described resources for pharmacists to sponsor wellness services directly on site in collaboration with other community health providers (Ciardulli & Goode 2003). Community staff could include public health nurses, parish nurses, dietitians, exercise therapists, and the like. They recommended using the calendar of health themes distributed by the federal Office of Disease Prevention and Health Promotion as a structure to select topics. They also noted that patient education materials could be obtained from national health organizations such as the American Heart Association, the American Cancer Society, and others. Examples of services were given, including blood pressure screening, influenza vaccinations, and classes on nutrition and exercise.

Spiritual Program for Oncology Center

The staff of an ambulatory oncology center in a secular hospital recognized the need to address spiritual issues with their patients. They sought out three churches to develop a spiritual program for twelve hundred cancer survivors, their families, and their friends (Dann & Mertens 2004). Clergy of each church presented prayer, scripture reading, music, and litany, while patients contributed testimonials. The majority of the attendees reported that they found the services helpful, and especially appreciated that their clinicians attended their churches.

Mental Health Needs

With regard to mental health, the role of faith groups in providing services is affected by attitudes toward mental illness. In a metropolitan area of Connecticut, pastors of nearly all the African-American churches were interviewed to explore the nature of their mental health services (Young, Griffith, & Williams 2003). Ninety-nine pastors described the most frequent issues they encountered, as well as their interventions. Common types of problems included spiritual distress, physical illness, family issues, addiction, financial hardships, and grief. They described their main interventions as listening, giving support, prayer, and sharing scripture. They also noted a reciprocal referral process with mental health professionals. Almost half reported receiving referrals from professionals in health care agencies, especially social workers, and the majority felt comfortable in referring their members to a community mental health center.

A second study of faith groups and mental health care found some similarities but also identified potential barriers (Dossett, Fuentes, & Wells 2005). Forty-two organizations in the Queenscare Health and Faith Partnership Network of Los Angeles completed a survey about attitudes toward mental illness and services. The majority believed that their congregations needed services and stated that they offered informal counseling and referrals to community providers. But they cited barriers to care as well, from limited budget and staff to lack of staff training. Half of the respondents were unwilling to work with a local government agency to provide services. Some expressed the belief that mental illness was a moral or spiritual problem and was not responsive to the medical model of illness and treatment.

One example of a successful faith-based mental health program is Celebrate Recovery, a modification of the twelve-step program of Alcoholics Anonymous (Baker 1998). Founded by a pastor who is a recovering alcoholic, this program revised the original twelve steps by substituting scripture quotations for each step, and defining Jesus Christ as the Higher Power (see Table 11–2). There is a structured training manual for lay leaders who then conduct weekly group meetings on site in the church. The program also goes beyond substance addiction to address other distressing habits or beliefs in members.

Table 11–2　Comparison Between 12 Steps of Alcoholics Anonymous and Celebrate Recovery

Alcoholics Anonymous	Celebrate Recovery
1. We admitted we were powerless over alcohol—that our lives had become unmanageable.	I know that nothing good lives in me, that is, in my sinful nature. For I have desire to do what is good, but I cannot carry it out. (Romans 7:18)
2. We came to believe that a power greater than ourselves could restore us to sanity.	For it is God who works in you to will and to act according to his purpose. (Philippians 2:13)

(table continues)

(Table 11–2 continued)

Alcoholics Anonymous	Celebrate Recovery
3. We made a decision to turn our will and our lives over to the care of God, as we understood Him.	Therefore, I urge you brothers, in view of God's mercy, to offer your bodies as living sacrifices, holy and pleasing to God—this is your spiritual act of worship. (Romans 12:1)
4. We made a searching and fearless moral inventory of ourselves.	Let us examine our ways and test them, and let us return to the Lord. (Lamentations 3:40)
5. We admitted to God, to ourselves, and to another human being the exact nature of our wrongs.	Therefore, confess your sins to each other and pray for each other so that you may be healed. (James 5:16)
6. We were entirely ready to have God remove all these defects of character.	Humble yourselves before the Lord, and He will lift you up. (James 4:10)
7. We humbly asked Him to remove all our shortcomings.	If we confess our sins, He is faithful and will forgive us our sins and purify us from all unrighteousness. (1 John 1:9)
8. We made a list of all persons we had harmed, and became willing to make amends to them all.	Do to others as you would have them do to you. (Luke 6:31)
9. We made direct amends to such people wherever possible, except when to do so would injure them or others.	Therefore, if you are offering your gift at the altar and there remember that your brother has something against you, leave your gift there in front of the altar. First go and be reconciled to your brother; then come back and offer your gift. (Matthew 5:23–24)
10 We continued to take personal inventory and when we were wrong, promptly admitted it.	So, if you think you are standing firm, be careful that you don't fall. (1 Corinthians 10:12)
11. We sought through prayer and meditation to improve our conscious contact with God, as we understood Him, praying only for knowledge of His will for us and the power to carry that out.	Let the word of Christ dwell in you richly. (Colossians 3:16)
12. Having had a spiritual awakening as the result of these steps, we tried to carry this message to alcoholics, and to practice these principles in all our affairs.	Brothers, if someone is caught in a sin, you who are spiritual should restore him gently. But watch yourself, or you may be tempted. (Galatians 6:1)

Source: Alcoholics Anonymous World Services, Inc. (2001, 10–11).

Summary

As noted through the examples above, partnerships between faith groups and health care providers can lead to effective and rewarding outcomes for all participants. There are many resources available to those who are interested in exploring or developing programs specific to their own congregations—see the list at the end of the chapter (Hale & Koenig 2003). Hale and Bennett (2000) surveyed doctors, nurses, social workers, clergy, and congregations to identify a "Top Ten" list of health care topics for starting a health ministry (see Box 11–4). Pattillo and colleagues (2002) came up with five factors useful in forging effective alliances between faith groups and other community agencies. Although their focus was on nursing networks, these recommendations are applicable to all disciplines.

1. Create a formal structure with a mission statement, common goals, defined values, and objectives.
2. Provide credible leadership, especially to oversee policies and training related to nursing practice.
3. Determine the appropriate organizations to join the network—hospitals, community health facilities, colleges and universities, and government agencies.
4. Ensure that all participants are clear about shared values for health and faith.
5. Develop expertise in training volunteers.

Box 11–4 "Top Ten" List of Health Topics for a Health Ministry	
1. Coronary heart disease	6. Dementia
2. Hypertension	7. Advance directives
3. Cancer	8. Accidents and falls
4. Diabetes mellitus	9. Influenza and pneumonia
5. Depression	10. Medication management

Source: Hale & Bennett (2000, 25).

There are still challenges in forming these partnerships, which may act as barriers to successful outcomes. Government officials in local health or social services departments and faith leaders may express mutual distrust of one another, jeopardizing true collaboration. Access to federal funding requires navigating through complex regulations, testing the perseverance of first-time applicants. Members of one congregation may not have sufficient expertise to address certain needs, such as mental health, requiring additional training or sharing of resources with other faith groups. Finally, the leaders must take time at the outset to define a formal structure that will support shared values about health and faith among diverse participants.

There are certainly many obstacles to overcome in the drive to improve delivery of health care for all Americans. But it is equally true that creative partnerships with faith communities can multiply scarce health care resources to greatly benefit congregations and communities with unmet needs.

Reflective Activities

1. Can you identify one way that you were influenced by a faith group to develop good health?
2. If you were approached by a faith group to volunteer in a health fair, would you agree? Why or why not?
3. Think about your family or neighborhood. Do you see any unmet health needs that could be met through collaboration between a health agency and a faith community?
4. Would you feel comfortable collaborating with leaders of a faith group to plan a community health function?
5. Can you think of other health topics for a health ministry which would especially apply to youth?

Resources for Initiating a Health Ministry

Caring Communities Program
Duke Divinity School
3600 University Drive, Suite D
Durham, NC 27707
(919) 401-3737 ext 102
www.divinity.duke.edu

Center for Community Health
Ministry, Florida Hospital
2400 Bedford Road, 2nd Floor
Orlando, FL 32803
(407) 303-5574
www.parishnursing.net

Center for Spirituality, Theology
and Health
Box 3400
Duke University Medical Center
Durham, NC 27710
(919) 681-6633
www.dukespiritualityandhealth.org

Faith in Action
A National Program of the Robert
  Wood Johnson Foundation
Wake Forest University, School of
  Medicine
Medical Center Boulevard
Winston-Salem, NC 27157
(877) 324-8411
www.fiavolunteers.org

Health Ministries Association
980 Canton Street, Building 1,
  Suite B
Roswell, GA 30075
(800) 280-9919
www.hmassoc.org

Institute for Congregational and
Community Health
Stetson University, Campus
  Box 8272
Deland, FL 32723
(386) 822-7289
www.stetson.edu/icch

Local Initiative Funding Partners
A National Program of the Robert
  Wood Johnson Foundation
760 Alexander Road, P.O. Box 1
Princeton, NJ 08543
(609) 275-4128
www.lifp.org

Shepherd's Hope
4851 S. Apopka-Vineland Road
Orlando, FL 32819
(407) 876-6699
www.shepherdshope.org

Wheat Ridge Ministries
One Pierce Place, Suite 250E
Itasca, IL 60143
(800) 762-6748
www.wheatridge.org

Note

1. J. Winthrop, *Puritan Political Ideas, 1558–1794*, ed. E. S. Morgan (Indianapolis: Bobbs-Merrill, 1965), 92.

References

Adler, J., et al. (2005). Spirituality 2005 a special report. *Newsweek* (September 5, 2005): 48–64.

Alcoholics Anonymous World Services, Inc. (2001). *Alcoholics Anonymous*, 4th ed. New York: Author.

American Nurses Association & Health Ministries Association, Inc. (1998). *Scope and Standards of Parish Nursing Practice*. Washington, D.C.: American Nurses Publishing.

Baker, J. (1998). *Celebrate Recovery Leader's Guide*. Grand Rapids: Zondervan Publishing House.

Buijs, R., & Olson, J. (2001). Parish nurses influencing determinants of health. *Journal of Community Health Nursing* 18 (1): 13–23.

ADD Center on Budget and Policy Priorities. (2006). The number of uninsured Americans is at an all-time high. www.cbpp.org/8-29-06health.htm. Accessed March 16, 2008.

Chase-Ziolek, M., & Iris, M. (2002). Nurses' perspectives on the distinctive aspects of providing nursing care in a congregational setting. *Journal of Community Health Nursing* 19 (3): 173–86.

Ciardulli, L. M., & Goode, J-V. R. (2003). Using health observances to promote wellness in community pharmacies. *Journal of the American Pharmaceutical Association*, 43 (1): 61–68.

Dann, N. J., & Mertens, W. C. (2004). Taking a "leap of faith": Acceptance and value of a cancer program-sponsored spiritual event. *Cancer Nursing* 27 (2): 34–43.

Dossett, E., Fuentes, S., & Wells, K. (2005). Obstacles and opportunities in providing mental health services through a faith-based network in Los Angeles. *Psychiatric Services*, 56 (2): 206–8.

Habermeier, N. (2004). Collaboration in spiritual care. In K. L. Mauk & N. K. Schmidt (eds.), *Spiritual Care in Nursing Practice*, 277–87. Philadelphia: Lippincott, Williams & Wilkins.

Hale, W. D., & Bennett, R. G. (2000). *Building Healthy Communities through Medical-Religious Partnerships*. Baltimore: Johns Hopkins University Press.

Hale, W. D., & Koenig, H. G. (2003). *Healing Bodies and Souls: A Practical Guide for Congregations*. Minneapolis: Fortress Press.

Henry J. Kaiser Family Foundation. (2005). Medicare at a glance fact sheet. www.kff.org/medicare/upload/Medicare-at-a-glance-fact-sheet.pdf. Accessed March 16, 2008

Hugg, A. (2002). Undercover(ed) nursing. www.nurseweek.com/news/features/02-06/Clinics_print.html; accessed March 26, 2006.

Kelley, J. T. (1994). Five group dynamics in team ministry. *Journal of Pastoral Care* 48: 118–30.

Pattillo, M. M., et al. (2002). Faith community nursing: Parish nursing/health ministry collaboration model in central Texas. *Family Community Health* 25 (3): 41–51.

Schommer, J. C., et al. (2002). Interdisciplinary medication education in a church environment. *American Journal of Health-System Pharmacy* 59 (5): 423–28.

U.S. Department of Health & Human Services. (2006). The center for faith-based & community initiatives. www.hhs.gov/fbci/; accessed March 8, 2006.

Weis, D. M., et al. (2002). Parish nurse practice with patient aggregates. *Journal of Community Health Nursing* 19 (2): 105–13.

White House. (2001). Unlevel playing field: Barriers to participation by faith-based and community organizations in federal social services programs. www.whitehouse.gov/news/releases/2001/08/print/unlevelfield.html; accessed March 8, 2006.

Wilson, L. C. (2000). Implementation and evaluation of church-based health fairs. *Journal of Community Health Nursing* 17 (1): 39–48.

Young, J. L., Griffith, E. E. H., & Williams, D. R. (2003). The integral role of pastoral counseling by African-American clergy in community mental health. *Psychiatric Services* 54 (5): 688–92.

12

ETHICAL DECISION MAKING AND SPIRITUALITY

GARY BATCHELOR

> Speaking against abortion, someone has said, "No one should be denied
> access to the great feast of life," to which the rebuttal, obviously is that life
> isn't much of a feast for the child born to people who don't want it or can't
> afford it or are one way or another incapable of taking care of it and will one
> way or another probably end up abusing or abandoning it. And yet, and
> yet. Who knows what treasure life may hold for even such a child as that. Or
> what a treasure even such a child as that may grow up to become? To bear
> a child even under the best of circumstances, or to abort a child even under
> the worst—the risks are hair-raising either way and the results incalculable.
> There is perhaps no better illustration of the truth that in an imperfect world
> there are no perfect solutions. All we can do, as Luther said, is sin bravely,
> which is to say (a) know that neither to have the child nor not to have the
> child is without the possibility of tragic consequences for everybody yet (b)
> be brave in knowing also that not even that can put us beyond the forgiving
> love of God.
>
> —Frederick Buechner (1988, 1)

Introduction

Though many may consider abortion to be the quintessential issue with
which spirituality and ethics must engage in some kind of dialogue, this
chapter will not be about abortion or any other single issue. Instead, the

chapter will address the broader implications illustrated in this quote from Buechner: that ethical concerns and the decisions they call forth have an impact that may reach far beyond the immediate situation, that there are no perfect solutions in an imperfect world, and that spiritual issues are inextricably interwoven with the kinds of ethical decisions that confront health care professionals and those for whom they care. Those ethical issues run the gamut from dramatic decisions about discontinuing life-sustaining treatments to equally dramatic decisions about when life begins and what are appropriate interventions for nascent life. However, even more common are the "mundane" decisions about how best to respect the *person* in need of care when the caregiver has special knowledge, disproportionate power, competing allegiances, stressful workloads, and personal or cultural values that may be different from the one for whom she is caring. "Spirituality demonstrates that persons are not merely physical bodies that require mechanical care" (VandeCreek et al. 2001, 2). Therefore the comingling of spirituality and ethical decision making are not only appropriate but are vital in considering how a health care professional might best fulfill her calling.

Defining the Place of Ethics in Health Care

It seems appropriate to offer some explanation about the perspective from which this chapter is written. The author is a professional hospital chaplain whose knowledge and experience in dealing with ethical issues come from seventeen years of "front line" clinical ethics experience, including cochairing the hospital ethics committee and serving as ethics faculty for a family practice residency program. The focus of the chapter is on ethical reflection for individuals in critical illness or trauma situations—the kinds of "bedside ethics" that hospital ethics committees most often encounter. Though issues of organizational ethics and ethical considerations in mass casualty situations challenge those engaged in health care ethics to expand their scope beyond the bedside, such considerations are beyond the present scope. This chapter is offered as an overview, touching on only the most salient aspects of topics that are developed by others in book-length scholarly and research volumes. It is hoped that sections offering mere glimpses into complex topics or clearly indicating a lack of in-depth exploration will serve as a stimulus for the reader to delve more deeply.

Let us consider exactly what meaning we shall give to the broad term ethics. To begin with, let us dispel several misconceptions about ethics in the health care arena. These misconceptions include the idea that ethics is primarily a judicial process, that ethics is nothing more than glorified second-guessing, that ethics is an exercise in moralizing, and that ethics is a matter of mere opinion—one opinion being as good as another.

A most distressing misunderstanding of ethics—ethics as judicial process—is heavily influenced by connotations that come from the political arena. How often do we read about a state or federal "ethics commission," which is charged with the task of reviewing questionable behavior and determining some sanction or punishment for the wrongdoer? Meting out punishment becomes a primary task when ethics is understood within a judicial metaphor. Clearly the issues that concern health care matters have an element of determining right and wrong, but not with the purpose of punishing wrongdoers nor of inflating the stature of those who decide "rightly." Lacking a clear rejection of the punitive connotation, health care professionals are likely to be guarded or hostile, rather than cooperative, when ethical questions come to the fore.

When some clinicians hear the word "ethics," they fear that yet another person is going to second-guess some practice by the clinician. Furthermore, that second-guesser is feared to be someone far removed from the situation, and having little or no responsibility for the actual outcome. Especially for physicians, who have seen multiple encroachments into realms of decision making that were once exclusively their domain, the thought of having their judgment questioned from yet another perspective is highly unappealing! It is one of the challenges to those concerned with ethical issues in health care to be sure that they are willing to undergo the necessary discipline and training to develop firsthand knowledge of these matters, rather than pontificating based on mere theories from the ivory tower of academia.

Acknowledging that any significant ethical issue involves some level of moral decision making about right and wrong, it does not follow that ethics is mere moralizing. The understanding of moralizing being rejected here is that of authoritarian activity by a so-called expert, or, even worse, a designated paragon of virtue, who makes pronouncements from some figurative place on high. Expertise may indeed be displayed through knowledge or virtue exhibited through respected character, but always with humility and respect for all parties involved in the issue at hand. When an ethical issue formally comes before an ethics committee, all parties are to be heard and all valid concerns taken seriously. When the kind of ethical reflection offered in this chapter is the standard of ethical caring, no dominant person or perspective has the authority to dictate an outcome.

The final misunderstanding to be considered and discarded is the idea that, because of the complexity and frequent ambiguity of ethical decision making, ethics is mere opinion. If ethics is but opinion, in a pluralistic society, one opinion is as authoritative as any other. It would therefore follow that there really are no grounds for considering some ethical decisions to be "better" than others. Oftentimes, ethical dilemmas do not lend themselves to a final and unanimous decision about what action should be taken or avoided. Those who seek the clarity of mathematical or logical precision will certainly be frustrated by that! It is the purpose of this chapter to delineate elements of theory and practice, of precedent and knowledge, of compassion and of courage that will distinguish ethics as a spiritual practice of careful and wise deciding in difficult situations. Such practice is far removed from the mere proffering of one superficial opinion to another.

Having described several inadequate understandings of ethics, it is now time to offer a working definition. For the purposes of this writing, ethics will be considered as a coherent and structured way of making moral choices related to the issues and practices of health care. This definition consists of three elements that reflect the basic questions to be raised in ethical reflection. The first question is: "What is the best choice in the situation?" This question recognizes that the clinician does not have the luxury to not decide (Jonsen 1991) and that the decisions may be about seeking good or about avoiding harm—related but sometimes very different goals. A "best" choice, or one of several acceptable choices, may be all that can be identified because there will likely not be a single, obvious choice in the specific situation. The second question is "Who decides?" In the Western world of the twenty-first century, it is presumed that the individual affected must decide, if necessary in an existential and solitary manner. However, the question quickly becomes complicated if the patient is unconscious or otherwise lacks decision-making capacity or if the patient and family come from a culture with differing values than the dominant rationalistic individualism characteristic of most American health care. Finally, this question arises: "How are decisions to be made?" The how and who questions together address the "coherent and structured" portion of our definition. There are multiple issues and multiple perspectives that must be considered if a good process is to be followed; likewise, poor ethical decisions are almost inevitable consequences of making snap ethical judgments without following sound methodology.

Ethics, Philosophy, and Spirit

When this author was recognized for contributions to health care ethics in Georgia, a colleague combined gentle teasing with congratulations when he commented that he was glad to know that the award went to an "ethical chaplain." His comment reflects the almost instinctive reaction of many that the field of ethics is about the behaviors and character of individuals. In reality, that perspective has a long and storied history in health care ethics. When in need of care from another, we want that other to be a person of good character. Arguably, the seminal document in the field is the venerable Hippocratic Oath, a statement of principles to guide the physician in his practices, probably dating from the fifth century BCE (Fletcher et al. 1997, 289). The famous injunction attributed to Hippocrates, "First do no harm," is not primarily for the purpose of weighing what actions might do direct or indirect harm, but is for the purpose of defining and declaring the character of the one making the decisions.

Though the term "paternalism" has taken on negative connotations in our time, prior to the twentieth century medicine was almost exclusively a paternalistic pursuit. The physician had the specialized knowledge and training, employed ideally for the greatest benefit to the patient, and the physician made the decisions. The current concerns with issues such as patients' rights and informed consent were simply not imagined in the nineteenth and early twentieth centuries. In this context of greatly disproportionate power between patient and physician, it was most important for the physician to be a person of trustworthy and ethical character. Over the years, various codes of ethics have served as means to describe and regulate the practices of physicians and to assure the patient of the physicians' faithfulness to the expected professional conduct.

When the American Medical Association met for the first time in 1847, one of the first items for consideration was establishing a code of ethics (Fletcher et al. 1997, 290). Even as paternalism has waned, revisions of that code still prominently set standards of ethical behavior for modern physicians. Moreover, as other professions have established themselves in modern health care, they, too, have offered codes of ethics. The Code for Nurses was adopted in 1950 and has been revised periodically since (Brody & Engelhardt 1987, 395). The American Association for Respiratory Care, the National Association of EMTs, and the Association of Professional Chaplains are other professional organizations of health care providers whose codes of ethics clearly set forth the expectations that those practitioners will be "ethical" in the very best sense when they offer care to one in need. In all these instances, a code of ethics may be understood in a very restricted sense as nothing more than describing behaviors. However, it is the contention of this author that the appeal to character is fundamentally an issue of spirit, for it is ultimately an appeal to the caregiver as a humane and caring person who brings specialized skills and training to that humanity held in common with the receiver of the care.

As important as are character-based ethics and their concomitant codes of ethics, there are other very powerful influences in modern health care that have necessarily expanded the accepted realm of ethics. The most dominant of those influences is the rise of technology. As health care decisions became more complex, it became apparent that being of good character was not sufficient in itself. With the rise of technological possibilities came both a great concern about increasing emotional distance between physician and patient and an ever-increasing number of dilemmas about availability and appropriate usage of these technologies. In the current environment of diagnoses by lab tests and radiology procedures, it seems amusing to recall that the stethoscope was resisted when it was first introduced in 1816 because of the distance it put between doctor and patient. Later, the Frankenstein story represented in fiction a fear of medical technology and its grandiosity (Jonsen 1991). Both early examples foreshadow even more dramatic changes!

It was during the 1950s and 1960s that the revolutionary advances in technology first dramatically impacted health care and the role that ethical reflection might play. The opening shot in the revolution was the iron lung, the precursor of the modern ventilator, developed during the polio epidemic of the '50s. A technology had become available that was clearly lifesaving for those for whom it could "buy time" for the body to recover respiratory function. For those who did not recover respiratory function, decisions loomed about whether to continue treatment. Distinctions between heroic and nonheroic measures of treatment, growing in large part from Roman Catholic moral theology of the time, were suggested. Then came the advent of kidney dialysis and the fact that far more people needed treatment than there were machines to treat them. Precursors of modern ethics committees were formed to make decisions about who would and would not have access to the lifesaving dialysis. The committees were known, likely with both derision and anxiety, as "God Squads" because they literally made life and death decisions. On the heels of these technologies and the issues they raised came the development of intensive care units (ICUs), CPR, brain death determinations, advance directives, numerous end-of-life concerns, and questions of equal access to care. Increasingly, ethical dilemmas and their resolution became the dominant meaning of ethics in the health care arena, and ethics of character was relegated to a role of secondary importance.

With the technological intrusions and the ethical dilemmas that resulted, the health care field increasingly looked to philosophical ethics to offer a framework to guide reflection and decision making. Rational categories and thought processes became the vehicles for health care ethics. Classical systems of thought and classical philosophers were consulted for guidance. Two broad categories of ethical thought have been frequent foundations for ethical reflection applied to specific situations. These categories, teleological theories (weighing burdens and benefits) and deontological theories (duty ethics), will be introduced at this point.

The term "teleological ethics" is derived from the Greek telos, or "end." This category of ethics looks to the outcome of actions as the determinant of good/bad, right/wrong. A popularized and overly simplified phrase of the 1960s referred to situational ethics (taking the term "situation ethics" from a book by that title, written by Joseph Fletcher). In the typical language currently used in medical ethics, the relevant questions for ethical reflection are about burdens and benefits of a particular choice. For example, it is common knowledge that chemotherapy and/or radiation therapy are treatments for cancer and that those treatments frequently have negative side effects. It is also common knowledge that the ability to predict how any single person will respond to any treatment or which side effects that person may experience is not at all precise. In deciding upon treatment plans, the physician is expected to describe both the possible good and bad that might come from the treatment so the patient can weigh these anticipated consequences in light of the patient's values. Benefits and burdens become a more pronounced ethical dilemma for a patient who cannot speak for himself (that is, someone who lacks decision-making capacity) and for whom the possible treatment options may be very unpleasant. It is from this kind of situation that concerns arise about quality of life. For example, a particular treatment may briefly prolong the life of a critically ill patient (benefit) but create much suffering (burden) as a consequence. Does the treatment "prolong life" (benefit) or merely "forestall death" (burden)? The evaluation of that balance is a question asked from the perspective of teleology.

Another dimension of teleological ethics may be consideration of the greatest good for the most people or the least harm to the fewest. From this perspective, a decision is considered ethical if good is maximized or bad minimized. For example, most would consider that good is maximized in amputation of a gangrenous limb in order to save a life. Experimental protocols for medications or treatments will recognize that some percentage of those involved in the experiment will probably experience some degree of harm—or, at the least, no help. However, the ethical reflection that reviews the protocol will seek ways to ensure an absolute minimal amount of harm. Allocation of resources issues surface in this context. At a policy level, are health care dollars better spent to ensure minimal levels of health care for all (universal inoculations for children, for example) or to ensure pediatric intensive care beds to "rescue" the sickest children from life-threatening circumstances? At an extreme, a kind of triage ethics can result, with drastic and arbitrary decisions to treat some and not others. Concerns about pandemic diseases or bioterrorism raise questions of quarantine—recognizing that some will be left to knowingly die in order to save as many others as possible. Whatever ethical reflection that accompanies thoughts of quarantine will seek maximum good and minimum bad. Finally, a particularly troublesome version of triage ethics is the indirect triage of economics that allows limited access to health care resources because of cost concerns (no insurance) or living conditions (rural patients with no transportation to a doctor or hospital).

Whether or not we favor the ethical balancing that is inherent in teleological ethical systems, it is important to recognize another very different approach to making ethical decisions. The term "deontological ethics" is derived from the Greek *deon*, or "duty." In simple terms, deontological systems are based on the premise that some things are "right" in and of themselves and some things are "wrong." It therefore becomes the duty of an ethical person to align with the right and to refuse to engage in the wrong. Whereas teleological thought seeks comparisons and the weighing of relative good versus relative evil, adherents of deontology take a firm stand in certitude and will likely be repelled by the relativity of teleology. It is easy to see that religious belief systems are often the foundation for deontological ethics. We can also draw an easy correlation between deontology and character-based ethical approaches and codes of ethics. The ethical code lays out right and wrong behavior, and the deontologist is duty-bound to follow.

Few health care practitioners will care to ponder long whether they think ethics should be defined as either teleological or deontological. In fact, many will think, "Who cares?" It is important, however, to be aware of the two systems because people make presumptions about situations; by definition, presumptions are not examined. Problems arise when people approach situations from very different perspectives. By way of illustration, it is the opinion of this author that a major and so far unbridgeable chasm in thought makes the abortion debate so intractable. A strong "pro-life" position argues from a deontological perspective—abortion is wrong. It is the duty of ethical people to refuse to participate in the procedure, and indeed, to make it impossible for others to participate in it because it is patently wrong. To argue benefits and burdens of fetal life and maternal choice is irrelevant at best and inflammatory at worst. And yet, it is exactly the valuing of choice and the asking of benefit and burden questions that characterize the strong "pro-choice" position. At this point, the reader is challenged to return to the quotation from Frederick Buechner with which the chapter begins and to read it as if pro-life and pro-choice were arguing in Buechner's mind. The two sides cannot reach agreement because they argue from different basic premises, which can only be convincing to someone who shares similar premises. To make clear ethical discourse even more problematic, without a determined effort to consistently appeal to the same ethical system, it is far too easy to change systems when the question is changed. Consider the pro-life proponent who opposes abortion and supports capital punishment while the pro-choice abortion activist opposes capital punishment "because it is wrong."

In the health care arena, issues of ethical theory and practice and ethical conflict play themselves out in the lives of patients, families, and the health care professionals who care for them. A physician, nurse, or therapist may believe herself insulated from the considerations suggested here. That practitioner may scoff at ethical methodology, yet she inevitably will encounter situations in which it is simply not obvious what course of action is right or wrong. The dilemmas are fostered and complicated by technology and by forces completely outside the control of the health care professional. A practitioner who is most comfortable operating from (a probably unspoken and/or unrecognized) deontological style will encounter a dementia patient in an ICU and have to make some choice about whether a treatment option will do more good than harm. Another practitioner will experience great frustration in the apparent lack of some colleague's ability to operate except out of expediency, as if truly nothing were ever right or wrong. Difficult decisions will have to be made because the clinician does not have the luxury to not decide when a patient's well-being is at stake. Therefore, we need a method of ethical reflection that evolved to help consider the complex issues of modern medicine and to seek a consensus of opinion from professionals of differing viewpoints and personal beliefs. In the experience of this author, the discipline sometimes known as clinical ethics is the one most frequently practiced "in the trenches" of decision making for and with health care professionals.

Precedent-Setting Cases

Clinical ethics looks to cases, as surely as does medicine itself, in order to understand ethical quandaries. Cases are the juncture of real life with the theory and dispassionate reasoning of the philosopher. Cases are about people, so clinical ethics must review, learn from, and occasionally resolve cases. A relative handful of high-profile cases have largely defined the issues that most dramatically and most often are involved in the need to resolve some ethical dilemma. (Note: The choice of these particular cases reflects the Health Care Ethics Consortium of Georgia's "Report of the Task Force on Futility.")

Karen Ann Quinlan

Karen Ann Quinlan was a twenty-one-year-old woman living in New Jersey in 1975. She was hospitalized after an alcohol/drug overdose. Due to anoxic brain injury, Ms. Quinlan was nonresponsive, and remained so even though her hospitalization ran the technological gamut from an admission through the Emergency Room to intensive care treatment that ultimately included mechanical ventilation and a feeding tube. After several months, her family requested that the ventilator be removed in the hope that Ms. Quinlan would "die with dignity," as the phrase later came into increasing usage. However, the standards of practice at the time did not easily allow for this decision to be made. The physicians involved and the hospital agreed that it was not appropriate to remove this life-sustaining treatment from Ms. Quinlan and allow her to die. They considered it tantamount to killing her, and thus completely unacceptable morally and legally. Initially, lower courts agreed, and it was only a ruling by the New Jersey Supreme Court that allowed the ventilator to be turned off (Fletcher et al. 1997, 159). She was weaned from the ventilator with the expectation that she would die when the ventilator was finally removed. However, she did not die; she actually lived another ten years in a nursing home.

Quinlan is important for two reasons: First of all Ms. Quinlan's is the first high-profile media "case." Newspapers, radio, and television were eager to cover this tragic yet controversial human interest story. Second, the Quinlan case gave great impetus to the developing movement that would become known publicly by terms such as "right to die" and "death with dignity." The key issue from Quinlan that powerfully impacts future ethical reflection is this "right to die." It was the health care establishment that insisted on continued aggressive treatment with the ventilator and the family who battled to allow the death they considered as the natural and compassionate choice in the situation. With the final decision to remove the ventilator, a line was crossed in ethical consideration and a new standard of practice was considered acceptable ethically and legally. It has been the personal experience of this author as a hospital chaplain that from the time of Quinlan, decisions to remove ventilators are not casual but neither are they resisted and feared as "wrong" beyond question by the health care team. Ms. Quinlan's suffering and her family's persistence were largely responsible for ushering us to this point in our practice. The turmoil around Ms. Quinlan served as an impetus to the advent of biomedical ethics committees as referred to periodically in this chapter. Those committees typically include physicians, nurses, and non-clinical professionals such as chaplains, social workers, lawyers, and/or community representatives. The ethics committee co-chaired by this author for many years adopted such a structure and adopted goals suggested by the Health Care Ethics Consortium of Georgia to include: 1) education, 2) policy review, and 3) case consultation (Kinlaw 1996).

Before moving to the next precedent-setting case, it is instructive to identify some of the cross-currents of change and influence that rapidly and increasingly became entangled in the development of clinical ethical considerations. The issues of rights had taken a very powerful place in the mind of the American public with the social upheaval of the 1960s. Beginning at that time, rights concerns came into the culture's vocabulary and the practice of medicine in a powerful new way—hence the connection of Quinlan with right to die and the elevated right to privacy that was identified by the New Jersey Supreme Court in their ruling on Quinlan (Fletcher et al. 1997, 159). Correspondingly, patients' rights were being elevated while the paternalism practiced by physicians was being increasingly challenged. Paternalism was closely aligned with long traditions of medicine, as earlier identified, that viewed the physician as the authority to whom the patient deferred with little question. Elisabeth Kübler-Ross's classic *On Death and Dying* was published in 1969. Among its tenets was an indirect challenge to paternalism because she believed that dying patients should be given information and a decision-making role in their treatment. This was in stark contrast to the silence and evasion that was more standard practice among paternalistic physicians. Finally, this was a time in which living wills first appeared on the scene, as a way to address issues around the prolonged maintenance of a patient on life support when the patient was considered "terminal." It is the contention of this author that Quinlan was both a result of these issues and an impetus to bring them even more prominently into public attention. Health care professionals were increasingly practicing in an environment where these issues would need more and wiser attention.

Another excursus is warranted here against the backdrop of the increasingly public nature of ethical dilemmas in health care. The role of the news media in granting widespread attention to these issues raises concerns about a number of issues that are in themselves ethical in nature. First are issues of privacy. When the Quinlan case moved into the courts, it was no longer a matter of privacy among patient, family, and physician. In short order, anyone in the world with minimal interest knew all about the very personal issues surrounding the Quinlans and their caregivers. As can readily be seen from Quinlan up to the more recent Schiavo case, the intrusiveness of media is devastating to the privacy and dignity of the vulnerable, and opens attempts to regain that lost privacy to charges of secrecy and evasion. The "Inquiring minds want to know" mentality is elevated to an unquestioned right to turn private tragedy into public spectacle. Also, the involvement of lawyers and judges transfers these decisions to an arena of potential punishment for wrongdoing that raises the stakes for all concerned. Whatever caution has been displayed is heightened in the litigious environment of modern health care. Decision makers are afraid of being sued, and maintaining the status quo is less likely to incite the feared legal action. Therefore, when a situation becomes controversial or highly publicized, honest values of the parties and disagreements about the most appropriate course of treatment are increasingly difficult to separate from a mode of "Don't make waves." Finally, media involvement inevitably oversimplifies issues and degrades language. Sound bites do not adequately capture sound ethical reasoning nor agonizing personal decisions. In popular culture, terms like brain death, terminal illness, vegetable, euthanasia, and living will are all bandied about, but rarely with clarity or clinical precision. Even health care professionals too often misunderstand and/or misuse these and similar terms, though it is especially incumbent on those professionals to be clear and precise in their understanding and usage of terms and concepts in ethical reflection.

Nancy Cruzan

In 1983, at the age of twenty-five, Nancy Cruzan was involved in a serious traffic accident. The Missouri woman "survived" the accident but was nonresponsive even after prolonged intensive treatment. There were definite similarities with Karen Ann Quinlan's situation. Ms. Cruzan also had an anoxic brain injury. She also was initially on a ventilator and in intensive care. However, at some relatively early point in her prolonged treatment odyssey, she was diagnosed as being in a persistent vegetative state. Whereas the removal of the ventilator was the crux of the decision making for Ms. Quinlan, it was not so for Ms. Cruzan, largely because the issue had been addressed in the Quinlan case. After the initial intensive treatment, Ms. Cruzan was able to breathe on her own without ventilator assistance. However, she could not eat and after twenty-five days of hospitalization she was given a gastrostomy tube for artificial nutrition. She was transferred to a rehab center after nine months in the hospital. After some four years, her parents asked to have the feeding tube removed, stating that "Nancy did not want to live this way." A long odyssey of hearings in various courts ensued, ultimately ending in a 1990 ruling by the U.S. Supreme Court (the only major case involving biomedical decision making to be actually heard by the Supreme Court). The High Court ruling set two major guidelines in cases like these:

1. A competent person can refuse any life-sustaining treatment, including artificial nutrition and hydration. By implication, this allows for an understanding that artificial nutrition and hydration are medical treatments that are no more or less "artificial" than a ventilator or any other medical intervention that is not effective or not desired by the patient (or the patient's surrogate).
2. States can require "clear and convincing evidence about the person's expressed decision while competent" and individual states can determine those standards.

After another six months of controversy following the Supreme Court decision, Ms. Cruzan's feeding tube was removed in December 1990 and she died thirteen days later (Fletcher et al. 1997, 165–67). Once again, the news media were very eager to keep the story in the public eye. Included in the public controversy was a major role played by "right to life" protestors who considered the decision to remove the feeding tube a cruel form of "starving [Ms. Cruzan] to death." Right-to-life groups asked for injunctions, picketed, and a protestor even allegedly broke into Ms. Cruzan's room and tried to offer her a drink of water. (In a great irony, had he been successful, the likelihood of her aspirating that drink was very high, an understanding lost on the protestor.)

The significance of Cruzan for the evolution of health care ethics is threefold. First, and arguably most important, is the issue of artificial nutrition and hydration. Though the strong emotional attachment to food and water as basic human care persists, the Cruzan decision specifies that artificial nutrition and hydration are not in a sacrosanct category of medical treatments that must be carried out no matter what. They, too, can be forgone. Despite "common sense" understanding on the part of many inside and outside the health care profession that it is unconscionable to "starve someone to death," Cruzan offers powerful legal and ethical grounds that a choice to forgo is acceptable. (The reader is also encouraged to seek hospice and other end-of-life literature evaluating the actual experiences that accompany choices for and against artificial nutrition and hydration.) The second significant consequence of Cruzan is the expanded availability and encouraged usage of advance directives to clarify patient preferences (meeting the "clear and convincing evidence" requirement of the High Court). The Patient Self Determination Act of 1992, requiring health care facilities to aggressively develop policies about advance directives, was passed in large part to address the controversies aroused by Cruzan. The third consequence is the ever-growing intrusion and influence of the public into the formerly private realm of health care decision making. The media coverage and intrusiveness was arguably much greater in Cruzan than in Quinlan. Correspondingly, the right to life movement showed dramatically increasing strength, involvement, and media savvy in addressing their concerns about end-of-life issues.

Helga Wanglie

Helga Wanglie was an eighty-six-year-old Minnesota resident. In 1991 it was determined that she was in a persistent vegetative state and suffering from multiple medical problems. Her family, based on their religious beliefs, insisted that the patient be kept alive by any and all medical means. On the other hand, her physicians believed that she would not benefit from aggressive treatment and that such treatment should be considered futile. Furthermore, the physicians did not believe that Mr. Wanglie, her husband, really understood the medical facts nor that he had his wife's "best interest" at heart. When physicians and Mr. Wanglie could not agree, the hospital in question requested a court-appointed independent conservator to make decisions instead of Mr. Wanglie. That request was denied by the court, and Mr. Wanglie was affirmed as the appropriate decision maker for his wife. Mrs. Wanglie ultimately died several months later, still on the ventilator (Fletcher et al. 1997, 161).

The key issue in the Wanglie case is the emergence of disagreements about medical futility, or the more benign term for futility, medically inappropriate treatment. With futility issues, the dilemmas made possible by technology reach a kind of paradoxical climax. Whereas in the Quinlan and Cruzan cases, family members were challenging the medical establishment to cease aggressive treatment, roles have now been reversed. In the Wanglie case, it is now physicians and the hospital, and no doubt nursing staff, who are asking to call a halt to treatment and the family who are fighting to maintain it. Some would see that the "rights" issues and the autonomy issues of the patient and family (more on autonomy later) have now swung so far into dominance that other valid considerations are hopelessly muted.

In medical futility concerns, the question for physicians and health care professionals becomes "Do we have to do any treatment the patient or family demands, no matter how little the likelihood of success?" CPR and emergency resuscitation are violent procedures. Staff who must perform CPR, especially on frail patients, know that they may well break ribs when they do chest compressions. Statistically, patients who are resuscitated rarely recover sufficiently to leave the hospital. When a patient does survive a code, she may lose so much physical and/or mental capacity as to never regain consciousness. If she does regain consciousness, what level of physical, emotional, and spiritual pain must she endure? If the patient indeed survives and becomes the long-term recipient of intensive care treatment and cascading treatment modes, the financial burden may become staggering—for the family and for the hospital. Allocation of resource issues may surface if too many ICU beds are occupied by a "futility" patient and are not available for trauma victims or others who have a much greater likelihood of a good response to treatment. With all this in mind, it is small wonder that physicians and staff may find themselves in a situation of moral distress where they must act against their own principles (Dixson 2006). Staff frequently will describe such a situation of moral distress as having to "torture the patient." In part to relieve their own feelings and in part to truly seek understanding, physicians and staff also frequently make the same queries that were made of Mr. Wanglie. Does the family really understand? (Very frequently they do not, but emotional issues are powerful in superseding rational understanding.) Does the family have the best interest of the patient at heart? (Again, strong emotional components come into play as well as values issues about the nature and sanctity of life.)

Baby K

Baby K, an infant born in Virginia in October 1992, brings another aspect to reflections on futility. Before birth, Baby K was diagnosed as having anencephaly, a congenital malformation of the brain that results in a lack of any brain tissue except the brain stem. "The infant is permanently unconscious and presumably cannot experience pain" (Fletcher et al. 1997, 174). Though there was no expectation that Baby K could survive, his mother refused to have an abortion and requested maximal treatment. Her reasons were based on her religious beliefs about the value of all human life and her belief that God could work a miracle if it were God's will. Presumably, the fact that her nine-year-old daughter had died in the same hospital only one year before that from injuries sustained in an automobile accident had some emotional bearing on the mother's decisions. The fact that the baby's father did not agree with the mother's decisions carried no decision-making weight.

After birth, ventilator support was required, and the use of the ventilator became the crux of the dispute over subsequent months. Physicians considered use of the ventilator futile; the mother considered it basic care. Various efforts were made, including an ethics consultation, to resolve the dispute between the mother's wish for maximal treatment and the medical interpretation that aggressive treatment was futile. In July 1993, a federal judge ruled that the hospital must provide full medical care, including use of the ventilator, basing his decision on interpretation of EMTALA (Emergency Medical Treatment and Active Labor Act) and ADA (Americans with Disabilities Act) laws. Legal disputes continued in various venues and Baby K shuffled from nursing home to hospital as her medical condition waxed and waned. She finally died in April 1995 in spite of attempted resuscitation (Fletcher et al. 1997, 175).

The key issues in the Baby K case seem to confound resolution. From the perspective of the health care professionals involved, aggressive treatment of anencephaly is, by definition, futile. Yet, the court interpretations seem to be inconsistent with the trend toward recognizing a "right to die." The medical interpretation that aggressive treatment for Baby K was futile and prolonged the baby's suffering was not given legal standing. Instead, the court found other legal interpretations more compelling. The court referred to EMTALA laws, and raised questions about what emergency treatments should be available to patients who are "terminal" (Fletcher et al. 1997, 174). Also, though EMTALA laws seem to hold sway, the introduction of questions about disability and application of the ADA to Baby K's situation opened the door for disabilities activists to voice concerns. In simple terms, the inclusion of disability concerns adds another element of debate about the value of life and about the claim that "death with dignity" may be camouflage for a belief that certain lives "are not worth living" because they are so lacking in "quality."

Terri Schiavo

The case of Terri Schiavo is perhaps the most high-profile and publicly disputed case yet involving issues of health care ethics. Terri Schiavo was twenty-six in February 1990 when she collapsed at home. She died in March 2004 after years of intensive treatment, long-term supportive treatment, and finally the highly disputed cessation of treatment. Her case was marked profoundly by family disagreement and dissolution. In the early years of treatment, her parents and her husband seemed to have a very good relationship and to agree on the direction of Mrs. Schiavo's treatment. In later years, their bitter estrangement led to legal and ethical disputes that gained worldwide attention. At issue was whether or not Mrs.

Schiavo was in a persistent vegetative state and would never recover or if she were severely disabled but cognizant and possessing some potential for rehabilitation. When her husband accepted the diagnosis of persistent vegetative state and asked that her feeding tube be removed to allow her death, her parents vehemently disagreed and sought custody of Mrs. Schiavo. Ultimately, the feeding tube was removed and she died.

The key issues in the Schiavo case are minimally issues of health care ethics, as narrowly defined, but primarily about the environment in which ethical decisions are made. Previous decisions were not applied when they well could have been. The questions about removing a feeding tube seem to be very closely allied with the issues from Cruzan years before. Did the resolution of Cruzan have no relevance to Schiavo? The commonsense position that "a person should not be starved" was powerful at the time of Cruzan and is no less so now. The emotional connection to food and water as the most basic of human caring responses are not easily overcome by counterarguments from medical and ethics professionals who may be easily cast as uncaring or unscrupulous. Did the parties involved consider and/or invoke Cruzan in a significant way in their reflections? And yet, had they done so, what impact would be given when there was dispute about whether, indeed, Schiavo was in a persistent vegetative state? Certainly, supporters of Schiavo's parents raised disability issues—Mrs. Schiavo was disabled and deserved treatment—reminiscent of Baby K. Also missing, at least to general public knowledge, was the decision in Wanglie that affirmed the patient's spouse as the legitimate decision maker, even if disputants think the spouse does not have the patient's best interest at heart. While the arguments based on the value of human life to aggressively support Mrs. Schiavo seem very similar to arguments for aggressive support of Baby K, this more socially conservative perspective was not consistent with other social conservative values because it also disputed the role of the spouse as the appropriate surrogate decision maker.

It was the blatant politicizing of ethical reflection that is the most significant issue in Schiavo. Health care professionals know that agonizing treatment decisions are made daily in institutions throughout the country. Ethical disputes have typically been resolved as much as possible privately in a collaboration between the patient, the physician, and the patient's immediate family. On occasion, other parties—chaplains, patient representatives, social workers, mediators, or ethics committees—become involved to try to resolve conflicts. Typically, respect for patient dignity and privacy have been powerful forces in keeping disputes from becoming publicized and politicized. Complex information and personal interactions are more appropriate to conversation and relationship than to posturing and position statements by those less involved or less well informed. Schiavo, instead, became a public and political battleground. Politicians from Florida to the U.S. Senate majority leader made public statements and took public positions. Courts reviewed and appealed and appealed appeals. The pope made a statement in favor of prolonging Mrs. Schiavo's life, a statement that seems to this writer to be at variance with previous Roman Catholic understandings on end-of-life treatment issues. Mrs. Schiavo's personal privacy and dignity were cast aside by those who broadcast videos of her profoundly disabled and wasted body. Family disagreements became grist for talk shows and strangers to choose sides. Health care professionals and Mrs. Schiavo's hospice bore the brunt of vicious accusations that they were heartless and cruel. The presumed sanctity of marriage and the unquestioned expectation that a spouse is the best surrogate decision maker was challenged repeatedly by Mrs. Schiavo's parents and their supporters. Through it all, Terri Schiavo became more and more a pawn in a power struggle among those who claimed to care about her.

In reviewing these precedent-setting cases, we must acknowledge that the effort to maintain privacy has consequences as well. Perhaps the degree to which the Schiavo issues were publicly distressing is as much a reflection on the ubiquitous nature of media and politicized power groups as on the issues themselves. The fact is that each case presented here became quite public and distressing. People who are unfamiliar with the kinds of ethically demanding decisions that result in high-tech medical situations must consider at some level how they might respond for themselves or a loved one, and those reflections are extremely uncomfortable. Activists of all stripes aside, people of good conscience have differing and often strongly held opinions about the kinds of issues highlighted in these precedent-setting cases. In the same way, people of strong religious or moral conviction will come to different conclusions about how their beliefs should apply to the complexities of treatment decisions in an environment overwhelmed by specialists and specialized knowledge. Even for the activists, there will be soul searching and differing approaches on the degree to which public opinion or political intervention should be brought to bear in perceived defense of the weak or in a challenge to powerful individuals or groups. It is, in part, for these reasons that we previously considered ethical theories. Without some consistent theoretical framework, acknowledged or not, ethical reflection is little more than a matter of personal preference or even prejudice. One may advocate for a position in one situation based on a "right/wrong" argument, only to completely switch reasoning on another issue by adopting a "benefit/burden" argument. It is also in recognition of the distress inherent in this kind of reflection, that it is now time to move to considering a methodology for dealing with complex ethical issues. Though the methodology cannot remove the challenges, it will offer a framework for weighing multiple factors. In the experience of those in ethics committees who have used this or a similar methodology, this framework also offers the very real possibility for people of good conscience to arrive at consensus-based decisions, even if they use differing avenues in their reflection and in arriving at the final decision itself.

A Methodology for Ethical Decision Making

Two things should be very clear by this point. First of all, the circumstances and consequent decisions that may be encountered by health care professionals and those they care for clearly do not lend themselves to simplistic or predetermined responses. Second, the ethical systems and understandings that have evolved to address these issues do not speak with a unified voice. Ethical systems have different starting points and different values by which they make judgments. These systems have changed over time and are strongly influenced by societal values that have also changed. How, then, are we to find a way through the maze to the necessary task of making decisions?

Dr. Al Jonsen defines the term "clinical ethics" as a "practical discipline that provides a structured approach to assist physicians in identifying, analyzing, and resolving ethical issues in clinical medicine" (Jonsen et al. 1998, 1). During the first day of the Fourth Annual Summer Seminar in Health Care Ethics (1991), Dr. Jonsen explained that an academic ethicist may well have the luxury of extended reflection on a thorny problem and may indefinitely delay making a clear decision. A health care professional, on the other hand, does not have the luxury to not decide—a patient's well-being awaits her decision. To illustrate, he displayed a sculpture of a hot air balloon and a bicycle. The perspective from the balloon is broad, quiet, and comprehensive, but distant from the ground. Ethical theory operates well from the balloon. The bicycle is in touch with every bump of the road. It is close to the action; it not only can but must see and respond to details in its course. The bicycle is the practical reality of clinical practice and clinical issues. A person may see a potential crash from the balloon that the bicyclist cannot anticipate; hence the need for theory and reflection. On the other hand, the bicyclist alone can know the precise responses needed to negotiate each immediate section of the road, and the cyclist is the one who bears the consequences of a bad judgment along the way. In seeking to combine the best of both theory and practical experiences, clinical ethics will be the framework from which this chapter will proceed to suggest a viable way to make wise and compassionate ethical decisions.

The methodology of clinical ethics is grounded in the classic work by Beauchamp and Childress (1983), *Principles of Biomedical Ethics*. Even the most cursory consideration must note the significance of this work by a philosopher and an ethicist working together at Georgetown University. As stated in the Preface to the second edition, their goal is to offer "a systematic analysis of the moral principles that should apply to biomedicine" (ix). After two chapters on ethical and moral theories, the bulk of the book focuses on four major ethical principles: beneficence, autonomy, nonmaleficence, and justice. For Beauchamp, Childress, and their myriad followers, these principles may be applied in dynamic interplay around specific situations. They also deal with philosophical concepts about how "rules" may be required for a moral life to guide and interpret the proper interplay of the principles (43ff.) and about the roles of ideals and virtues (255ff.). However, they are best known for the four principles. There has even been a respectfully teasing reference used by many health care ethicists that adhering to the four principles in ethical decision making is following the "Georgetown Mantra."

Beneficence

Beneficence is the principle of actively seeking to do good for another. For many health care professionals, a major source of meaning and spiritual fulfillment in their work derives from the desire to help people. Patients and their families are seeking someone to help them, so the confluence of need and desire to help in health care settings is obvious. The virtue-based ethics from various codes of ethics are heavily concerned with defining the ways to do good and avoid harm in the helping professions. The concept of physician paternalism was referred to earlier, the notion that the physician knew what was best for the patient and could be trusted without question. Though not popular in contemporary individualistic, Western cultures, paternalism's roots are in the very positive soil of beneficence. The specialized knowledge that health care professionals, especially physicians, offer is foundational in identifying appropriate treatment goals and means. With the sheer amount of knowledge to be applied to the task and the interplay of complex variables to be considered, it is hard to imagine ways in which the patient would not be heavily dependent on a beneficent cadre of health care professionals eager to offer expert help.

Autonomy

Autonomy refers to the patient as the decision maker. This principle recognizes that it is the patient who must bear the consequences of any decisions made about his treatment, so it is the patient who should have the final decision about his course of treatment. The idea of "informed consent"—the patient must know as clearly as possible all important relevant information so he can weigh all possible consequences and personal values before agreeing to a procedure or medication—is based on the principle of autonomy. Issues of decision-making competence (actually a legal determination rather than an ethical one) and decision-making capacity are grounded in a valuing of autonomy and a commitment to ensure that autonomy is not violated. Autonomy can be extended beyond the patient's consciousness or cognitive impairment through completion of some form of advance directive to state treatment preferences or to name a surrogate decision maker.

The individualism of Western cultures places great value on autonomy (non-Western cultures often do not share this vision of the patient-provider relationship, leading to potential conflict in some cross-cultural situations). In fact, it is argued that the rise of medical futility issues (see Precedent-Setting Cases, earlier in this chapter) shows that the pendulum has swung so far in favor of autonomy and individualism that autonomy is too often an unquestionable "trump card." With a powerful admixture of "rights" language, especially in the social foments of the 1960s, autonomy has taken almost unquestioned precedence over other ethical principles. Add the contemporary situation of limitless information from the Internet and pervasive advertising by pharmaceutical companies, and health care professionals often believe that their expertise is too easily dismissed in favor of the patient's rights. Therefore, we might well ask whether, in the current context, the patient is served or harmed by the degree of autonomy presumed in our culture.

Nonmaleficence

Nonmaleficence refers to the time-honored medical dictum to "first do no harm." Whereas beneficence seeks positive good, nonmaleficence requires the avoidance of intended or unintended hurtfulness. We might recall incidents where a drug, perhaps effective for the purpose for which it was prescribed, caused significant harm in some other way. Thalidomide in the 1960s, prescribed for morning sickness and other pregnancy-related illness, caused severe birth defects. Popular drugs for the treatment of arthritis in the early 2000s were withdrawn when evidence surfaced that they greatly increased cardiovascular risks. Certainly, at first blush, these medication fiascoes exemplify the principle of nonmaleficence not being honored. In the context of ethical reflection, the principle is often applied to questions surrounding aggressive and/or unproven treatment modalities with known or potential negative side effects. *Quality of life* may become a shorthand term to address concerns about side effects of treatment. Examples that are commonly raised in professional and nonprofessional realms are chemotherapy and radiation for cancer. It is well known that side effects of both can be devastating, so people consider "Is it worth it?" or "Will I live longer but be miserable?" Whether identified as such, these are questions of quality of life, based on the concern about avoiding harm. The person who must consider treatment options for herself will have the recourse to autonomy in weighing benefits and burdens of the treatment. Professionals who prescribe or provide treatments with strong side effects must consider that their advice may weigh very strongly indeed with the patient. When a patient is incapacitated in some way, the weight of the decision for the professional dramatically heightens the need to adequately consider the principle of nonmaleficence.

A strong disclaimer must be made about quality of life considerations. Many readers have commented in the face of some suffering or disability, "I would not want to live like that. . . ." The relatively healthy may too easily consider a disability of some kind to be more undermining of quality of life than does the person with that disability. Striving, successful, active people may think life would not be worth living if they could not maintain the levels of achievement to which they are accustomed. An accident, illness, or infirmity may require drastic adjustment in lifestyle, but many such victims go on to lead very meaningful lives. Advocates for disabled people are quick to warn against the devaluing of lives once we invoke a simplistic mantra about "poor quality of life." Therefore, as a principle, nonmaleficence must be considered carefully. Cautious scrutiny is necessary to ensure that factors like circumstances, prognosis, and individual values are considered when quality of life concerns are invoked.

Justice

Justice is the principle of treating everyone the same. Jonsen and his colleagues (1998) link the principle of justice to a broader set of issues they call "contextual issues" (see Table 12–1). Status, wealth, race, gender, or any other social criteria should, if justice is considered, have no determining effect on how a patient is treated. In the egalitarian political system of American life, it seems obvious that equality of access to treatment and quality of that treatment would be the norm. In the earliest days of ethics committees, so-called "God Squads" were created to determine who would receive kidney dialysis when there was far greater need than there was capacity for treatment. To the extent that preference for treatment was granted to those with "more to offer" society, a backlash developed that demanded a more "just" approach. It became increasingly unacceptable

Table 12–1

Medical Indications	Patient Preferences
1. What is the patient's medical problem? history? diagnosis? prognosis?	1. What preferences has the patient expressed about treatment?
2. Is the problem acute? chronic? critical? emergent? reversible?	2. Has the patient been informed about benefits and risks? Does he understand them, and has he given consent?
3. What are the goals of treatment?	3. Is the patient mentally capable and legally competent? What is the evidence of incapacity?
4. What are the probabilities of success?	4. Has the patient expressed prior preferences, e.g., advance directives?
5. What are plans in case of therapeutic failure?	5. If he is incapacitated, who is the patient's appropriate surrogate? Is the surrogate following appropriate standards?
6. In sum, how can this patient benefit from medical and nursing care, and how can harm be avoided?	6. Is the patient unwilling or unable to cooperate with medical treatment? If so, why?
	7. In sum, is the patient's right to choose being respected to the greatest possible extent in ethics and law?

Quality of Life	Contextual Features
1. What are the prospects, with or without treatment, for a return to the patient's normal life?	1. Are there family issues that might influence treatment decisions?
2. Are there biases that might prejudice the provider's evaluation of the patient's quality of life?	2. Are there provider issues (that is, issues confronting physicians and nurses) that might influence treatment decisions?
3. What physical, mental, and social deficits is the patient likely to experience if treatment succeeds?	3. Are there financial or economic considerations?
4. Is the patient's present or future condition so dire that continued life might be judged undesirable by her?	4. Are there religious or cultural considerations?
5. Is there any plan or rationale to forgo treatment?	5. Is there any justification to breach confidentiality?
6. What plans for comfort and palliative care are there?	6. Are there problems of allocation of resources?
	7. What are the legal implications of treatment decisions?
	8. Is clinical research or teaching involved?
	9. Is there any provider or institutional conflict of interest?

to presume, for example, that a white male businessman was more "valuable to society" and thus automatically granted priority access to lifesaving treatment than was a poor Native American woman. More recently, liver transplant priorities that considered alcoholics as automatically ineligible for transplant have been challenged and largely rejected as unjust.

Less obvious justice issues surface in health care ethics when issues of economics are introduced. Access to care for those with insufficient insurance or personal finances and allocation of resources for institutions with limited funds are both issues that fall into the realm of the justice principle. It is not treating everyone equally to have a system that may deny a treatment based on the patient's ability or inability to pay; yet at some point absurdity and bankruptcy loom in the attempt to provide every possible treatment option to everyone. Hospitals may be put in great financial jeopardy if they have too large a percentage of patients who cannot pay or if they must maintain too many critical care beds filled with long-term patients who cannot be transferred to nursing homes or other facilities. At the level of individual patient and family, justice issues may take the form of the heart-wrenching decisions that expensive treatment for one family member may deprive other family members of any number of economic opportunities in the present or future. Justice, then, is a noble and important principle, but a very complex one when applied to the realities of health care decision making and health care ethics. As with other principles, it must be considered in dynamic interplay rather than as a static rule.

In a health care facility, a situation in which the best decision possible is not clear may result in an ethics consult being requested. The specifics of how such a consult might be done and who might do it vary from facility to facility. However, a fictional consult situation is a good way to consider exactly how the previous information about ethical principles and method might be applied. Consider a set of circumstances that is not uncommon:

> An elderly dementia patient is admitted to a hospital from a nursing home. The patient has shown progressive loss of appetite and weight loss over the past three weeks. He has a temperature of 101.5 (38.6°C) and a nonproductive cough. Decisions must be made about aggressiveness of treatment. What ethical issues are significant?

In considering Beneficence, what *good* might be done medically for this patient?

1. Would a ventilator for respiratory support be appropriate?
2. Would a feeding tube for nutrition be appropriate?
3. Would surgery for a life-threatening condition be appropriate?
4. Would IV antibiotics be appropriate?

In considering Autonomy, what are the *patient's wishes?*

1. Does the patient have the mental capacity to make informed decisions?
2. Is there an advance directive?
3. Are there immediate family members to make decisions?
4. What considerations (substituted judgment about patient's wishes versus "best interests" of the patient) are important if someone must make decisions for the patient?

In considering Nonmaleficence, what *harm* might be avoided?

1. Quality of life issues may be considered: Whose values will decide what constitutes "quality of life" for this patient?
2. How will benefits and burdens of treatment be weighed?
3. What degree (if any) of physical or mental deficit will be considered as an unacceptable quality of life?
4. Should comfort care and/or Do Not Resuscitate orders be instituted?
5. If a feeding tube is not inserted, or if a tube in place is considered for removal at some future time, does this constitute "starving the patient to death"?
6. On the other hand, will aggressive treatment only prolong the natural progression of his body toward death while introducing discomfort and likely medical complications?

In considering Justice and contextual issues, what is *fair and just* for all parties?

1. What family issues (economic stress, interpersonal conflict) impact on the treatment decisions?
2. Are there religious or cultural issues that affect treatment decisions?

3. Are there issues that relate to keeping or breaking of confidentiality?

4. Are there allocation of resources issues (scarce ICU beds, indigent status of the patient, consideration of transplantation of scarce organs)?

5. Are there legal issues (no legal decision-maker, patient a ward of the state)

6. Are there issues of conflict of interest among family members (does a next-of-kin have a potential motive to halt care—say, for financial gain—if the patient dies)?

For either an ethics committee or an individual ethics consultant, these are the kinds of reflections that must be made in completing an ethics consult. Table 12–1, called the "Four Boxes" by many proponents, offers a summary guide for an ethics consult following the methods and procedures outlined here. Though at one level, the attempt to apply ethical principles may be seen as a merely cerebral exercise, it is in reality an effort to become highly attuned to values of patients and of those directly involved in relationship to that patient. In this attention to values and relationships, ethical decision making and spirituality intersect.

Current and Future Issues

Because the health care ethics perspective presented here has developed in large part over the past fifty years, let us consider the kinds of issues that are most currently pressing and those that present particular challenges for the immediate future. As with other sections, the goal is to be suggestive only because whole volumes could be written on any of these issues. Furthermore, predicting the future is a notoriously unreliable exercise. However, it is the opinion of this author that much of the focus for health care ethics will be on the following:

1. End-of-life issues.
2. Costs, access, and effectiveness of health care.
3. Genetics applications.
4. A clash of competing perspectives.

End-of-Life Issues

End-of-life issues continue to be the focus of a great number of ethics consults and of ethics considerations. That is largely because of the obvious fact that they are so final. The prevailing sentiment is to err, if at all, on the side of life because life, once gone, cannot be recalled. The routine experience of making critical decisions related to life and death is a familiar occurrence in the lives of physicians, nurses, and other clinicians. By contrast, those kinds of experiences are very unfamiliar to the patients and families who are receiving care. When a physician treating a critically ill patient suggests that the patient should be offered "comfort care" and should not be resuscitated, it is from a base of both knowledge and experience that she does so. The physician has likely seen similar patients in similar situations numerous times. She sees little "good that can be done," significant "harm to avoid," and the likelihood of impending death. It is, however, likely the first time the patient and family have ever been in such a situation. Furthermore, it is a loved one for whom the family must consider the decision. They may well see the physician "giving up," "lacking faith," or "hastening death." The prospect of death for their loved one is foreign, frightening, and sad. There is a virtual chasm of different perspectives to be bridged for this hypothetical end-of-life decision to be made. It is not terribly difficult to understand that the family may grasp for "any chance" and desire/demand aggressive treatment in the hope of saving their loved one. It is also not terribly difficult to understand that clinicians and those concerned about the costs of care focus in the same situation on the inappropriateness of aggressive treatment and the "futility" of the situation. Consider further any of several educational or cultural divides—language barriers, different cultural expectations, lack of comprehension of basic anatomy and body function—and the opportunities balloon for conflict around making the decision.

Finally, changing patterns of physician/patient relationship impact the ways ethical decisions may be confronted. Increasingly, patients sick enough to be hospitalized are likely to receive their care from one or more physicians who are strangers to them—the patient's primary care physician likely will be only an outpatient practitioner. The care within the hospital may be excellent in technical application but splintered among specialists focused on organs and organ systems rather than on the whole person.

Patient and family values may be unrecognized or discounted; communication may be limited or fragmented. Yet life and death decisions will loom. Given the noted concerns, it is clear that end-of-life decisions will remain of immediate concern for ethical consideration. Because the issues grow increasingly complex, it seems likely that the resolution of end-of-life decisions will only grow more difficult in the future.

Costs of and Access to Treatment

Costs of treatment and access to that treatment come together to raise especially thorny issues around the principle of justice. In simple terms, can we claim that the principle of justice is honored when the cost of health care so frequently overwhelms families with bills or when limited income means that prescribed medications are forgone because of their expense? What will we accept as limits in considering the costs of care? Arguably, high-cost treatments at an early stage of illness may be less expensive than even more costly ones needed later on if treatment is neglected. For example, long-term medical treatment for hypertension is almost always less expensive to patient and society alike than is treatment for a severe stroke. Yet stories are common of patients on a fixed or limited income who simply cannot afford the prescribed medications. It is not an uncommon experience to see in a convenience store or a fast food restaurant a jar with a picture and a note requesting funds for a family who has been hard hit by medical expenses. Other organized community events are frequently means for friends or family to seek funds for costly procedures such as organ transplant, long-term treatment of illness, or traumatic injury. However much such efforts may help an individual, they are almost assured of being inadequate for the needs even while they raise the question whether the ability to garner attention is a "just" way to address issues of cost and access to treatment.

The ideal and goal of American health care is for patients to receive needed treatments regardless of their ability to pay for it, and in many instances we come close to that ideal. Yet the perspective of a hospital whose patient base is heavily uninsured or underinsured may be that some patients are referred after receiving a "wallet biopsy" (Does the patient have insurance?) at a competing facility with stringent requirements about payment. It is common knowledge that there are gaping holes in the medical insurance coverage available to Americans and that the costs of insurance continue to rise dramatically. In a competitive economic climate, businesses bemoan the expense of health care, citing exorbitant health insurance costs as a stumbling block in their ability to compete, especially with foreign businesses. At the same time, because such a large percentage of American health insurance is offered through workplaces, employees are very concerned when insurance availability is threatened. For both business and workers, cost pressures on the piecemeal system currently in place promise no respite in the immediate future.

Issues of access to treatment and costs surface in other ways as well. As economic pressures on hospitals, clinics, and other health care providers become more intense, a cycle of increasingly limited access to care may develop. There is much concern about the poor overburdening emergency rooms by using them as their primary source for health care, but all too often the emergency room is the only care available. Private physicians who require insurance or payment at the time of service are simply not an option for poor people, whereas an emergency room must at least evaluate a patient who comes into the ER. Similar situations exist with babies born with little or no prenatal care, at least in part because Mom could not afford or had limited access to that care. So the emergency room may well become the point of entry, and the labor room of the hospital that provides indigent care the birthplace for this baby and mother who are both poorly prepared for their new life together. If an inner-city hospital closes its emergency room, or worse yet closes as an institution, those who had been cared for must find other sources of care. In rural areas, similar dynamics are at work, and patients may have to travel out of town or out of county to get care when "their" hospital cannot keep its doors open.

Genetics Applications

Genetics applications seem to offer a Pandora's box, twenty-first-century style. The possibilities for good are limitless, but the potentials for unanticipated consequences or for frankly evil outcomes are equally limitless. With the human genome project completed, efforts abound to develop commercial applications of the knowledge that has been catalogued to this point. With those efforts comes great hope, both for sufferers and for their loved ones. Who could not be pleased at the prospect that a prevention or cure might be found for any of the multitude of debilitating and fatal diseases of our time? Perhaps genetics research might wipe out one of the scourges that affect so many—cancer, AIDS, diabetes, or Alzheimer's disease. Perhaps it might provide a solution to the problems associated with there being far too few organs available for transplantation for the numbers of those in need of transplanted organs. On the other hand, perhaps a disaster of unfathomable proportions could be unleashed accidentally or intentionally by a lethal virus or the introduction of a new species of plant or animal into the ecosystem. Do genetics research and applications have the potential to redefine life itself, to dramatically improve life as we know it, or to destroy it? Unquestionably, research will continue and the outcomes of that research will find their way into the diagnosis and treatment of patients. We must fervently hope that insightful ethical reflection will keep pace with scientific study.

Ethical reflection about genetics applications must include the "seek good/avoid harm" concerns that will closely question new technologies and will not be overly swayed by either humanitarian concerns (make it available to "help" even if we don't know the long-term consequences) or of market concerns (seek a large return on investment even if little or no actual benefit to patients is established and/or potential risks must be artificially minimized in order to proceed to market). Though other technologies have passed through phases of promised help well before actual benefit is available, this concern may be a particularly urgent one in the field of genetics technologies. The constant propensity for media and/or marketing to trumpet new "discoveries" before there is reliable data on the actual benefit or the potential risks opens a door for the desperate or the gullible to embrace the discovery prematurely. Early indicators of genetic links to a disease or syndrome are rarely able to claim with certitude whether there are actually multiple factors underlying the disease and to know how those factors may interact. Furthermore, breakthroughs in diagnosis will almost surely precede breakthroughs in treatment. Profound ethical questions are inherent in the possibility of learning that we will be stricken with a terrible malady at some time years in the future, but that there is no way to prevent it from happening. Do we really want to live the ensuing years waiting for a tragic outcome? Some will answer a resounding "yes"; others an equally resounding "no." Many will look to the health professional who has and understands the information to make a decision as to whether or not to disclose it. Therefore, health professionals are wise to consider in advance their own ethical understandings and boundaries in terms of how they will determine what information they seek from a patient and what information they are ethically bound to share with the patient.

This author claims no expertise in the specific issues surrounding cloning, especially the cloning of human life, or stem cell research aimed at repairing or replacing dysfunctional organs. It is indeed a stretch to even cite the two in conjunction. However, it seems that they have in common the ethical issues raised by possible genetics-assisted human replacement parts. At face value, it would seem that either one holds the potential to unleash a Frankenstein's monster, with truly mind-boggling consequences for humanity. Aside from the ethical issues regarding how to incorporate a cloned "human" into family and society (consider a "Four Box" set of questions relative to cloning an individual), a less obvious issue remains. If, as some proponents of human cloning suggest, a benefit of cloning would be to provide organs, blood, or other biological means to combat a physiological problem, what are the consequences of facilitating the manufacture and distribution of human "parts" as commodities? What are the consequences if it becomes possible to progressively replace failing organs and increase an individual's life span by years, or even decades? Though stem cell research seems immediately less dramatic than cloning, it also seems more likely to make significant breakthroughs in the shorter term than human cloning. The contention made here is that the ethical questions relating to both issues seem very similar because of the concerns about body parts as commodities. It is troubling to recognize that, despite declarations by government or professional groups, research can proceed outside of guidelines or proscriptions. Perhaps there is no way to ensure that research at the controversial extremes of genetics will not continue until it is successful somewhere.

At the level of society, ethical concerns about genetics technologies also cluster around cost and information sharing. How will costly treatments be justly made available in conjunction with other societal priorities? Undoubtedly, there will be discoveries of lifesaving but very expensive treatments, treatments similar to those that have changed AIDS from an unwavering sentence of early death to a chronic illness. With medical insurance participation and costs of health care in general already issues of great concern, who will benefit from these treatments and who will be denied treatment based on cost? The other great societal concern revolves around how information might be used with or without a person's knowledge to dramatically impact financial or personal concerns. In a nightmare scenario, insurance companies could abuse information obtained in genetic testing to deny insurance coverage to people genetically predisposed to particular illnesses. For example, if it is possible in the near future to test for one or more predispositions to serious illness during a routine blood test, how would that information be used and shared? Might a baby be denied medical coverage because parental genomes may mean the child will develop a disease? Even more troubling, might the genome of an uncle or grandparent or sibling be made the basis for determining likely health hazards for an individual or his children? Clearly, these issues are replete with uncertainty, speculation, and questions. However, it would be ethically irresponsible not to think them through as clearly as possible in advance, seeking to avoid problems whenever possible, rather than to try to repair damage after the fact. Repeatedly, this chapter has emphasized that a dominant aspect of ethical reflection in health care is to consider difficult issues and to raise questions about benefits and burdens.

Competing Perspectives

Competing perspectives, at a simplistic level, would simply reinforce the recognition that ethical issues are complex and that there are often no obvious wrong answers. However, in the context suggested here, the competing perspectives are potentially so profound as to risk dramatic disconnects in the process. The intensity of interest and restricted focus coming from the right to life perspective has already been alluded to. An earlier section of this chapter pointed out that a system for ethical reflection might be broadly based on either a "duty" ethic (deontology) or a "benefits/burdens" ethic (teleology). A duty ethic needs clarity, perhaps to the point of requiring black-and-white alternatives. It should be clear, however, that the system developed here is based on teleology. It is the contention of this author that the complexity and the "real world" urgency of decision making are powerful forces, requiring the give-and-take perspective of benefits/burdens. If that basic presupposition cannot be reasonably sustained among the parties involved, it is extremely difficult to maintain dialogue. Duty and teleology do not readily find common ground. Issues of abortion and end-of-life issues lumped (inappropriately) together as euthanasia have galvanized a segment of religious and political concerns and activists. The understanding of "life" from this perspective is known as vitalism, and locates the most basic understanding of human life at the biological level. In relation to abortion, vitalism contends that life begins at conception, so it follows that any intentional intervention that harms an embryo after conception is unacceptable. At the other end of the spectrum, vitalism rejects the validity of quality of life concerns. Thus, a persistent vegetative state is still life and should be aggressively maintained. Furthermore, the discontinuation of aggressive treatment, such as use of a ventilator, kidney dialysis, or especially artificial nutrition and hydration, can be considered only in the most extremely limited cases or not at all. In our discussion of precedent-setting cases, reference was made to a family belief system based on vitalism (Wanglie) and to right to life proponents vehemently protesting discontinued treatment for Cruzan and Schiavo. Should the proponents of vitalism continue to gain activist power through public sympathy, media, and political channels, health care ethics may be thrust into very differing modes than those offered here.

Another major challenge for the future of health care ethics comes from issues raised by diversity and multiculturalism. The methodology for ethical reflection offered here is a reflective model that seems to presume a high degree of formal education. It is heavily influenced by Western and Enlightenment presuppositions. Many health care professionals have these presuppositions and perspectives in common. However, many of the recipients of care do not necessarily share them. Even in areas where there is limited ethnic or cultural diversity, there is still likely a very large educational gap between caregivers and many of the patients and families. Crucial concepts, such as brain death, persistent vegetative state, and futile or medically inappropriate treatment, are very difficult to grasp for even well-educated people not in a medical field; it becomes exponentially more difficult for poorly educated people to understand these concepts. How effective may a conversation be when a decision maker does not have minimal understanding of anatomy or disease process or the vocabulary to comprehend the terms used to clarify them? In such a case, when an ethical dilemma arises, how effective can a consult and hoped-for resolution be by superimposing even more foreign words and concepts onto the confusion? What about the almost inherent social intimidation an undereducated person feels in the presence of doctors or perhaps several health care professionals?

When the conversations take place between those of very different cultural and/or ethnic backgrounds, even more complications are introduced. The powerful role of autonomy in the ethics process becomes very ambiguous indeed if the patient does not share with the health care team a high value on Western individualism. For cultures that value group decision making or look to a designated person other than the patient as the ultimate authority, consent and information sharing take on very different manifestations. Typically Latino and Middle Eastern cultures follow such patterns, and both groups are bringing increasing numbers of patients into most health care systems. In none of the cases noted is there an automatic inability to communicate and resolve, but certainly there are factors that will challenge the communication and respectfulness required for ethical reflection. Though most would abhor a descent into mere political correctness, an honest recognition of and concern for cultural value differences is absolutely incumbent for health care workers and systems. Especially if we are to approach ethical reflection in a manner respectful of spiritual concepts and values, we must do so with as open an attitude as possible.

Ethics, Spirituality, and Technology

Ethics, spirituality, and technology intersect most obviously at a bedside in a hospital, in a physician's examining room, in a research lab, or in a program educating health care professionals. Reference has already been made to the many ways in which technological innovation has been the driving force behind developing ethical issues and dilemmas. Typically, the scientific perspective, which creates new technology, and the spiritual perspective, which seeks value and meaning in relationships, have coexisted uneasily at best and have been in open conflict at worst. It is clearly the intent of this book to foster respectful dialogue between the two rather than conflict. It is the contention of this author that spiritual issues are never absent from health care, though they are all too often ignored or discounted in importance.

For the patient and family entering the health care system, the need is for both "high tech" and "high touch." Patients assume they will be the recipients of the latest medical technology and that the technology will be a benefit in diagnosis and treatment. However, they come to diagnosis and treatment with their very personal hopes and fears. Life-changing bad news may come in the form of test results or the fearsome phone call to come to the emergency room because a loved one has been in an accident. Despite dramatic changes in the doctor-patient relationship, with the declining numbers of primary care physicians who do hospital work, patients still want "their" doctor. The wise physician also continues to recognize the importance of trust and openness between patient and physician. At the very least, the technological tools must be understood by physicians and explained to patients, along with what the findings from those high-tech tools mean. An increasingly large body of research identifies multiple important roles of religious and spiritual experiences in recovery from health crisis and/or in coping when a cure is not forthcoming. Because this confluence of issues presumes the need for evaluating and deciding among options, an ethical stance and a methodology like the one presented here can offer guidance that bridges the divide between technology and spirituality.

In considering ethical decision making and spirituality for the needs of health care professionals themselves, terms such as stress and burnout are freely bandied about. A term that increasingly appears in the literature is compassion fatigue. It is a term that is largely self-explanatory, applying to those whose caregiving activities have begun to exhaust them because of too many demands on their psychic energies. The model of critical incident stress recognizes the need to wisely intervene at times when a particular incident overwhelms people's normal coping ability, leaving them vulnerable to the toxic effects of the stress and perhaps to post-traumatic stress disorder. Caregivers working during 9/11 and the immediate aftermath, and those who have spent extended time caring for victims of natural disasters, immersed themselves in stress and risked becoming victims themselves. Obviously, the health care professional who invests emotional energy over long periods is at risk, and those who frequently deal with trauma, death, or other crises are at special risk.

Closely related to compassion fatigue, and even more directly aligned with considerations of ethical decision making, is the concept of moral distress. According to Chaplain Dan Dixson, moral distress "is generally seen in situations where a person must go against one's own principled beliefs because of imposed constraints" (Dixson 2006). Nursing personnel, in particular, may find themselves in such situations when they are required to administer treatments that, in their view, will inflict inappropriate suffering on the patient. (A common situation of moral distress is the need to administer CPR on a frail, dying patient with the concurrent likelihood of fracturing ribs in the course of chest compressions.) The American Association of Critical Care Nurses includes in its position paper on moral distress (www.aacn.org) a reference that states that "in one study 1 in 3 nurses experienced moral distress" (Redman & Fry 2000). In another, nearly half the nurses studied left their units or nursing altogether because of moral distress (Millette 1994). Clearly there is great potential for the quality of ethical decision making to have a dramatic impact on staff for good or for ill. Having the conceptual tools and the support of colleagues in addressing ethical dilemmas may help limit the stresses inherent in caregiving. Furthermore, acknowledging through professional or organizational codes of ethics that the detrimental effects of stress on health care professionals constitute an issue that requires sensitivity and responsiveness also links a spiritual perspective with good ethical decision making.

A final consideration in reflecting on ethical decision making and spirituality is that of meeting the emotional and spiritual needs of patients and families. It goes without saying that the primary goal of health care professionals is to help people deal with illness, trauma, and disability. However, in many or perhaps most situations, a patient presumes competent technical care and makes judgments about the perceived quality of care based on much more personal issues. "A physician who pays personal attention to the patient, who is respectful, compassionate and competent, that's what every patient wants," Dr. James T. C. Li of the Mayo Clinic College of Medicine in Rochester, Minnesota, said in a statement (Li 2006). It is no great stretch to include all health care professionals in this assessment. Specific to the role of good ethical decision making, the Joint Commission on Accreditation of Healthcare Organizations (JCAHO) recognizes the significance of nontechnical issues by including in its Hospital Accreditation Standards a chapter on "Ethics, Rights, and Responsibilities." Within that chapter are standards for putting in place an "ethics mechanism," a means of conflict resolution, and requirements for informed consent, the use of advance directives, good end-of-life decision making, and good communication (Hospital Accreditation Standards 2004, 99–116). In addition, the emphasis on patient satisfaction and patient service within health care organizations has seen the proliferation of service standards to better meet the emotional and spiritual needs of patients and families and of consumer surveys to assess exactly how well those needs are being met.

In reality, high-quality health care has always included attention to the whole person in need of help, not simply attention to a malfunctioning part of that person. The increasing interest in spirituality as it relates to health care issues is a creative and heartening move toward a more intentional focus on the inclusion of these issues in the training and practice of health care professionals. The inclusion of a chapter on ethical decision making and spirituality in this book offers reflection and information on how multiple issues have come together—past, present, and future—combining technology, decision making, and personal values in a sometimes volatile mix. With the inclusion of a proposed methodology for considering and weighing these issues and values, it is possible for health care professionals to develop confidence in dealing with people in crisis, which inevitably affects the physical, emotional, and spiritual dimensions of their lives.

Summary

In summary, this chapter begins with a conscious effort to distance popular misconceptions of "ethics" from the subsequent development of issues and methods in health care ethics. Though health care ethics is a moral enterprise, designed to seek good decisions in difficult situations, it does so with no punitive intent and with profound recognition of the complexity of the issues involved. The spirituality interwoven through the chapter expands the focus beyond technological interventions and detached mental exercises into the intensely personal realm of value-laden decisions that impact the meaning of life and death. The methodology offered begins with a threefold consideration of "best" choices in a particular situation, the significance of who makes the decisions, and the process by which those decisions are made. The method is further developed by identifying the role of character-based ethics that addresses the work of the health care professionals and of two theories by which ethical reflection may be organized. Teleological theories weigh benefits and burdens in ethical reflection; deontological theories emphasize that some things are inherently "right" or "wrong" and that we are duty-bound to act in accordance with what is right. After reviewing five precedent-setting cases, the case review method identified as the "Four Boxes" is described. In this method the four ethical principles of beneficence, autonomy, nonmaleficence, and justice are the basis for considering the dynamic balance of ethical concerns as they relate to a particular patient-care dilemma. Significant current and future issues are identified, with a discussion regarding the challenge of competing perspectives to the ethical system developed in the chapter. The chapter closes with a discussion of relationships in the health care setting as they are impacted by the confluence of ethics, spirituality, and technology.

Reflective Activities

1. Your father's physician recommends discontinuing life-sustaining treatment when he has developed multiple complications after a stroke. Your father is a widower. Your brother says, "No way"; you want to honor your father's stated wishes to "not live on a machine." How would you resolve the decision with your brother?
2. Under what circumstances would you want life-sustaining treatment to be discontinued for you?
3. Do you have an advance directive? If not, what stops you from completing one?
4. The news media have presented claims that health care professionals intentionally gave overdoses of medication to

debilitated patients in the wake of Hurricane Katrina. Does the perspective of this chapter offer sufficient help for making ethical decisions in cases of mass casualty or pandemic illness?

5. If you are a health care professional, to what extent does the term *compassion fatigue* describe your current spiritual and emotional state?

References

Beauchamp, T. L., & Childress, J. F. (1983). *Principles of Biomedical Ethics*, 2nd ed. New York: Oxford University Press.

Brody, B., & Engelhardt, H. T., Jr. (1987). *Bioethics Readings & Cases*. Englewood Cliffs, N.J.: Prentice-Hall, Inc.

Buechner, F. (1988). *Whistling in the Dark: A Doubter's Dictionary*. San Francisco: Harper & Row.

Dixson, D. (2006). Moral Distress in Clinical Staff. *Plain Views* 3, no. 5 (April 5). Available at: http://www.plainviews.org/.

Fletcher, J., Lombardo, P., Marshall, M., & Miller, F. (eds.). (1997). *Introduction to Clinical Ethics*, 2nd ed. Frederick, Md.: University Publishing Group, Inc.

Health Care Ethics Consortium of Georgia. (1997). Report of the Task Force on Futility.

Hospital Accreditation Standards. (2004). Oakbrook Terrace, Ill.: Joint Commission on Accreditation of Healthcare Organizations.

Jonsen, A. (1991). "Ethics and Clinical Decisions." Lecture, August 5. Fourth Annual Summer Seminar in Health Care Ethics. Seattle, Wash.

Jonsen, A., Siegler, M., & Winslade, W. J. (1998). *Clinical Ethics*, 4th ed. New York: McGraw Hill Health Professions Division.

Kinlaw, Kathy. (1996). "Organizing an Ethics Committee." Lecture, April 4. Floyd Medical Center, Rome, GA.

Li, J. (2006). Reuters from http://www.msnbc.msn.com/id/11947169/; accessed 2006.

Millette, B. E. (1994). Using Gilligan's Framework to Analyze Nurses' Stories of Moral Choices. *Western Journal of Nursing Research* 16(6): 660–74.

Redman, B., & Fry, S. T. (2000). Nurses' Ethical Conflicts: What Is Really Known about Them? *Nursing Ethics* 7(4): 360–66.

VandeCreek, L., & Burton, L. (eds.). (2001). *Professional Chaplaincy: Its Role and Function*. Schaumburg, Ill.: Association of Professional Chaplains.

13

SPIRITUALITY WITHIN EDUCATIONAL AND WORK ENVIRONMENTS

ELIZABETH ARNOLD

> When God made the earth,
> He could have finished it, but He didn't,
> He left it as raw material to tantalize us,
> To start us thinking and experimenting,
> And risking and adventuring,
> And therein lies life's greatest meaning.
> God gave us an unfinished world
> So that we might share with Him
> The joy and satisfaction of creation.
> —Alan Stockdale (Bach 1962)

Introduction

In previous chapters, meeting the spiritual needs of patients and their families in health care settings was the focal point. This chapter focuses on meeting the spiritual needs of the nurse in educational settings and work environments. Without regular reflection on the spiritual nature of the work itself in nursing, and the reciprocal impact that nurses and the organizational culture have on patient care, the subject of spirituality in nursing is one-sided and incomplete. It is difficult to conceptualize how nurses can be truly sensitive to clues that their patients are struggling with spiritual issues unless they themselves are leading a spiritual life.

Our spiritual nature resides in the soul, sometimes referred to as the human spirit, and considered the noblest part of humanity (Nee 1968). As an embodied spiritual being, the spiritual aspects of self cannot and should not be considered a separate part of the holistic human health service provider. Genuine spirituality works in tandem with the psychological and physical parts of self to fulfill each individual's destiny. Spirituality modulates the spiritual hunger within the self for an ultimate truth and purpose beyond human desires, money, physical characteristics, and intellectual endowment. The human soul illuminates a personal philosophy of living to effectively direct the care and commitment of our service to others: patients and families in health care settings, students, and collaborative health care team members. The outward expression of the soul is evidenced through a disciplined life, moral reasoning, and compassion toward self and others.

Spirituality represents an empowered understanding of the Divine found in diverse images of God, nature, the self, and life itself. This understanding is intuitive, and connected with personal worth, dignity, and respect for others. Spiritual growth ideally results in a sense of inner peace, consistent with the eight Cs, described by Schwartz (2001) as calmness, clarity, curiosity, compassion, confidence, courage, creativity, and connectedness. Spiritual experiences emphasize finding meaning in life, whereas religions represent organized faith communities, emphasizing specific beliefs and behavioral codes (Tisdale 2007).

Although Western and Eastern philosophical approaches to the development of the spiritual self differ in focus, both perspectives can contribute to our understanding of spirituality in professional health care settings. From a Western viewpoint, the spiritual nature of a human being is defined as a transcendent force, a way of life centered on a human connection with God (Sulmasy 1997). This alliance is with a Higher Purpose which connects us with an enduring sense of self and with our personal destiny.

An Eastern pantheistic worldview does not define a personal God, arguing that it is not possible to conceptualize a phenomenon so beyond all limits, and existing in all things. All of life's activities are infused with a spiritual dimension. From an Eastern perspective, each individual is part of a larger world family, and is considered inseparable from a larger universal consciousness. Acknowledgment of a personal reality directly connected to all other living things is referred to as beingness.

Eastern spirituality emphasizes a metaphysical approach to knowing the spiritual self through the heart rather than the head. Eastern perspectives recommend developing an authentic detachment from the rush of life with its habitual ways of thinking, feeling, and doing. Accomplished best through meditation and/or chanting, when practiced daily, these spiritual practices enhance the unity of mind needed for wisdom and inner peace. Dorn (2006) suggests that "in a sense, the personal self is expanded through belief in a common underlying consciousness and universal interdependence, so that doing good to others is in fact, a service to one's own self" (159). By losing the self, we gain the self and are better able to perceive the real meaning of our situation and our destiny. As with all other culturally influenced aspects of the self, there is significant diversity in people's specific spiritual beliefs, and traditions within a culture and across cultures. How each one of us interprets the meaning of our spiritual attitudes reflects our own uniqueness (Marques 2005).

Our spiritual nature as nurses benefits from both Eastern and Western perspectives. Both views are concerned with a realization of human potential more fully expressive of a person's higher self, which is aligned with a Higher Purpose and community.

Both worldviews agree that there is an eternal law or principle that rules the nature of life. By accepting a measureless order or unifying principle, which buttresses a seemingly chaotic, perpetually changing universe, people are better able to trust in their ability to make sense of it, whether directly identified with a personal God, or not. Despite significant differences in the conceptual understanding of spirituality, cultural integration in a global society is creating an awakening of consciousness and an acceptance of the impact of Eastern influence on Western spirituality among contemporary Western religious leaders and scholars (Oldmeadow 2004).

Frankl (1968) describes spirituality as those mental activities involved in transforming base instincts into productive actions, the capacity to exercise free will, to make reasoned choices, to grapple with moral decisions, and to determine personal values in pursuit of finding meaning. Although Frankl's spirituality stemmed from a humanistic worldview, his exploration of a broader meaning of what is transpiring in our life, which transcends the strictly objective meaning of a particular life event, seems relevant. Every important occurrence in life potentially offers us a unique opportunity to refine the understood meaning of objective life circumstances—no matter how undesired or traumatic the situation appears to us at the moment—in a constructive way.

Developing the Spiritual Self

Spirituality as a transformational concept in health care organizations begins with an individual's search for, and realization of core spiritual values, which can then be applied to the work environment (Biberman, Whitty, & Robbins 1999).

Although intimately connected, spiritual knowing differs from, and enhances intellectual and emotional knowledge in that it is intuitive, concerned with a pattern recognition process that explores how the different pieces of our lived experience fit together as a coherent whole. Spiritual knowing surpasses human reasoning and does not depend on our external senses for origin or validity. Conceptualized as a carrier of knowledge about the inner creative possibilities of life, our human soul radiates an intrinsic vitality, and enriches our life by attaching meaning to its content. This, in turn, influences our behavior both consciously and unconsciously. Peppers & Briskin (2000) state that "the essence of soul work is gathering up the pieces of ourselves and holding opposite forces in tension long enough for new possibilities to emerge" (89). Honesty with self is the foundation of soul work, and is critical to the development of a spiritual presence in the work environment (Guillory 1997). Through soul work, individuals can listen to the dissonance created by inevitable life transitions; make sense of them with guidance from a Higher Power (God), and live a fulfilled life with no regrets. Questions you can ask yourself to tap into this type of spiritual knowing might include: "What inspired me today?" Or "What surprised me today about myself?" Or "What moved me?"

Applications

Spiritual Development in Professional Education

Incorporation of spirituality into nursing ideally begins with the nurse's professional education, where faculty provide a framework for integrating spiritual and moral considerations into course content. Gough (1998) refers to an observation by Ralph Waldo Emerson that the goal of academic learning requires more than book knowledge; it also requires "helping students use their newly acquired ideas and theories to become good, decent, and responsible human beings" (49).

Professional education, conducted in colleges and universities, offers the most formative and visible form of spiritual development for nurses, directly through course content and objective, compassionately delivered feedback to students about their clinical performance. For a relatively short period of structured time, faculty join with their students as a community of scholars exploring the concepts of nursing. Unlike other forms of education, students must learn skills in the art of healing as well as prescribed content. This requires developing an awareness of the mystery of life inherent in their work, and respect for the self-determined personhood of their patients. Integrated into their educational experience are important transcendent values about life, care of the self, and interacting patterns of connectedness with concrete scientific knowledge in a seamless tapestry of educational content and process. Hargreaves (1997) suggests that excellent teaching is "infused with pleasure, passion, creativity, challenge and joy" (12), characteristics often associated with spiritual values.

There are three primary sources of knowledge that most educational formats in health care cultivate, regardless of content specifics. These are intellectual knowledge, emotional knowledge, and self-knowledge. Spiritual development offers a unique intersection in which these sources of knowledge can connect, through the creation of meaning and life purpose. Vaclav Havel is quoted as saying, "Every education is a kind of inward journey" (Moyers 1993, xi). Courses and/or specialty-based content applications, specifically designed to help students in nursing apply spiritually based work principles to specific clinical cases, should be a part of the nurse's educational curriculum. Providing intellectual knowledge to students without focusing on character-inspired applications limits the effectiveness of the teaching.

Schwartz (1996) notes that "Wisdom recognizes that you can be connected because of that part of you which is not different from others" (55). Human wisdom connects us to the rest of the world in developing common understandings about the nature of reality, the world, and ourselves.

Infusing spiritual values into the education experience of nursing students occurs largely through example. When students observe excellent ethical character and compassion, which resonates with eternal truth, in professors and clinical mentors, they are more likely to incorporate these values into their own clinical work. Excellent teachers teach not only from textbooks, but from their own experience.

Faculty members serve as agents of support, role models, exemplars of accomplishment, and sources of inspiration to novice nurses as they learn to negotiate health care issues under less than ideal conditions. Students need faculty and clinical mentors who can be lovingly objective about their performance and open to working with students in their quest for self-discovery in a complex, everchanging health care environment.

Students learn certainly as much, and perhaps more, about ethical conduct and spiritual presence by observing the behaviors of their faculty and clinical mentors. The importance of example cannot be underestimated. Gough (1998) writes:

Every life is a profession of faith and exercises an inevitable and silent influence. . . . He is as it were, a beacon which entices a ship upon the rocks if it does not guide it into port. . . . His conduct is an unspoken sermon, which is forever preaching to others. Such is the high importance of example. (112)

Faculty often are in the best position to help their students connect the dots in developing ways to humanize the illness experience. Faculty who really listen to their students as they relate their struggles with performance in the clinical arena and who support them in developing insights that humanize and personalize the health care experience for individuals and their families are a critical educational resource. Sharing relevant, personal experiences with struggle and failure can strengthen a nursing student's perspective.

Spirituality in the Health Care Work Environment

Leonard and Murphy (1995) suggest that "all those engaged in a serious calling—whether scientist or nurse, artist or contemplative—are strengthened in that calling by a sustainable philosophy that supports their work" (169). The development of this inner philosophy originates in the soul and acts as a tangible foundation for all our professional and personal actions. Ideally, the development of this inner philosophy is a result of a deliberative reflective process concerned with cultivating awareness and compassion for the self that we are now, and the one we wish to become. Bloch and Richmond (1998) propose that spirituality and work are connected when

Workers view their work as a calling.

There is a strong belief that a person's work has a valuable purpose.

People work in environments consistent with their values.

There is a sense of community with others at work.

Walsh (1999) refers to spirituality in our lives as "the direct experience of the sacred" (3). Spirituality in health care is not value-neutral. Inasmuch as the work that physicians; nurses; social workers; physical, occupational, and speech therapists; psychologists; and ancillary health care workers represents a committed service to others, God is always present, either bidden, or unbidden (Pierce 2005) as the ultimate healer. Although adherence to the particular beliefs of a religious faith provides an important personal framework for the practice of spirituality, members of all the major world faiths—Protestant, Catholic, Jewish, Buddhist, Hindu, Muslim, and others—can offer their own affirmation of spiritual possibility, easily recognized by others in a spiritually based work environment (Mitroff & Denton 1999).

In this context, spiritual faith continually evidences itself as "a total and centered act of the personal self, the act of unconditional, infinite, and ultimate concern . . . an act in which both the rational and the non-rational elements of his being are transcended" (Tillich & Gorman 1985, 16, 17).

Spirituality in spiritually infused work environments focuses on the values and ethics of an organization, and is strongly linked to good moral habits, honesty, loyalty, trustworthiness, and honor in its employees (Cavanagh & Bandsuch 2002, Hartman 1998, Weston 2002). Spirituality in nursing is about developing purpose, values, and meaningful relationships with others in our work environment, which enrich the soul and enhance productivity through the best use of its human resources. Creating a meaningful, spiritually infused work culture has direct and indirect effects that enhance patient coping, as evidenced in a growing number of research studies (Duchon & Plowman 2005, Koenig 2005).

Wheaton and Baird (2002) also note that a synergistic spirituality occurs when personal spiritual values influence the ethics and organizational culture of a workplace setting. For both leaders and employees, this process enables them to find renewed meaning in their work, inspired commitment, and deeper work relationships (Neal & Banner 1999). This holistic commitment to these values in a spiritually infused work community supports and enriches personal spirituality through a reciprocal transformative process (Mirvis 1997).

Developing a spiritual outlook helps us reframe and defuse problems great and small that stand in the way of professional growth and personal fulfillment in the workplace. This disciplined approach does not magically eliminate troubles, but rather enables us to face them honestly, to examine their relevance in our lives from a broader perspective, and to know that we have a Higher Power to help guide us in courageously working through them. Peppers and Briskin (2000) wrote that it is by "delving directly into the gritty realities of contradiction and uncertainty at work that one is able to bring spirituality into work life" (13).

Management and human resources personnel can play an important role in the development of a spiritually infused organizational culture by hiring the right people for the appropriate job; providing workers with the tools, incentives, and training required for job effectiveness; and working with their employees to ensure a creative balance between work and outside life responsibilities (Marques 2005).

Challenges to Developing Spiritual Work Practices in Nursing

Instability in health care work settings occasioned by hospital closings, cross-training that changes specialists into generalists, a litigious society, managed care, and shortened hospital stays create some of the same spiritual hungers present in other workplaces (Sulmasey 1997). Building spirituality in health care settings is both a personal and a collective imperative.

In nursing, the spirituality of the caregiver provides an important bridge through caring stewardship, even when circumstances are most difficult. It helps explain how an ordinary nurse embraces a sacred energy, which reaches beyond the common intellectual knowledge of an everyday world to bring hope, healing, and comfort to patients and families. Often referred to as the "art" of nursing, this inner energy enables nurses to embrace the ultimate virtues of life in the form of hopefulness, courage, faith, honor, love, acceptance, caring, and meaningful encounter with death in working with vulnerable patients and families. Accepting the finiteness of human existence as a reality without becoming discouraged or denying its inevitability sharpens our sensitivity to our patients as we share in their pain; in the process, we perhaps discover its special meaning in our own lives.

Health care settings do not always support the full tenets of ethical practice, resulting in moral distress for nurses as well as compromised health care for patients. For example, Hardingham (2004) recalled a work experience she had as a young nurse in which she felt she failed to question the substandard, disrespectful care given to a patient, because of the culture in the clinical setting. She stated, "I knew what the right thing to do was. I simply didn't have the courage to do it" (129). In many cases, this fear is highly realistic, so it becomes a consideration for even the most committed health professional. Secondary stress—related to managed care reimbursement policies, its misaligned incentives, threats of litigation, and time constraints—tests the integrity of nursing practitioners in championing the needs of their patients while recognizing the reality of having less funding for quality health care on a regular basis (Pattison 2006). Over time, it results in moral fatigue.

A genuine sense of humility, together with a sense of higher purpose without ego or pride, is a characteristic associated with leaders in spiritually infused organizations (Marsh & Conley 1999).

The Soul and the Shadow

Briskin (1998) tells us that "to include soul in our view of organizational behavior necessitates recognition of its shadow" (52). While the ego represents the conscious side of self, the shadow represents the unconscious. Integrating the shadow side of self with the ego is an important component of the spiritually evolved self. Originally described by Carl Jung as consisting of all the denied, neglected, or disowned parts of the experienced self, the shadow is also characterized as a moral problem that requires significant effort to acknowledge and accept (Jung 1938, Dunne 2000). According to Jung (1938), there is a capacity within each of us to act from dark or unpleasant impulses as well as from altruistic, spiritually evolved principles. Jung stresses the importance of acknowledging that we are all capable of doing things we are not proud of and suggests that "the less it is embodied in the individual's conscious life, the blacker and denser it is" (131). Knowledge of the shadow allows flexibility in choosing a higher path to achieving goals. The Arasini Foundation (2007) further notes, "Trying to grow spiritually while not dealing with our shadow side is like trying to walk through a dark room filled with objects—chances are we will become very frustrated, and repeatedly trip and fall."

Ego pride, as a common presentation of the shadow side of self, is one of the most powerful saboteurs of creating and sustaining a spiritually infused work culture in health care. Health professionals are particularly vulnerable to the development of unrecognized ego pride. Their patients usually revere them because of well-deserved confidence in their clinicians' abilities. Over time, professional health practitioners can lose sight of the fact that their talents are God-given, and that their efforts and their conduct in a truly noble profession represents a stewardship for which they will be held accountable. When reality gets misinterpreted through the rose-colored glasses of a person's ego pride, it often results in poor clinical judgment. Taken to an extreme, a person can begin to act in a blind, instinctive way, blaming others for her own shortcomings, and compromising quality care as her desire to protect the image of her public self becomes a primary goal. Not being able to transcend the self or to identify with a worthy purpose often results in boredom and/or burnout.

Ego pride stunts spiritual growth not only for the person, but also in the larger organization. Briskin (1998) suggests that often the individual experience of the shadow in the workplace mirrors a larger organizational shadow, which can be even more threatening to uncover. For example, many times the people we experience as hardest to deal with have a need to exert control, a need for recognition, a competitive drive, and the like, that we ourselves also possess. Knowing this about ourselves allows us to take a kinder, gentler approach to people who annoy us.

Helping others achieve their goals is a worthy endeavor, but it can turn into control behaviors when the rights of patients to self-determination are not fully considered. Becoming comfortable with our assets and talents, and working to master our vulnerabilities, can help unleash our creative capacities in a more holistic, humane manner. This self-understanding allows us to become all we can be, and frees our patients to seek and claim their own meanings and potential. Reflecting on the existence of these polarities, that is, the potential for good and evil within each of us, and respecting their presence in other people, enhances our understanding in ways that show the way both to spiritual healing and to leading an authentic life (Zweig & Wolf 1997). Integration of the dark side of our personality provides a stronger awareness of the sources of interpersonal conflict between ourselves and others, and a deeper respect for the fullness of the human experience.

Living a Spiritual Life at Work

In their landmark text, Mitroff & Denton (1999) offer scientific data recognizing spirituality as a significant determinant of successful organizational performance. These authors identified five models of spirituality found in organizations. While they differed in structure and focus, common conceptual threads of "caring, heart, love and trust" (10) were found across all models. For health care professionals, the connection between these identified work-related spiritual values and their importance in the provision of health care delivery should be striking.

Groen (2001) found the following to be characteristics of a spiritually infused work organization:

People have a sense of vocation and a passion about their work.

The workplace culture encourages creativity and risk taking through training and career development.

The workplace balances both work and home by having supports and programs in place that foster outside commitments.

Baseline wages and benefits are in place, which demonstrate the organization's willingness to invest in its workforce.

There is a sense of community both within and beyond the workplace, which is reflected in its operational and decision-making practices.

The articulated values of the organization are infused into its day-to-day practice. (20)

Living a spiritual life at work is not easy, but it is a rewarding enterprise.

Guillory (1997) insists that it is actually an essential ingredient in high-performing competitive work settings. In health care, spirituality strengthens our application of the ultimate virtues of life. It is found in the form of hope, courage, faith, honor, love, acceptance, and meaningful encounter with death—often on a daily basis. Spiritually infused organizations are characterized as being purpose-driven, and as providing opportunities for supportive relationships to develop among its workers.

Finding Purpose

Peppers and Briskin (2000) state that "Purpose in work takes on a transcendent nature when we link inwardly with what is most true and natural for ourselves, and outwardly with something of importance larger than ourselves" (123). Finding a purpose that affirms our spiritual energy requires effort and focused attention on what each of us most values about the work we do. Reframing work so that each activity we perform becomes an opportunity to make a contribution to the health and well-being of another human being, claiming each opportunity to make what we do a work of art, and a chance to enhance our work environment through our full and authentic presence are reflections of a spiritual orientation to life. Encountering every moment is an opportunity to be fully present to life.

Building Relationships: Community and Spirituality

Ministering to others can be an isolating, intense experience unless there are opportunities for regular and intentional conversation with trusted colleagues in the work environment. Duffy (2006) notes that "The current conception of spirituality as it relates to the workplace has less to do with a support based definition tied to a higher power or powers and more to do with systems and community. Spiritually infused work cultures are fortified through community with others" (54). Formal exchanges can also take place through compassionate supervision (Lambie 2006). Each nurse trusts that support will be given when needed and that the work will be accomplished to everyone's mutual satisfaction.

A spiritually infused community in work settings refreshes, strengthens, and renews commitment. A holistic way of being—with professional colleagues, patients, and patients' families—enables people to connect on the level of the spirit. This creates energy—the strength of new ideas, the power of respect, the support of diversity within community, and the presence of the moment.

Passion is the outward evidence of spirit and heart combined with competence in the workplace. Passion about our work is contagious! A common characteristic of a spiritually infused work culture, conspicuous but difficult to measure empirically, is the collective excitement people have about their work. Duchon and Plowman (2005) assert that workplace spirituality is recognizable when employees seem to have an inner sense of self-esteem, which nourishes and is nourished by meaningful work accomplished in community with others. People who are passionate about their work and consider it a vocation inspire others to greater effort. When people in a work setting respect and value each other's work, it is a pleasure to go to work, even when there are significant problems to be resolved. The trust they evince in each other can deepen the sense of meaning about the value and purpose of the work itself for health care professionals.

In health care, a spiritually infused organization demonstrates an ongoing quest for better patient care, with practitioners seeking the best for their patients in clinical settings, and faculty seeking the best for their students in health education settings. Spiritually infused health organizations want the best for their professional colleagues and make the commitment to put resources in place to accomplish this goal. For example, Toni, a veteran nurse on a research nursing unit, commented that at the monthly meetings of the clinical staff, her nurse manager had a habit of commenting on something good or special she had noticed each of her nurses doing that month. Toni observed, "I don't know how she did it, but she managed to do this for each person at each meeting. It means a lot to have your efforts noticed."

One of the more exciting paradigm shifts in health care is that physicians, nurses, and social workers tend to more thoroughly respect each other's work as equal contributors to the patient's well-being. Fostered by an emphasis on interdisciplinary collaboration, there is a creative tension in relationship with other health care team members, which helps people acknowledge their strengths and limitations and learn from one another and their experiences, rather than being crushed by them. The connectivity of the interdisciplinary relationship becomes spiritual when it altruistically serves the higher purposes of quality health care.

Burnout as a Spiritual Issue

Freudenberger (1980) described *burnout* as a state of mental and physical exhaustion related to unrelieved work stress, and attributable to long-term role strain or conflict. Most at risk are people who care about and value their work. Virtually all health care professionals are at risk of developing burnout because caring permeates their every activity. In addition to caring about their work, their professional effectiveness requires a strong personal and professional commitment to caring for others. Maslach and Leiter (1997) refer to burnout as the high cost of caring. This is particularly troubling for individuals in the caring professions who typically view their work as a calling or vocation, something of great existential purpose and value (Skovholt 2001)

Closely allied with a loss of meaning in one's work are work environments offering little social support and a lack of control over one's work. Labor practices that are unjust or inconsistent with values strongly held by an individual, and inequitable compensation are work factors that can lead to employees experiencing burnout (Maslach & Leiter 1997). Although more commonly defined as a psychological condition, burnout has a spiritual aspect. Maslach and Leiter (1997) suggest that burnout "represents an erosion in values, dignity, spirit and will—an erosion of the human soul" (17). Spiritual depletion, with its accompanying "malaise of the spirit," is said to occur when the spirit is pitted against a reality that cannot be changed. The symptoms of burnout reflect a blockage of the spirit, evidenced in generalized tension, fatigue, confusion, inability to concentrate, irritability, and a temporary lessening of energy and loss of interest in previously satisfying work. The sources of conflict of the spirit in clinical practice lie both in the people experiencing them and in the situations they encounter. Men and women who choose to make nursing a career make an ongoing commitment to a ministry of helping others. Most nurses do not adhere to a nine-to-five work schedule. Because health care activities are viewed as a committed service profession, everyone involved with the health care process upholds an ideal image of the health professional, totally dedicated to caring for others and never challenging the physical, emotional and spiritual toll this often takes on the caregiver. Caring is considered a hallmark of excellence across all health care professions. Health professionals want to make a caring difference in their patients' lives, and they are educationally prepared to do so.

Regrettably, the tangible evidence of pain, poverty, illness, violence, and people's inhumanity to one another continues to confront us despite extraordinary advances in technology and closer attention to ethical issues in clinical practice. Unlike many other professions, health care is intimately involved with critical life and death issues on a daily basis. Although it is an exciting profession, in which high drama and climactic events proliferate, pain, suffering, and negative outcomes occur with unrelenting regularity despite the valiant struggle. The reality of the job is that some patients will get sicker and die, despite our best efforts. A medical student commented after his clinical rotation on a bone marrow transplant unit, that he would never choose to specialize in an area where so many patients died. The dual loss of meaning and purpose in a service-oriented profession can bring one's professional life to a standstill.

Although most professionals are distressed by symptoms of burnout, they often are skeptical that making changes in the way they approach their work or life situation will make much of a difference in their circumstances. The ABCs of burnout prevention presented below, when practiced as a whole, can reduce the sense of separation from one's spiritual core that often occurs under prolonged stress or exceptional stressful circumstances.

Awareness

Gough (1998) notes that "The only mirror for the spirit is wise self-reflection" (21).

Since the working operations of the mind, spirit, and body are so closely integrated, fatigue, self-doubt, and physical or emotional symptoms serve as reliable indirect cues for the need for self-reflection. Self-reflection allows us to explore the full truth about ourselves, to examine our place in the work environment, and the reality of our relationships with others (Duff 2003). The personal energy that comes from looking at what is important to us, and letting go of those activities and things that get in the way of our life goals, can replenish our spirit.

Awareness also benefits from conversations with others. We don't always see ourselves as others see us, and their perceptions can offer useful insights. Health care professionals can and should sharpen their thinking and validate their conclusions through conversations with a soul friend, a compassionate colleague, or a professional, such as a cleric or chaplain. With an awareness of the strength and limits of our personal coping skills come opportunity and challenge. Walsh (1999) asserts that "the ultimate aim of spiritual practices is awakening; that is, to know our true self and our relationship to the sacred" (4).

Awareness should be focused. Focused awareness takes in all aspects of a situation. Much of what happens in our work life escapes observation unless it directly demands our attention. Bender (1996) uses the image of an empty bowl to describe the open attitude needed for focused awareness. "Each day a monk goes out with his empty bowl in his hands. Whatever is placed in the bowl will be his nourishment for the day. . . . Like the monk going out with his empty bowl, I set out to see what each day offered" (5, 6). Taking critical time to listen attentively to the inner self allows health professionals to better understand the basic essentials of life. Examining inner motivations critically within the light of faith and acknowledging base instincts—the shadow side of the self—allows for more flexibility in response. Being true to our self and our deepest values allows us to be true to our work, our patients, and our purpose in life. Having the courage to see problems as they exist in reality, coupled with the humility to accept the implications of our role, allows us to take needed personal responsibility for our actions.

Seaward (1997) identifies four processes to raise awareness:

Centering: Making a time of solitude to tune into the voice of God or our Higher Power as each person defines their Higher self.

Emptying: Cleansing the mind and soul of anything claiming our attention for the moment.

Grounding: Humanizing our intellectual and imaginative powers by correlating these understandings with the reality of a situation.

Connecting: Sharing the insights gained in the grounding of self, with others.

This inner work helps us discover and respond to an inner authentic drive to serve others, and to honor the self within. It allows us to open more fully to life, to reaffirm our purpose, to work more constructively with difficult life situations, and to resolve feelings that hurt or make us angry. Awareness brings into view those parts of life that are out of balance, and allows professionals to make choices consistent with their values and a higher life purpose. As Jung (2000) asserts, a satisfying, self-realized life is one which is both earth rooted and spiritually centered.

Balance

Walking in balance is a critical dimension of burnout prevention. Simple habits, such as taking time for yourself, not working unnecessarily long hours, eating well and regularly, and keeping a sense of perspective, help people maintain a balanced healthy lifestyle. As Thurman (1984) observes, "We must stop for the quiet replenishing of an empty cupboard." It is as important to develop and maintain interests and relationships outside the work environment as it is to sustain them within it. People committed to their work need to make and protect "quality time" with family and friends, as well as for meaningful leisure activities.

One of the best ways to achieve balance in our lives is to develop a clearer understanding of our limits and to appreciate our personal and professional boundaries. It takes self-discipline to say "no" to unreasonable demands, to deliberately choose moderation, and to cultivate a needed balance between work responsibilities and time spent on family or leisure activity. When the legitimate care of self consistently receives little attention, an individual loses inner perspective and important allies in developing a lifestyle that fits his inner needs as well as his outer persona. Accepting too much responsibility can be just as imprudent as inertia in meeting the complex demands of life. Sometimes, something quite drastic has to occur before we are willing to pay attention to the lack of balance in our life. A loss of energy, a physical illness, or the sudden awareness of a lost relationship with someone important to our sense of self may alert us to feeling off-balance. As unsettling as it is, personal chaos and conflict frequently serve as useful stimulants for change.

Lack of balance should be suspected whenever the amount of effort expended is significantly disproportionate to the outcome achieved by those efforts. For example, Marge is an assistant head nurse on a busy medical unit that is badly understaffed. Marge has been working double shifts at least once a week. She feels responsible for seeing that the unit is covered because of her position. After doing this for two months, Marge finds she has little time to spend with her family; she neglects her spiritual practices of prayer and attending church services; she pulls back from the charitable activities that give her such pleasure. Marge does not understand why the other nurses seem angered by her easy compliance with the charge nurse's excessive demands on her time and views their protection of personal boundaries as less desirable than her commitment (ego pride). A bout with the flu finally forces the issue of the long-overdue need for balance and a respite from an untenable situation. Paradoxically, the other nurses seem to pick up the slack and the charge nurse suddenly seems able to hire more staff. In Marge's case, as in our own lives, there needs to be a vigorous interplay between self-care/self-renewal activities that nourish our spirits, thereby putting energy into devising a creative response to each day's challenges. Setting aside time for these activities actually helps the overtaxed health care professional accomplish more, rather than less, in the responsible discharge of professional duties. Include time to review your values and goals and make scheduled time for family, spiritual activities, self, and community.

Choice

Everyone has choices, but professionals who experience burnout characteristically feel they have few if any choices left, other than to leave a bad situation. Sometimes this is the best choice, but not always. There are other choices we can make that help free us from previous ways of dealing with difficulties by expanding our range of possible responses. When combined with faith and awareness, the choices a person makes in the throes of burnout can be life-changing, purpose-driven, and meaningful. Occasionally, our choice is simply to acknowledge and accept circumstances that objectively cannot be changed and to use the experience productively as yet another step in personal growth. But even then, as Assagioli (1974) notes, there are choices.

I could rebel inwardly and curse; or I could submit passively, vegetating; or I could indulge in the unwholesome pleasure of self pity and assume the martyr's role; or I could take the situation in a sporting way and with a sense of humor, considering it a novel and interesting experience . . . or finally, I could make it into a spiritual retreat. (114–15)

There is a natural ebb and flow to all human experience. If we are willing to go with the flow and integrate the higher internal resources within ourselves with the reality of external situational forces, the choice process ultimately can prove enriching as well as more empowering. Making the choice to go beyond what you think you can do in a quest of higher values and deeper meanings is a powerful antidote to the attitudes that set the stage for burnout.

The choice process relates to the spiritual dimensions of burnout in several ways. Combating burnout invariably requires changes in attitude and the way a person conducts her life for resolution. Although the precise facts leading to burnout remain the same, making positive choices allows for opportunities not previously available, and the development of new skills. For example, a nurse educator trained in psychiatric nursing was reassigned to teach in a different clinical specialty, maternity nursing. Although the change was difficult to accept at first, she blended her psychiatric nursing skills into her new assignment and learned the required skills for maternity nursing. A significant part of her ability to accept this change was her deep spiritual connection to God and her regular use of prayer. In the process, she developed a new clinical expertise that resulted in some gratifying professional experiences she never would have had without the unplanned change in direction.

Appropriate use of free will works hand in hand with making reliable, reasoned choices. Experienced as an unwavering dedication to a particular enterprise despite obstacles and ambivalence, as a persistence in light of fear and vulnerability, or as a spontaneous and genuine response arising from our convictions, free will is not the same as having the license to do whatever we want regardless of the circumstances. Merely trying harder when a different type of interpersonal strategy is called for or behaving in any manner we may choose without considering the rights and values of others is not the same as making a reasoned choice.

Even when the circumstances objectively seem harsh and unyielding, choices can be the basis for making meaning. A young lawyer, diagnosed with terminal cancer just as he was about to start his first job with a prestigious law firm, spoke not of his recent marriage, the birth of his first son, or his law school achievements, but of his coping with terminal illness as his greatest accomplishment. In the eyes of his friends, his courage in planning for his family, his loving concern that this be a special time with his family, and his unqualified acceptance of his fate were indeed his greatest achievements—a legacy well worth remembering. He was able to transform his impending loss into a force for good through a belief in God's mercy and a trust in God's promise that "All things work together for the good." It was a conscious choice on his part.

Detachment

To speak of detachment as an integral part of spiritual growth sounds like a contradiction in terms. However, detachment in the spiritual sense provides distance, not from other persons but from excessive ego involvement, personal ambition, and expressive acts that momentarily gratify our own needs at the expense of another's.

Detachment incorporates concern for others, but does not focus on a linear outcome. It refers to doing the best we can at the moment, without worrying about the future or the past, neither of which is fully under our control. The concept acknowledges the contributions of the past as an informational resource and gives hope for the future. Not to be confused with indifference, detachment as an element of concern allows for a different perspective on the rhythm and essence of an experience. A problem or situation can sometimes be like a Chinese puzzle: The more we try to force a solution or become mired in it, the more entangled it seems to become.

Freeman (1986) suggests using meditation as a spiritual strategy to enhance genuine detachment. The meditator assumes a relaxed position in a quiet place twenty to thirty minutes a day, closing his eyes gently and repeating a single word (mantra) without thinking. When distractions intrude, he forces his full attention back to the mantra, a word originating in prayer, poetry, or philosophy. Although it can be any one word that has meaning to him, maranatha, an ancient Aramaic word meaning "Come Lord," pronounced slowly in four syllables, seems particularly fitting on a spiritual pilgrimage to the inner self (Freeman 1986). Using a mantra or symbolic word over and over silences the perplexing thoughts and conflicting feelings that threaten to destroy the inner spirit, if not put into their proper perspective. Cultivating a proper attitude gives us a different perspective on the rhythm and essence of an experience in our lives. Turning over a problem to a Higher Power allows us to view it from a different vantage point. Appealing to a Higher Power to enter our lives as a support, instead of dictating what form the Power needs to take in order to be helpful, allows us to fully experience the mystery and synchronistic coincidences of a guided life. Both self-understanding and the accompanying actions are completed in stages, with care and compassion.

Detachment from ego involvement can be an important component of making good choices. Deliberately choosing to move with the flow of life as it is experienced in the present moment requires a conscious effort to let go of all preconceived ideas and expectations of how life should be and how people should act, coupled with an acceptance that the rules of life are relative in many respects. This can be a difficult axiom to embrace for those who seek definitive rules in life to guide their every action, but it also can be quite invigorating. With a heart open to the spirit, unfettered by regrets or wishful thinking, a person is free to make a more creative use of her talents and personal gifts in a unique way. Waiting to see how life unfolds while still feeling very connected with the present often presents new possibilities.

Detached concern is an especially crucial attitude in clinical situations. For example, in a support group for nurses on a bone marrow transplant oncology unit, the nurses were very upset when a youngster with a long-term illness suffered a relapse, and the parents wanted the child moved to intensive care because "The nurses on the ward couldn't take care of him anymore." The ward used a primary care model, and during the six months Danny was in the unit a strong bond developed between the nurses, Danny, and his parents. Although the physician privately agreed with the nurses that Danny should remain in the unit, he moved the child to intensive care at the parents' request. This action further disturbed the nurses because it implied that their nursing care had been less than competent.

After discussing their concerns in the support group, the nurses decided to put aside their anger and to attend to their primary mission of providing the best possible care for Danny and his parents. Instead of avoiding his parents, the nurses frequently visited Danny in the intensive care unit when they were there. They spent time showing the ICU nurses the special ways Danny liked to be suctioned and, whenever they were able to, they continued engaging in a relationship with Danny. The rapport that developed between Danny's frightened parents and the transplant nurses became a source of strength for all of them.

When Danny lay dying, the nurses from the unit were called to be with him. If these nurses had chosen to focus only on their past relationship with Danny or on speculating about what the future would hold should they remain involved, the shared meaning in this human encounter might never have taken place. With their efforts refocused on the task of making this child's final days as memorable and comfortable as possible, they stopped worrying about whether their efforts would be appreciated, and their nursing practice as a task and an art merged together in an unexpectedly meaningful way. "Man should not ask what he may expect from life, but rather understand that life expects something from him" (Frankl 1968, 92). It is only in losing our need to be perfect, to reach some impossible ideal, that we can begin to find ourselves.

Altruistic Egoism

Part of developing a stronger sense of a self, connected with a Higher Purpose operating in one's life includes cultivating a sense of altruistic egoism. When we appreciate ourselves, we are better able to appreciate and love others (Seaward 1997). Individuals entering the health care professions usually have natural empathy and a strong predisposition to helping others. As with the other self-renewal approaches described in this chapter, there needs to be a healthy balance between energetically confronting difficult issues and temporarily withdrawing from involvement with outward activities, taking time to "smell the roses" and finding a center of restfulness within the self. Health care professionals are often reluctant to provide the same quality time for themselves that they so willingly extend to others. Helping others feels legitimate; extending the same care to oneself feels foreign and uncomfortable. Often the best clue as to whether enough time is being given to oneself is to ask oneself the following questions: "When was the last time I took time to do something just for myself, something I wanted to do?" "When was the last time I took time to feed my own spirit?" If you cannot find an answer to these questions as you mentally scan your activities over the past week, it is only a matter of time before the reserve supply of comfort and understanding for others will be empty.

A useful exercise is to write down some activities that were meaningful at a different time in life—for example, praying, reading scripture, attending worship services, spending time with friends, having fun, engaging in pleasant conversation, sharing a meal with a friend.

Once you identify these activities, it is important to make sure that you include in the next week some of these activities that not only refuel your emotions and relational connections but also nourish your spirit. For example, when asked to do this exercise, a social worker at a day care center for elderly patients came up with the following activities. He used to start his day with prayer but because of his busyness, he was rushing into the activities of the day without this soul feeding. Once he resumed this important activity, he felt an immediate spiritual refreshment. The other enjoyable activity that came to mind was a good conversation. It surprised him that this activity came to mind, but when it did, he made active plans to deliberately arrange to have a conversation with a friend the following week. Until he did the exercise, he said, he had not been aware of how isolated and lonely he felt despite his daily work contacts.

Faith

One of the certainties in life is that there will be bad times as well as good in each person's lifetime. Faith is a powerful resource in burnout prevention that people don't always think about immediately. It is not necessarily the property of a particular religious belief system, but rather a quality of living that enables people to find a stable meaning in their lives even in the midst of chaos (Smith 1998). Faith that each of us has a unique destiny within the larger universe helps stabilize us when we don't know what is going to happen next. Faith is particularly important when, despite our best efforts, we lose a job, we fail to get a promotion, a project fails, or changes in a work environment turn a previously enriching work culture into a toxic one. New conditions may require different choices. Faith can help us. Faith requires us to trust in a Higher Power or Purpose to show us the next step, or the next direction, when it is unclear what we should do next. Duffy (2006) notes that people who feel supported by their faith are often better able to develop an optimistic worldview, and experience less depression and emotional distress. An exceptional exemplar of a professional who lived by faith is Dr. Viktor Frankl. He sustained faith that his life had meaning and worth even in a concentration camp. Frankl lived his life accordingly both as a physician and as a prisoner in horrific circumstances, serving as a beacon of hope to others and ministering to all those in need, including his captors. Connecting with spirit through faith lets us continue with our internal struggle to resolve inner conflicts. By challenging the feeling that what happens in life is determined by circumstances completely beyond our control, we are applying one of the best antidotes to the malaise of the spirit associated with burnout.

Faith as a component of burnout prevention can offer tangible support in difficult times. The reality that God or a Higher Power is both transcendent as well as immanent and, as such, is always with us is a tremendous comfort and resource. Mother Teresa was fond of saying, "Work like it all depends on you, but pray as if it all depends on God." Continually confronting the inner self with courage, seeking spiritual guidance, choosing to change and to grow—that is what keeps the spirit within us alive and healthy. Faith allows a person to confront obstacles and to work through them confident that God or a Higher Power will direct the activities needed to achieve important life goals for ourselves and our patients.

Goals

Without goals in life, we travel blindly. Our goals direct the type of effort and the nature of the activities we need to achieve inner harmony. They represent a coherent ground plan for accomplishing what is important for self-realization. Selye (1976) argues that man needs goals to exercise his innate capacities and feel worthwhile as a person.

Goal setting is the active phase of productive living and burnout prevention. Insights, no matter how relevant and powerful, are useless without action. Without developing practical applications to accept and work through personal issues, we are not utilizing our faith. We hold others accountable for their actions, but not ourselves. It is small wonder that, without realistic goals we make little forward progress. Frustration occurs when others block our goals, either because they are not realistic, they are out of line with our capabilities at the time, or they interfere with another person's right to achieve his personal goals. The development of professional and personal goals requires a concentrated investment of time and effort. Ideally, our goals should be in line with our personal strengths, and capabilities as well as our needs and the larger purpose of our work.

Goals need to be realistic. Performance standards that are too high inevitably lead to burnout. The need to appear perfect requires, in part, a superficial appearance of flawless control. Outwardly, a health care professional may act as if she has control of a situation, accomplishing tasks with an efficiency that is truly impressive. No one is really aware of the clinician's personal struggle to appear competent in every action, relationship, and therapeutic encounter. When the clinician collapses physically or overreacts emotionally to a situation, colleagues frequently are shocked. They do not know how to respond appropriately, for they had no idea there was a problem.

In this situation, the clinician's innermost needs and values have been overlooked. With impossible goals, health care professionals are doomed to failure before they begin, because perfection is impossible in most human service professions. There simply are too many variables to control. Furthermore, a person's spirit eventually will rebel against the absurdity of trying to achieve all these goals.

Other goals that clearly are within the realm of possibility sometimes fail to materialize despite our best efforts. When sufficient efforts have been made and achievement of a particular goal still eludes us, it is sometimes useful to "retreat in place" to allow for the spiritual guidance that is always available to us if we only listen to it. Waiting patiently for a more opportune time or a different set of circumstances is sometimes more productive than trying to crash through gates forcibly closed against us at the time.

Two steps are required to develop realistic goals. The first is to focus on the inner gifts that might help us achieve our aims. It is a good idea to ask a friend or advisor to help you with this part of the process. Oftentimes, it is difficult to discern our own potential assets without feedback, particularly in times of emotional turmoil. The second step is to realize that we will need the help and cooperation of others, including our Higher Power, to realize any important aim in life. Knowing what we wish to accomplish and figuring out how to achieve it may call for two different processes. Input from others in sharing groups, one-to-one relationships with friends, spiritual directors, or mentors provides fresh perspectives, solutions, and ideas that would otherwise never cross our mind. More important, a sense of community generates hope.

Hope

Biberman, Whitty, and Robbins (1999) note that "Hope is found in the human spirit" (244). Hope often considered to be a spiritual virtue is an important element in burnout prevention, a gift from God. But it operates in tandem with carefully chosen professional and personal goals. A hopeful attitude does not just happen. Hope is intentional and involves taking action. Viewing barriers as challenges to be solved rather than as endpoints stimulates hope. Snyder (1994) suggests that the development of hope goes hand in hand with setting goals, and determining the actions needed to reach those goals. Hope helps provide the inner determination to use abilities and behaviors to meet important goals and to figure out strategies when we are not sure that a positive outcome is possible.

The spiritual aspect of hope needs to be acknowledged in our carefully chosen goals, and in our hearts there needs to be a deliberately willed openness to accepting the love and guidance of a Higher Power. Without it, we can easily fall prey to the circular reasoning of expecting that no one will care. Consequently, we are less willing to share our innermost thoughts and feelings in ways that allow other important people in our lives to respond. The resulting feelings of anger and frustration continue unabated, and in our interpersonal relationships we begin to engage in a cyclical process of offering others inadequate information about our emotional state and lamenting our unmet needs. Burdens—spiritual, emotional, or physical—need to be shared if they are to be lightened.

Other people can play a vital role in stimulating and sustaining hope. Building relationships or changing ways of encountering life always involves risk, and to some extent a leap of faith. Co-workers can encourage and recognize our contributions as well as provide feedback and suggestions. Spirituality is nurtured through a way of life that involves shared vision, and hope in the company of others. Today, it may come as no surprise that personal involvement and interpersonal connectedness within a larger health care community form the essence of commitment and meaning for the health care professional.

The nurturance of a hopeful attitude as a function of the soul has a second role. Life's journey is best described as a process—an uncertain searching in which each step on a road we create through our own efforts becomes a necessary prerequisite for understanding and advancing to the next. Every individual has different but equally important assets and limitations. All are needed in combination with each other for the successful functioning of the whole. The most effective approach is to use our assets to the best of our ability and to acknowledge our limitations while working diligently within their constraints. This way we invite all kinds of opportunities for the formative development of a strong spiritual orientation to life.

Hope is the soul's attribute that allows us to experience the possibility of our own worth in the larger scheme of things. At the end of each person's life, this worth will be measured not by the number or quality of our accomplishments but only by how well we have loved and by our stewardship of the talents and gifts given freely to us. In 1967, Frankl advised nurses that it will be the gift of the self that will be most meaningful as they look back on the validity of the nursing profession as their life choice.

And what about the work of nurses . . . ? They sterilize syringes, carry bedpans, and change bedding—all necessary acts but scarcely enough in themselves to satisfy the human spirit. But when a nurse does some little thing beyond her more or less regimented duties, when say, she finds a personal word to say to a critically ill person, then and only then is she giving meaning to her life through her work. (96)

Integrity

Symbolically, Rodin's sculpture *The Hand of God* illustrates the joining of the sacred with the human in development of self-integrity. The sculpture reveals the human form of man and women emerging out of an unformed mass of material with much of the form still incomplete. Held or supported by the hand of God, the hand is open, not closed around the figures. Substance still to be formed shows through the open spaces between the fingers, suggesting that the creative possibilities for refinement of the figures are left to the imagination of the human figures. So too, it is left to us to determine the precise design and application of meaning of our lives with the support of a Higher or Greater Power.

Health professionals with self-integrity embrace life, work, and play with their entire being. A spiritual person is one who lives an authentic, principled life. Health care professionals can experience a reawakening of spirit and the renewed purpose essential for a spiritually infused practice. People with integrity are clear about who they are and demonstrate this self-understanding through their values and behavior. The sense of mastery that comes from making choices that support a personal philosophy of self as well as being feasible in a particular clinical setting can be particularly empowering for an individual. People who allow themselves to become spiritually infused conduct their lives from an integrated core of inner strength and personal energy that is dynamic and creative. Their integrity is manifested in meaningful human relationships with their fellow humans, and a clear relationship with God, however they may conceptualize their Higher Power to be.

Our spiritual connection allows us to tap into a knowledge resource that expands intuitive and conventional wisdom to include an understanding of what is meaningful to the human soul. In health care situations where feelings of doubt, fear, or uncertainty often occur, a humanistic approach infused with the spiritual nature of human existence helps nurses to negotiate and make choices consistent with fundamental beliefs and value systems, both their own and those of their patients. No matter how difficult the situation, or how demanding the patient is, this caregiver is able to consistently see beyond outward appearances and behaviors to the inner struggle each person brings to understanding the meaning his or her life holds for self and others. In health care settings, these issues are particularly poignant for both patients and professional health care providers. Take John for example. As a hospice nurse, he is the one constant in Barbara's life. When she panics as her condition worsens, John never takes personally her verbal abuse or suspicions that he is not caring enough. And when she is grateful for his ministrations, he is able to accept this with equal equanimity. Is this tough to accomplish? Of course, but with the inner resource of a personal God to give him strength and a different deeper way of looking at all things, John is able to offer a level of care that enriches the soul as well as cares for Barbara's physical and emotional needs.

Summary

Chapter 13 focuses on the spiritual needs of the professional nurse in educational settings and work environments. The nature of spirituality among health care providers presents visible evidence in their caring health care stewardship. Finding meaning in one's life and work is intimately associated with the development of a spiritual sense of self.

Western and Eastern philosophical approaches to the development of the spiritual self both contribute to our understanding of spirituality in professional health care. Spirituality connects us with a wider sense of self, and with our individual destiny. The soul is intimately involved in developing the spiritual self because our spiritual nature resides in the soul. Through soul work, individuals can listen to the dissonance created by inevitable life transitions, make sense of them with guidance from a Higher Power, and live a fulfilled life with no regrets.

Professional education offers the most formative and visible form of spiritual development for health care practitioners. Practicing spiritual values as professionals in health education settings entails more than transmitting knowledge. Students need faculty and clinical mentors who can be lovingly objective about their performance and open to working with students in their quest for self-discovery in an uncertain and complex health care environment.

Spirituality in health care is not value-neutral. Developing spiritual practices in health is about developing purpose, values, and meaningful relationships with others in our work environment, which enrich the soul and enhance productivity through the best use of its human resources. Living a spiritual life at work is not easy, but it is a rewarding enterprise, which includes recognizing and working with the shadow side of self. Learning to live a principled spiritual life at work is associated with developing a meaningful purpose, and a connection with others and a Higher Power. Developing the spiritual self and preventing burnout requires awareness and directed actions to achieve a sense of balance, making responsible choices, practicing detachment, taking care of self, having faith in oneself and the future, and developing goals and sustaining hope, completed in stages, with care and compassion. Health professionals with self-integrity embrace life, work, and play with their entire being.

Reflective Activities

1. Make a commitment to spend fifteen to twenty minutes at the start or end of each day contemplating the mystery of life lived in faith. This process can be enhanced through the use of appropriate devotional materials or structured sharing groups.

2. Reflect on the gifts you have been given and identify one way in which you can share a particular talent or gift. Who would you like to reach out to, and what would be important to share this particular day?

3. Resolve to select one activity that you really enjoy, and take the necessary actions to make it happen within the next week.

4. Using a relaxation technique, imagine yourself having greater freedom from the situation, project, idea, or person with whom you have the greatest attachment. What parts of your ego are bound up in the outcome? Think of one way you could decrease your own ego involvement in the outcome.

5. Carefully list your present responsibilities and obligations. Name two ways you could achieve inner balance between your obligations to self and others. Who else would have to be involved to help you achieve this goal? How would you go about enlisting help?

6. Picture yourself at the end of your life. Ask yourself what you want to be thinking and feeling about yourself, and how you have lived as you prepare to leave this earth. What will you be proud of? What will you regret? What will you wish you had done differently?

REFERENCES

Assagioli, R. (2007). *The Act of Will.* London: Penguin, Viking Press.

Arasini Foundation. (2007). Awakening the Self: Our Shadow Side. http://www .ahealingplace.org/arasini/arasini.html. Accessed March 9, 2007.

Bender, S. (1996). *Everyday Sacred: A Woman's Journey Home.* San Francisco: HarperCollins Publishers.

Biberman, J., Whitty, M., & Robbins, L. (1999). Lessons from Oz: Balance and wholeness in organizations. *Journal of Organizational Change Management* 12(3): 243–55.

Bloch, D. P., & Richmond, L. J. (1998). *Soul Work: Finding the Work You Love, Loving the Work You Have.* Palo Alto, Calif.: Davies-Black.

Briskin, A. (1998). *The Stirring of the Soul in the Workplace.* San Francisco: Berrett-Koehler Publishers, Inc.

Cavanagh, G., & Bandsuch, M. (2002). Virtue as a benchmark for spirituality in business. *Journal of Business Ethics* 38: 109–17.

Conger, J. A. (1994). *Spirit at Work. Discovering the Spirituality in Leadership.* San Francisco: Jossey-Bass Publishers.

Duchon, D., & Plowman, D. (2005) Nurturing the spirit at work: Impact on work unit performance. *Leadership Quarterly* 16(5): 807–33.

Duff, L. (2003). Spiritual development and education: A contemplative view. *International Journal of Children's Spirituality* 8(3): 227–37.

Duffy, R. (2006). Spirituality, religion and career development: current status and future directions. *The Career Development Quarterly* 55: 52–64.

Dunne, C. (2000) *Carl Jung: Wounded Healer of the Soul.* Sandpoint, Idaho: Morning Light Press.

Frankl, V. (1967). *The Doctor and the Soul,* 2nd ed. Translated by R. and C. Winston. New York: Alfred A. Knopf.

———. (1968). The humane dimension. In J. Fabry, *The Pursuit of Meaning.* Boston: Beacon Press.

Freeman, L. (1986). *The Light Within.* New York: Crossroads.

Freudenberger, H. (1980). *The High Cost of Achievement.* New York: Anchor Press.

Giacalone, R., & Jurkiewicz, C. (2003). *Handbook of Workplace Spirituality and Organizational Performance.* New York: ME Sharpe, Inc.

Gough, R. (1998). *Character Is Destiny: The Value of Personal Ethics in Everyday Life.* Rockland, Calif.: Prima Publishing Co.

Groen, J. (2001). How leaders cultivate spirituality in the workplace: What the research shows. *Adult Learning* 12(3): 20–21.

Guillory, W. (1997). *The Living Organization: Spirituality in the Workplace.* Salt Lake City: Innovations International Inc.

Hardingham, L. (2004). Integrity and moral residue: Nurses as participants in a moral community. *Nursing Philosophy* 5: 127–34.

Hargreaves, A. (1997). Rethinking educational change. Going deeper and wider in the quest for success. In A. Hargreaves (ed.), *Rethinking Educational Change with Heart and Mind.* Reston, Va.: Association for Supervision and Curriculum Development.

Hartman, E. (1998). The role of character in business ethics. *Business Ethics Quarterly* 3 (July): 547–59.

Jung, C. G. (1938). "Psychology and Religion." In *CW* 11: *Psychology and Religion: West and East.* New Haven: Yale University Press.

King, S., & Nichol, D. (1999). Organizational enhancement through recognition of individual spirituality: Reflections of Jaques and Jung. *Journal of Organizational Change Management* 12(3): 234–42.

Koenig, H. (2005). Religion, spirituality and medicine: The beginning of a new era. *Southern Medical Journal,* Special Section: Spirituality/Medicine Interface Project 98(12): 1233–35.

Lambie, G. (2006). Burnout prevention: A humanistic perspective and structured supervision activity. *Journal of Humanistic Counseling, Education and Development.* 2: 32–44.

Leonard, G., & Murphy, M. (1995). *The Life We Are Given.* New York: Jeremy Tarcher/Putnam.

Maslach, C., & Leiter, M. (1997). *The Truth about Burnout: How Organizations Cause Personal Stress and What to Do about It.* San Francisco: Jossey-Bass, Inc.

Marques, J. (2005). HR's crucial role in the establishment of spirituality in the work-place. *Journal of American Academy of Business* 7(2): 27–32.

Marsh, F., & Conley, J. (1999). The fourth wave: The spiritually-based firm. *Journal of Organizational Change Management* 12(4): 292–301.

Mirvis, P. (1997). "Soul work" in organizations. *Organization Science* 8(2): 193–206.

Mitroff, I., & Denton, E. (1999). *A Spiritual Audit of Corporate America: A Hard Look at Spirituality, Religion, and Values in the Workplace*. San Francisco: Jossey-Bass, Inc.

Neal, J., & Banner, D. (1999). Spiritual perspectives on individual, organizational and societal transformation. *Journal of Organizational Change Management* 12(3): 175–87.

Nee, W. (1968). *The Spiritual Man*. New York: Christian Fellowship Publishers.

Oldmeadow, H. (2004). *Journeys East: 20th Century Western Encounters with Eastern Religious Traditions*. Bloomington, Ind.: World Wisdom, Inc.

Pattison, M. (2006). Finding peace and joy in the practice of medicine. *Health Progress* 87(3): 22–24.

Peppers, C., & Briskin, A. (2000). *Bringing Your Soul to Work: An Everyday Practice*. San Francisco: Berrett-Koehler Publishers.

Pierce, G. (2005). *Spirituality Work: 10 Ways to Balance Your Life on the Job*. Chicago: Loyola Press.

Selye, H. (1976). *The Stress of Life*. New York: McGraw-Hill.

Stockdale, A. (1962). In M. Bach, *Make It an Adventure*, 142. Englewood Cliffs, N.J.: Prentice Hall.

Schwartz, R. (2001). *Introduction to the Internal Systems Model*. Oak Park, Ill.: The Center for Self Leadership.

Schwartz, T. (1996). *What Really Matters: Searching for Wisdom in America*. New York: Bantam Books, Doubleday Dell Publishing Group, Inc.

Seaward, B. (1997). *Stand Like Mountain, Flow Like Water: Reflections on Stress and Human Spirituality*. Deerfield Beach, Fla.: Health Communications, Inc.

Skovholt, T. M. (2001). *The Resilient Practitioner: Burnout Prevention and Self-Care Strategies for Counselors, Therapists, Teachers, and Health Professionals*. Boston: Allyn and Bacon.

Smith, W. C. (1998). *Faith and Belief: The Difference between Them*. Oxford, U.K.: Oneworld Publications.

Snyder, C. R. (1994) *The Psychology of Hope: You Can Get There from Here*. New York: Free Press.

Sulmasy, D. (1997). *The Healer's Calling: A Spirituality for Physicians and Other Health Care Professionals*. New York: Paulist Press.

Thurman, H. (1984). *For the Inward Journey*. Cleveland: Harcourt Brace Jovanovich.

Tillich, P., & Gorman, M. (eds.). (1985). *Psychology and Religion: A Reader*. New York: Paulist Press.

Tisdale, E. (2007). In the new millennium: The role of spirituality and the cultural imagination in dealing with diversity and equity in the higher education classroom. *Teachers College Record* 109(3): 531–60.

Walsh, R. (1999). *Essential Spirituality: The 7 Central Practices to Awaken Heart and Mind*. New York: John Wiley & Sons.

Weston, S. (2002). Faith at work: Managing the spiritual renaissance. *New Zealand Management* 49(3): 28.

Wheaton, A., & Baird, C. (2002). Synergistic Spirituality: The Intersection of Spiritual Values, Organizational Culture and Ethics. Paper presented at the Sixty-second Annual Meeting of the Academy of Management, Denver, Colorado.

Zweig, C., & Wolf, S. (1997). *Romancing the Shadow: A Guide to Soul Work for a Vital, Authentic Life*. New York: Ballantine Books.

CONTRIBUTORS

Elizabeth Arnold, PhD, PMHCNS-BC, is a retired associate professor and former graduate behavioral specialty coordinator at the University of Maryland School of Nursing. She is also an ANCC seminar speaker, a psychiatric mental health nursing clinical specialist, and coauthor of *Interpersonal Relationship: Communication Skills for Nursing* (AJN Book of the Year, 2008).

Gary Batchelor, DMin, BCC, has been chaplain at Floyd Medical Center in Rome, Georgia, since 1975. He is board certified by the Association of Professional Chaplains. He and his wife Rosalind, a retired public school teacher, have two adult children and one granddaughter. He was named a Hero in Healthcare Ethics by the Healthcare Ethics Consortium of Georgia in April 2006.

Andrea L. Canada, PhD, is assistant professor of behavioral sciences at Rush University Medical Center in Chicago. She holds a PhD in clinical psychology and specializes in psychosocial oncology.

Verna Benner Carson, PhD, APRN/PMH is the director of mental health for skilled nursing and assisted living facilities at Erickson Retirement Communities. She is also the president of C&V Senior Care Specialists, Inc. Prior to these positions, she was the national director of behavioral health and Alzheimer's care at Tender Loving Care Home Health Services for eleven years. In addition, she was an associate professor of psychiatric nursing at the University of Maryland School of Nursing for twenty-one years. She is the author of eight books, including *Spiritual Dimensions of Nursing Practice.* Dr. Carson lives in Fallston, Maryland, with her husband.

Thomas E. DeLoughry, EdD, is executive director of the Center for Health Management, an agency that develops mind-body-spirit programs for individuals, organizations, and communities. His interest in mind-body-spirit programs parallels the twelve years he worked as a counselor; the ten years he directed wellness and disease management programs for a large managed care organization; and the three years he spent directing a Franciscan retreat center. He is the creator of the American Lung Association's national program, called Help Patients to Better Breathing. He received the National Award for Excellence in Quality Management from the American Managed Care Association for his program on Primary Care Quality Management. He served as assistant professor of Family Medicine at the State University of New York at Buffalo Medical School and as an assistant professor in the Health Services graduate program at D'Youville College in Buffalo.

George Fitchett, DMin, PhD, is associate professor and director of research in the Department of Religion, Health, and Human Values at Rush University Medical Center in Chicago. He is also an associate professor in Rush's Department of Preventive Medicine. He holds a PhD in epidemiology and is a certified chaplain (a member of the Association of Professional Chaplains) and pastoral supervisor (a member of the Association for Clinical Pastoral Education, Inc.).

Pat Fosarelli, MD, DMin, received her MD from the University of Maryland School of Medicine, her MA in theology from the Ecumenical Institute of Theology of St. Mary's Seminary and University, and her DMin from Wesley Theological Seminary. Currently, she is on the part-time faculty of the Johns Hopkins University School of Medicine (Department of Pediatrics) and the faculty of St. Mary's Ecumenical Institute of Theology (Departments of Spirituality and Practical Theology). Dr. Fosarelli is the director of religious education at Corpus Christi Church in Baltimore.

Miriam Jacik, RN, is a retired nurse, oncology specialist, and pastoral care counselor. She currently runs a bereavement support group for her parish in Greenbelt, Maryland.

Harold G. Koenig, MD, MHSc, completed his undergraduate education at Stanford University, his medical school training at the University of California at San Francisco, and his geriatric medicine, psychiatry, and biostatistics training at Duke University Medical Center. He is board certified in general psychiatry, geriatric psychiatry, and geriatric medicine, and is on the faculty at Duke as professor of psychiatry and behavioral sciences, and an associate professor of medicine. He codirects Duke's Center for Spirituality, Theology, and Health.

Patricia C. McMullen, PhD, JD, CNS, RNP, is the associate provost for academic administration at The Catholic University of America. She joined the School of Nursing at the Catholic University of America as associate dean of academic affairs in 2003. Prior to working in the School of Nursing, Dr. McMullen was the chair of the Department of Nurse Practitioner and acting associate dean at the Uniformed Services University of Health Science Graduate School in Bethesda, Maryland. Dr. McMullen was also a faculty member at the University of Maryland School of Nursing.

Patricia Murphy, RSCJ, MA, PhD, a Catholic sister, is an assistant professor in the Department of Religion, Health, and Human Values at Rush University Medical Center in Chicago, with a conjoint appointment in the Department of Psychiatry. She holds an MA in Christian spirituality and a PhD in pastoral counseling, and is a licensed clinical professional counselor and board-certified chaplain. She provides pastoral care for adult psychiatry inpatients and is the recipient of a George Washington Institute for Spirituality and Health grant for training psychiatry residents in the role of religion and spirituality for psychiatry patients.

Nayna D. C. Philipsen, JD, PhD, RN, CFE, FACCE, is associate professor and director of program development at the Coppin State University Helene Fuld School of Nursing. Prior to this position, she was the director of education, examination, research and communication at the Maryland Board of Nursing. Before working in professional regulation, Dr. Philipsen served on graduate and undergraduate nursing school faculties at universities in Texas, North Carolina, and Maryland. She is also a health educator at St. Agnes Hospital in Baltimore.

Nancy Christine Shoemaker is a psychiatric clinical specialist with more than thirty-five years' experience in psychiatric nursing. Most of her career has been in the public mental health sector, working with clients who have serious and persistent mental illness. She has contributed to various nursing textbooks and serves as a preceptor for graduate nursing students at the University of Maryland. She lives in Pasadena, Maryland, with her husband.

INDEX